Prioritization, Delegation, and Assignment in LPN/LVN Nursing

Practice Exercises for the NCLEX-PN® Examination

Prioritization, Delegation, and Assignment in LPN/LVN Nursing, 1e

Practice Exercises for the NCLEX-PN® Examination

Linda A. LaCharity, PhD, RN
Formerly, Accelerated Program Director
Assistant Professor
College of Nursing
University of Cincinnati
Cincinnati, Ohio

Candice K. Kumagai, RN, MSN
Formerly, Clinical Instructor
School of Nursing
University of Texas at Austin
Austin, Texas

Shirley Meier Hosler, BSN, MS, RN
Formerly, Critical Care Instructor
Santa Fe Community College
Santa Fe, New Mexico

ELSEVIER

ELSEVIER
3251 Riverport Lane
St. Louis, Missouri 63043

Prioritization, Delegation, and Assignment in LPN/LVN Nursing, FIRST EDITION   ISBN: 978-0-323-77916-6

Notices

Practitioners and researchers must always rely on their own experience and knowledge in evaluating and using any information, methods, compounds or experiments described herein. Because of rapid advances in the medical sciences, in particular, independent verification of diagnoses and drug dosages should be made. To the fullest extent of the law, no responsibility is assumed by Elsevier, authors, editors or contributors for any injury and/or damage to persons or property as a matter of products liability, negligence or otherwise, or from any use or operation of any methods, products, instructions, or ideas contained in the material herein.

ISBN: 978-0-323-77916-6

Senior Content Strategist: Brandi Graham
Senior Content Development: Laurie Gower
Senior, Content Development Specialist: Laura Goodrich
Publishing Services Manager: Shereen Jameel
Project Manager: Nadhiya Sekar
Design Direction: Renee Duenow

Printed in India

Last digit is the print number: 9   8   7   6   5   4   3   2   1

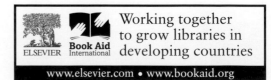

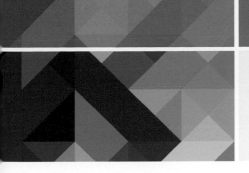

Contributors and Reviewers

CONTRIBUTORS

Martha Barry, MS, APRN, CNM IBCLC
Certified Nurse Midwife
OB Faculty Practice
Advocate Aurora Medical Group
Chicago, Illinois

Ruth Hansten, RN, MBA, PhD, FACHE
Principal Consultant and CEO
Hansten Healthcare
Santa Rosa, California

Mary Tedesco-Schneck, PhD, RN, CPNP
Assistant Professor
School of Nursing
University of Maine
Orono, Maine

REVIEWER

Kimberly Amos, PhD, MS(N), RN, CNE
Director
Foothills Nursing Consortium Associate Degree Nursing
Spindale, North Carolina

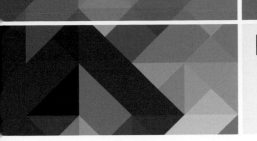

Preface

Prioritization, Delegation, and Assignment in LPN/LVN Nursing Practice Exercises for the NCLEX-PN® Examination is a new project focused on the key concepts of prioritization, delegation, and assignment from the perspective of the professional licensed practical/vocational nurse (LPN/LVN). It is a resource that spans general nursing knowledge while emphasizing management of care to assist students in preparing for the NCLEX® Examination. Our first edition includes many examples of practice questions for the new style questions (Nextgen) that will be added to the NCLEX examination. A second and equally important purpose of the book is assisting students, novice nurses, and seasoned nurses in applying concepts of prioritization, delegation, and assignment to nursing practice in a variety of today's patient care settings.

TO FACULTY AND OTHER USERS

Patient care acuity continues to be higher than ever with the essential added care of COVID-19 patients, while staffing shortages remain very real. Nurses must use all available patient care personnel and resources competently and efficiently and be familiar with variations in state laws governing the practice of nursing, as well as differences in scopes of practice and facility-specific job descriptions. Nurses must also be aware of the different skill and experience levels of the health care professionals with whom they work on a daily basis. Which nursing actions can be assigned to an experienced versus a new graduate LPN/LVN? What forms of patient care can the nurse delegate to an assistive personnel (AP)? Who should help the post-operative patient who has had a total hip replacement get out of bed and ambulate to the bathroom? Can the nurse ask APs such as nursing assistants to check a patient's oxygen saturation using pulse oximetry or check a diabetic patient's glucose level? When an LPN/LVN is assigned to monitor a patient after cardiac catheterization or to supervise an AP who takes vital signs, which parameters should be reported to the RN or healthcare provider? What patient care interventions and actions should **not** be delegated by the nurse? The answers to these and many other questions should be much clearer after the completion of the exercises in this book.

Exercises in this book range from simple to complex in terms of difficulty and use various patient care scenarios. The purpose of the chapters and case studies is to encourage the student or new graduate nurse to conceptualize using the skills of prioritization, delegation, and assignment, as well as supervision, in many different settings. Our goal is to make these concepts tangible to our readers.

The questions are written in NCLEX® Examination format, including new Nextgen styles to help faculty as they teach student nurses how to prepare for their licensure examination. The chapters and case studies focus on real and hypothetical patient care situations to challenge nurses and nursing students to develop the skills necessary to apply these concepts in practice. The exercises are also useful to nurse educators as they discuss, teach, and test their students and nurses for understanding and application of these concepts in nursing programs, examination preparations, and facility orientations. Correct answers, along with in-depth rationales, are provided at the end of each chapter and case study to facilitate the learning process, along with the focus/foci for each item. The faculty exercise keys include QSEN (Quality and Safety Education for Nurses) categories, concepts, and cognitive levels for each question, as well as IPEC (Interprofessional Education Collaborative) categories where appropriate.

On our Evolve site, you can find 8 additional case studies to be used as teaching tools for your class.

TO STUDENTS

Prioritization, delegation, and assignment are essential concepts and skills for nursing practice. Students and graduate nurses have told us of their difficulties with the application of these principles when taking program exit and licensure examinations. Nurse managers have told us many times that novice nurses and even some experienced nurses lack the expertise to practice these skills effectively and safely in real-world settings.

Although several excellent resources deal with these issues, there was still a need for a book that incorporates the management of these care concepts in real-world practice scenarios. Our goal in writing the first edition of *Prioritization, Delegation, and Assignment: Practice Exercises for the NCLEX-PN® Examination* is to provide a resource that challenges nursing students, as well as novice and experienced nurses, to develop the knowledge and understanding necessary to effectively apply these important nursing skills to examination preparation and real-world practice. The book focuses on important types of nursing, including medical-surgical, pediatrics, labor and delivery, psychiatric nursing, care of the older adult, and long-term care, as well as the role of the nurse in a variety of nonacute care settings. Additionally, we have stressed the current focus on evidence-based best practices, fundamentals of safe practice, COVID-19, and diabetes care. We also focus on pharmacology, an area that is problematic for many students, by adding more questions about medications. Drug-related questions have been added to most chapters, in addition to a pharmacology-focused chapter. Questions were added and revised throughout the book to broaden comprehension of key concepts and knowledge areas and to update current knowledge levels. We have also included Test Taking Tips in the rationales for the correct responses to the questions, to help students with choosing the best answers. Our first edition expands on all of these topics and incorporates examples of Nextgen questions formats to prepare students for the upcoming NCLEX changes.

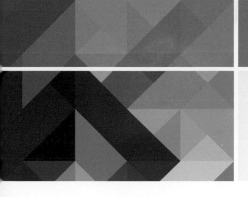

Acknowledgments

We would like to thank the many people whose support and assistance made the creation of the first edition of this book possible. Thanks to our families, colleagues, and friends for listening, reading, encouraging, and making sure we had the time to research, write, and review this book. We truly appreciate the expertise of our two contributing authors, Martha Barry (reproductive health) and Mary Tedesco-Schneck (pediatrics), who each contributed an excellent chapter related to their areas of expertise. Very special thanks to Ruth Hansten, whose expertise in the area of clinical prioritization, delegation, and assignment skills helps to keep us on track. Many thanks to the faculty reviewers, whose expertise helped us keep the scenarios accurate and realistic. Finally, we wish to acknowledge our faculty, students, graduates, and readers who have taken the time to keep in touch and let us know about their needs for additional assistance in developing the skills to practice the arts of prioritization, delegation, and assignment.

Linda A. LaCharity
Candice K. Kumagai
Shirley M. Hosler

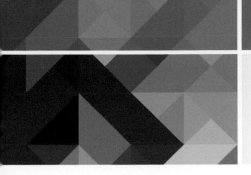

Contents

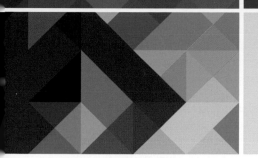

Guidelines for Prioritization, Delegation, and Assignment Decisions

*Ruth Hansten, PhD, MBA, BSN, RN, FACHE and
Linda LaCharity, PhD, MA, BSN, RN*

OUTCOMES FOCUS

Expert nurses have discovered that the most successful method of approaching their practice is to maintain a laser-like focus on the outcomes that the patients and their families want to achieve. To attempt to prioritize, delegate, or assign care without understanding the patient's preferred results is like trying to put together a jigsaw puzzle without the top of the puzzle box that shows the puzzle picture. Not only does the puzzle player pick up random pieces that don't fit well together, wasting time and increasing frustration, but also the process of puzzle assembly is fraught with inefficiencies and wrong choices. In the same way, a nurse who scurries haphazardly without a plan, unsure of what could be the most important, lifesaving task to be done first, or which person should do which tasks for this group of patients, is not fulfilling their potential to be a channel for healing.

Let's visit a change-of-shift report in which a group of nurses receives information about two patients whose blood pressure is plummeting at the same rate. How would one determine which nurse would be best to assign to care for these patients, which patient needs to be seen first, and which tasks could be delegated to assistive personnel (AP), if none of the nurses is aware of each patient's preferred outcomes?

Patient A is a 65-year-old woman who has been receiving chemotherapy for breast cancer; she has been admitted to this shift because of dehydration from uncontrolled emesis. She is expecting to regain her normally robust good health and watch her grandchildren graduate from college. Everyone on the health care team would concur with her long-term goals. Patient Z is an elderly gentleman, 92 years of age, whose wife recently died from complications of repeated cerebrovascular events and dementia. Yesterday while in the emergency department (ED), he was given the diagnosis of acute myocardial infarction and preexisting severe heart failure. He would like to die and join his wife, has requested a "do not resuscitate" (DNR) order, and is awaiting transfer to a hospice. These two patients share critical clinical data but require widely different prioritization, delegation, and assignment. A savvy charge nurse would make the obvious decisions: to assign a skilled nurse to the patient A and to ask AP to function in a supportive role to the primary care nurse.

The elderly gentleman (patient Z) needs palliative care and would be best cared for by a registered nurse (RN) or licensed practical nurse/licensed vocational nurse (LPN/LVN) and care team with excellent people skills. Even a novice nursing assistant could be delegated tasks to help keep Mr. Z and his family comfortable and emotionally supported. The big picture on the puzzle box for these two patients ranges from long-term "robust good health" requiring immediate emergency assessment and treatment to "a supported and comfortable death" requiring timely palliative care, including supportive emotional and physical care. Without envisioning these patients' pictures and knowing their preferred outcomes, the nurses cannot prioritize, delegate, or assign appropriately.

There are many times in nursing practice, however, when correct choices are not so apparent. Patients in all care settings today are often complex, and many have preexisting comorbidities that stump expert practitioners and clinical specialists planning their care. Care delivery systems must flex on a moment's notice when an AP arrives in place of a scheduled LPN/LVN; and agency, float, or traveling nurses fill vacancies, while new patients, waiting to be admitted, accumulate in the ED or wait to be transferred to another setting. AP arrive with varying educational preparation and dissimilar levels of motivation and skill. Critical thinking and complex clinical judgment are required from the minute the shift begins until the nurse clocks out.

In this book, the authors have filled an educational need for students and practicing nurses who wish to hone their skills in prioritizing, assigning, and delegating. The scenarios and patient problems presented in this workbook are practical, challenging, and complex learning tools. Quality and Safety Education for Nurses (QSEN) competencies are incorporated into each chapter and throughout the questions to highlight patient- and family-centered care, quality and safety improvement, and teamwork and collaboration concepts and skills (QSEN Institute, 2019). Patient stories will stimulate thought and discussion and help polish the higher-order intellectual skills necessary to practice as a successful, safe, and effective nurse. The Interprofessional Collaboration Competency Community and Population Oriented Domains from the Interprofessional Education Collaborative (IPEC) are applied to the questions in this book as appropriate (Interprofessional Education Collaborative, 2016, https://ipecollaborative.org). Domains include Interprofessional Teamwork and Team-Based Practices, Interprofessional Teamwork Practices, Roles and Responsibilities for Collaborative Practice, and Values/ Ethics for Interprofessional Practice. As reflected in the IPEC sub-competencies, especially crucial for patient outcomes is the role of the RN, armed with knowledge of scopes of practice, successfully communicating with team members to delegate, assign, and supervise (IPEC, 2016).

DEFINITION OF TERMS

The intellectual functions of prioritization, delegation, and assignment engage the nurse in projecting into the future from the present state. Thinking about what impact might occur if competing decisions are chosen, weighing options, and making split-second decisions, given the available data, is not an easy process. Unless resources in terms of staffing, budget, time, or supplies are unlimited, nurses must relentlessly focus on choosing which issues or concerns must take precedence.

Prioritization

Prioritizing is defined as "ranking problems in order of importance" or "deciding which needs or problems require immediate action and which ones could tolerate a delay in action until a later time because they are not urgent" (Silvestri & Silvestri, 2018). Prioritization in a clinical setting is a process that includes envisioning clearly patient outcomes but also includes predicting possible problems if another task is performed first. One also must weigh potential future events if the task is not completed, the time it would take to accomplish it, and the relationship of the tasks and outcomes. New nurses often struggle with prioritization because they have not yet worked with typical patient progressions through care pathways and have not experienced the complications that may emerge in association with a particular clinical condition. In short, knowing the patient's **purpose for care, current clinical picture,** and **picture of the outcome or result** is necessary to be able to plan priorities. The part played by each team member is designated as the nurse assigns or delegates. The "four Ps"—purpose, picture, plan, and part—become a guidepost for appropriately navigating these processes (Hansten, 2008a, 2011, 2014b; Hansten and Jackson, 2009). The four Ps will be referred to throughout this introduction because these concepts are the framework on which nurses base decisions about supporting patients and families toward their preferred outcomes, whether nurses provide the care themselves or work closely with assistive team members.

Prioritization includes evaluating and weighing each competing task or process using the following criteria (Hansten and Jackson, 2009, pp. 194–196):

- Is it life threatening or potentially life threatening if the task is not done? Would another patient be endangered if this task is done now or the task is left for later?
- Is this task or process essential to patient or staff safety?
- Is this task or process essential to the medical or nursing plan of care?

In each case, an understanding of the overall patient goals and the context and setting is essential.

1. In her book on critical thinking and clinical judgment, Rosalinda Alfaro-LeFevre (2017) suggests three levels of priority setting: The first level is **a**irway, **b**reathing, **c**ardiac status and circulation, and **v**ital signs and **l**ab values that could be life threatening ("ABCs plus V and L").
2. The second level is immediately subsequent to the first level and includes concerns such as mental status changes, untreated medical issues, acute pain, acute elimination problems, and imminent risks.
3. The third level is health problems other than those at the first two levels, such as more long-term issues in health education, rest, coping, and so on (p. 171).

Maslow's hierarchy of needs can be used to prioritize from the most crucial survival needs to those related to safety and security, affiliation (love, relationships), self-esteem, and self-actualization (Alfaro-LeFevre, 2017, p. 170).

Delegation and Assignment

The official definitions of *assignment* have been altered through ongoing dialogue among nursing leaders in various states and nursing organizations, and terminology distinctions such as *observation* versus *assessment*, *critical thinking* versus *clinical reasoning*, and *delegation* versus *assignment* continue to be discussed as nursing leaders attempt to describe complex thinking processes that occur in various levels of nursing practice. Assignment has been defined as **"the distribution of work that each staff member is responsible for during a given work period"** (American Nurses Association [ANA] et al., 2014, p. 22). In 2016, the National Council of State Boards of Nursing (NCSBN) published the results of two expert panels to clarify that **assignment** includes **"the routine care, activities, and procedures that are within the authorized scope of practice of the RN or LPN/LVN or part of the routine functions of the AP (Assistive Personnel)** (NCSBN, 2016b, pp. 6–7), and this definition was adopted by the ANA in 2019 in a joint statement with the NCSBN with the addition of the acronym **AP (Assistive Personnel)** (ANA & NCSBN, 2019, *National guidelines for nursing delegation*, p. 2). **Delegation** was defined traditionally as **"transferring to a competent individual the authority to perform a selected nursing task in a selected situation"** (NCSBN, 1995) and similar definitions are used by some nurse practice statutes or regulations. Both the ANA and the NCSBN describe delegation as **"allowing a delegate to perform a specific nursing activity, skill,**

or procedure that is beyond the delegatee's traditional role and is not routinely performed" (ANA & NCSBN, 2019, p. 2). However, the delegatee must be competent to perform that delegated task due to extra training and skill validation. The ANA specifies that delegation is a transfer of responsibility or assignment of an activity while retaining the accountability for the outcome and the overall care (ANA et al., 2014, p. 22).

Some state boards have argued that "assignment" is the process of directing an AP to perform a task such as taking blood pressure, a task on which assistive personnel are tested in the certified nursing assistant examination and that would commonly appear in a job description. Others contend that all nursing care is a part of the nurse's scope of practice and therefore such a task would be "delegated" rather than "assigned." Other nursing leaders argue that only when a task is clearly within the nurse's scope of practice, and not included in the role of the AP, is the task delegated. Whether the allocation of tasks to be done is assignment or delegation, in this book the term assignment will mean the "work plan" and it connotes the nursing leadership role of human resources deployment in a manner that most wisely promotes the patient's and family's preferred outcome.

Although the states vary in their definitions of the functions and processes in professional nursing practice, including that of delegation, the authors use the NCSBN and ANA's definition, including the caveat present in the sentence following the definition: delegation is "transferring to a competent individual the authority to perform a selected nursing task in a selected situation. The nurse retains the accountability for the delegation" (NCSBN, 1995, p. 2). Assignments are work plans that would include tasks the delegatee would have been trained to do in their basic educational program; the nurse "assigns" or distributes work and also "delegates" nursing care as she or he works through others. In advanced AP roles such as when certified medication aides are taught to administer medications or when certified medical assistants give injections, the NCSBN (2016) asserts that because of the extensive responsibilities involved, the employers and nurse leaders in the settings where certified medication aides are employed, such as ambulatory care, skilled nursing homes, or home health settings, should regard these procedures as being delegated and AP competencies must be assured (NCSBN, 2016b, p. 7). ANA designates these certified but unlicensed individuals as AP rather than unlicensed assistive personnel (UAP) (ANA & NSCBN, 2019). The differences in definitions among states and the differentiation between delegation and assignment are perplexing to nurses. Because both processes are similar in terms of the actions and thinking processes of the nurse from a practical standpoint, this workbook will merge the definitions to mean that RNs delegate or assign tasks when they are allocating work to competent trained individuals, keeping within each state's scope of practice, rules, and organizational job descriptions. Whether assigning or delegating,

the nurse is accountable for the total nursing care of the patient and for making choices about which competent person is permitted to perform each task successfully. Whether the nurse is delegating or assigning, depending on their state regulations, the expert nurse will not ask a team member to perform a task that is beyond the nurse's own scope of practice or job description, or a task outside of any person's competencies. In all cases, the choices made to allocate work must prioritize which allocation of work is optimal.

Delegation or Assignment and Supervision

The definitions of delegation and assignment offer some important clues to nursing practice and to the composition of an effective patient care team. The person who makes the decision to ask a person to do something (a task or assignment) must know that the chosen person is competent to perform that task. The nurse selects the particular task, given their knowledge of the individual patient's condition and that particular circumstance. Because of the nurse's preparation, knowledge, and skill, they choose to render judgments of this kind and stand by the choices made. According to licensure and statute, the nurse is obligated to delegate or assign based on the unique situation, patients, and personnel involved and to provide ongoing follow-up.

Supervision

Whenever nurses delegate or assign, they must also supervise. **Supervision** is defined by the NCSBN as **"the provision of guidance and direction, oversight, evaluation and follow up by the licensed nurse for accomplishment of a nursing task delegated to nursing assistive personnel"** and by the ANA as **"the active process of directing, guiding and influencing the outcome of an individual's performance of a task"** (ANA et al., 2014, p. 23). Each state may use a different explanation such as Washington State's supervision definition: **"initial direction… periodic inspection… and the authority to require corrective action."** (Washington Administrative Code 246-840-010, 2019, https://app.leg.wa.gov/wac/default.aspx?cite=246-840-010. The act of delegating or assigning is just the beginning of the nurse's responsibility. As for the accountability of the delegatees (or persons given the task duty), these individuals are accountable for (1) accepting only the responsibilities that they know they are competent to complete, (2) maintaining their skill proficiency, (3) ongoing communication with the team's leader, and (4) completing and documenting the task appropriately (ANA & NCSBN, 2019, p. 9). For example, AP who are unprepared or untrained to complete a task should say as much when asked and can then decline to perform that particular duty. In such a situation, the nurse would determine whether to allocate time to train the AP and review the skill as it is learned, to delegate the task to another competent person, to do it themselves, or to make arrangements for later skill training. The nurse's job continues throughout the performance and results of task completion, evaluation of the care, and ongoing feedback to the delegatees.

Scope of Practice for RNs, LPNs/LVNs, and APs

Heretofore this text has discussed national recommendations for definitions. National trends suggest that nursing is moving toward standardized licensure through mutual recognition compacts and multistate licensure, and as of October 2020, 31 states had adopted the nurse license compact (https://www.ncsbn.org/compacts.htm) allowing a nurse in a member state to possess one state's license and practice in another member state, with several states pending (NCSBN, 2019a). Standardized and multistate licensure supports electronic practice and promotes improved practice flexibility. However, each nurse must know their own state's regulations. Definitions still differ from state to state, as do regulations about the tasks that AP are allowed to perform in various settings.

For example, AP are delegated tasks for which they have been trained and that they are currently competent to perform for stable patients in uncomplicated circumstances; these are routine, simple, repetitive, common activities not requiring nursing judgment; for example, activities of daily living, hygiene, feeding, and ambulation. Some states have generated statutes and/or rules that list specific tasks that can or cannot be delegated. However, trends indicate that more tasks will be delegated as research supports such delegation through evidence of positive outcomes. Acute care hospitals' nursing assistants have not historically been authorized to administer medications. In some states, specially certified medication assistants (CMAs) administer oral medications in the community (group homes) and in some long-term care facilities, although there is substantial variability in state-designated certified nurse assistants (I) duties (McMullen et al., 2015). More states are employing specially trained nursing assistants as CMAs or MA-Cs (medication assistants-certified) to administer routine, nonparenteral medications in long-term care or community settings with training as recommended by the NCSBN's Model Curriculum (NCSBN, 2016a, p. 7). For over a decade Washington state has altered the statute and related administrative codes to allow trained nursing assistants in home or community-based settings, such as boarding homes and adult family homes, to administer insulin if the patient is an appropriate candidate (in a stable and predictable condition) and if the nursing assistant has been appropriately trained and supervised for the first 4 weeks of performing this task (Revised Code of Washington, 2012). Nationally, consistency of state regulation of AP medication administration in residential care and adult day-care settings has been stated to be inadequate to ensure RN oversight of AP (Carder & O'Keeffe, 2016). This research finding should serve as a caution for all practicing in these settings. Other studies of nursing

homes and assisted living facilities show evidence of role confusion among RNs, LPN/LVNs, and UAPs (Mueller et al., 2018; Dyck & Novotny, 2018). In ambulatory care settings, medical assistants (Mas) are being used extensively, supervised by RNs, LPNs (depending on the state), physicians, or other providers, and nurses are cautioned to know both the state nursing and medical regulations. In some cases (e.g., Maryland), a physician could delegate peripheral IV initiation to an MA with onsite supervision; but in some states, an LPN is prohibited from this same task (Maningo & Panthofer, 2018, p.2).

In all the states, nursing judgment is used to delegate tasks that fall within, but never exceed, the nurse's legal scope of practice, and a nurse always makes decisions based on the individual patient situation. A nurse may decide not to delegate the task of feeding a patient if the patient is dysphagic and the nursing assistant is not familiar with feeding techniques. A "Lessons Learned from Litigation" article in the *American Journal of Nursing* in May 2014 describes the hazards of improper nursing assignment, delegation, and supervision of patient feeding, resulting in a patient's death and licensure sanctions (Brous, 2014).

The scope of practice for LPNs or LVNs also differs from state to state and is continually evolving. For example, in Texas, LPNs have been prohibited from delegating nursing tasks; only RNs are allowed to delegate (Texas Board of Nursing, 2019, http://www.bon.texas.gov/faq_de legation.asp#t6), while in Washington state an LPN could delegate to nursing assistants (e.g., AP) in some settings (listed as hospitals, nursing homes, clinics, ambulatory surgery centers) (Washington State Department of Health Nursing Care Quality Assurance Commission, 2019, https://www.doh.wa.gov/Portals/1/Documents/6000/NCAO1 3.pdf). Although practicing nurses know that LPNs often review a patient's condition and perform data-gathering tasks such as observation and auscultation, RNs remain accountable for the total assessment of a patient, including synthesis and analysis of reported and reviewed information to lead care planning based on the nursing diagnosis. In their periodic review of actual practice by LPNs, the NCSBN found that assigning client care or related tasks to other LPNs or AP was ranked sixth in frequency, with monitoring activities of AP ranked seventh (NCSBN, 2019b, p. 156). IV therapy and administration of blood products or total parenteral nutrition (TPN) by LPNs/LVNs also vary widely. In some states IV therapy may be permitted along with IV drug administration when an approved course of study is completed by the LPN/LVN. Even in states where regulations allow LPNs/LVNs to administer blood products, a given health care organization's policies or job descriptions may limit practice and place additional safeguards because of the life-threatening risk involved in the administration of blood products and other medications. *The nurse must review the agency's job descriptions as well as the state regulations because both are changeable.*

LPN/LVN practice continues to evolve, and in any state, tasks to support the assessment, planning, intervention, and evaluation phases of the nursing process can be allocated. When it is clear that a task could be delegated to a skilled delegatee according to your state's scope of practice rules and is not prohibited by the organization policies, the principles of delegation and/or assignment remain the same. The totality of the nursing process remains the responsibility of the RN. Also, the total nursing care of the patient rests squarely on the RN's shoulders, no matter which competent and skilled individual is asked to perform care activities. To obtain more information about the statute and rules in a given state and to access decision trees and other helpful aides to delegation and supervision, visit the NCSBN website at http://www.ncsbn.org. The state practice act for each state is linked at that site.

ASSIGNMENT PROCESS

In current hospital environments, the process of assigning or creating a work plan is dependent on who is available, present, and accounted for and what their roles and competencies are for each shift. Assignment has been understood to be the "work plan" or **the distribution of work that each staff member is responsible for during a given work period**" (ANA et al., 2014, p. 22). Classical care delivery models once known as *total patient care* have been transformed into a combination of team, functional, and primary care nursing, depending on the projected patient outcomes, the present patient state, and the available staff. Assignments must be created with knowledge of the following issues (Hansten and Jackson, 2009, pp. 207–208; Hansten, 2020b):

- How complex is the patients' required care?
- What are the dynamics of patients' status and their stability?
- How complex is the assessment and ongoing evaluation?
- What kind of infection control is necessary?
- Are there any individual safety precautions?
- Is there special technology involved in the care, and who is skilled in its use?
- How much supervision and oversight will be needed based on the staff's numbers and expertise?
- How available are the supervising RNs?
- How will the physical location of patients affect the time and availability of care?
- Can continuity of care be maintained?
- Are there any personal reasons to allocate duties for a particular patient, or are there nurse or patient preferences that should be taken into account? Factors such as staff difficulties with a particular diagnosis, patient preferences for an employee's care on a previous admission, or a staff member's need for a particular learning experience will be taken into account.
- Is there an acuity rating system that will help distribute care based on a point or number system?

For more information on care delivery modalities, refer to the texts by Hansten and Jackson (2009) or access Hansten's webinars related to assignment and care delivery models at http://learning.hansten.com/and Alfaro-LeFevre (2017) listed in the References section. With surges of patients during a pandemic or emergency, nurses must flex their routine methods of assignment to adapt to temporary personnel and unfamiliar roles (Hansten, 2020a). Whichever type of care delivery plan is chosen for each particular shift or within your practice arena, the relationship with the patient and the results that the patient wants to achieve must be the foremost, followed by the placing together of the right pieces in the form of competent team members, to compose the complete picture (Hansten, 2019).

DELEGATION AND ASSIGNMENT: THE FIVE RIGHTS

As you contemplate the questions in this workbook, you can use mnemonic devices to order your thinking process, such as the "five rights." The *right task* is assigned to the *right person* in the *right circumstances*. The RN then offers the *right direction and communication* and the *right supervision and evaluation* (Hansten and Jackson, 2009, pp. 205–206; NCSBN, 1995, pp. 2–3, Hansten, 2014a, p. 70; NCSBN, 2016b, p. 8, ANA & NCSBN, 2019, p. 4).

Right Task

Returning to the guideposts for navigating care, the patient's four Ps (purpose, picture, plan, and part), the right task is a task that, in the nurse's best judgment, is one that can be safely delegated for this patient, given the patient's current condition (picture) and future preferred outcomes (purpose, picture), if the nurse has a competent willing individual available to perform it. Although the nurse may believe that they personally would be the best person to accomplish this task, the nurse must prioritize the best use of their time given a myriad of factors. "What other tasks and processes must I do because I am the only RN or LPN/LVN on this team? Which tasks can be delegated based on state regulations and my thorough knowledge of job descriptions here in this facility? How skilled are the personnel working here today? Who else could be available to help if necessary?"

In its draft model language for nursing AP, the NCSBN lists criteria for determining nursing activities that can be delegated. The following are recommended for the nurse's consideration. It should be kept in mind that the nursing process and nursing judgment cannot be delegated.

- Knowledge and skills of the delegatee
- Verification of clinical competence by the employer
- Stability of the patient's condition
- Service setting variables such as available resources (including the nurse's accessibility) and methods of

communication, complexity and frequency of care, and proximity and numbers of patients relative to staff

AP are not to be allocated the duties of the nursing process of assessment (except gathering data), nursing diagnosis, planning, implementation (except those tasks delegated/assigned), and evaluation. Professional clinical judgment or reasoning and decision-making related to the manner in which the RN makes sense of the patient's data and clinical progress cannot be delegated or assigned (ANA & NCSBN, 2019, p. 3).

Right Circumstances

Recall the importance of the context in clinical decision making. Not only do rules and regulations adjust based on the area of practice (e.g., home health care, acute care, schools, ambulatory clinics, long-term care) but patient conditions and the preferred patient results must also be considered. If information is not available, a best judgment must be made. Often nurses must balance the need to know as much as possible and the time available to obtain the information. The instability of patients immediately postoperatively or in the intensive care unit (ICU) means that a student nurse will have to be closely supervised and partnered with an experienced RN. The questions in this workbook give direction as to context and offer hints to the circumstances.

For example, in long-term care skilled nursing facilities, LPNs/LVNs often function as "team leaders" with ongoing care planning and oversight by a smaller number of on-site RNs. Some Eds use paramedics, who may be regulated by the state emergency system statutes, in different roles in hospitals. Medical clinics often employ "Mas" who function under the direction and supervision of physicians, other providers, and RNs. Community group homes, assisted living facilities, and other health care providers beyond acute care hospitals seek to create safe and effective care delivery systems for the growing number of older adults. Whatever the setting or circumstance is, the nurse is accountable to know the specific laws and regulations that apply.

Right Person

Licensure, Certification, and Role Description

One of the most commonly voiced concerns during workshops with staff nurses across the nation is, "How can I trust the delegatees?" Knowing the licensure, role, and preparation of each member of the team is the first step in determining competency. What tasks does a patient care technician (PCT) perform in this facility? What is the role of an LPN/LVN? Are different levels of LPN/LVN designated here (LPN I or II)? Nearly 100 different titles for AP have been developed in care settings across the country. To effectively assign or delegate, the nurse must know the role descriptions of coworkers as well as their own.

Strengths and Weaknesses

The personal strengths and weaknesses of everyday team members are no mystery. Their skills are discovered through practice, positive and negative experiences, and an ever-present but unreliable rumor mill. An expert nurse helps create better team results by using strengths in assigning personnel to make the most of their gifts. The most compassionate team members will be assigned work with the hospice patient and their family. The supervising nurse helps identify performance flaws and develops staff by providing judicious use of learning assignments. For example, a novice nursing assistant can be partnered with an experienced oncology nurse during the assistant's first experiences with a terminally ill patient.

When working with students, float nurses, or other temporary personnel, nurses sometimes forget that the assigning RN has the duty to determine competency. Asking personnel about their previous experiences and their understanding of the work duties, as well as pairing them with a strong unit staff member, is as essential as providing the ongoing support and supervision needed throughout the shift. If your father was a long-term care resident and his care provider were an inexperienced AP, what level of ongoing support and guidance would the AP need from the supervising nurse? Many hospitals and care facilities delegate only tasks and not overall patient responsibility, a functional form of assignment or delegation, to temporary personnel who are unfamiliar with the clinical area.

Right Direction and Communication

Now that the right staff member is being delegated the right task for each particular situation and setting, team members must find out what they need to do and how the tasks must be done. Relaying instructions about the plan for the shift or even for a specific task is not as simple as it seems. Some nurses believe that a written assignment board provides enough information to proceed because "everyone knows their job," but others spend copious amounts of time giving overly detailed directions to bored staff. The "*four Cs*" of initial direction will help clarify the salient points of this process (Hansten and Jackson, 2009, pp. 287–288; Hansten, 2021, p. 316). Instructions and ongoing direction must be clear, concise, correct, and complete.

Clear communication is information that is understood by the listener. An ambiguous question such as: "Can you get the new patient?" is not helpful when there are several new patients and returning surgical patients, and "getting" could mean transporting, admitting, or taking full responsibility for the care of the patient. Asking the delegatee to restate the instructions and work plan can be helpful to determine whether the communication is clear.

Concise statements are those that give enough but not too much additional information. The student nurse who merely wants to know how to turn on the chemical strip analyzer machine does not need a full treatise on the transit of potassium and glucose through the cell membrane. Too much or irrelevant information confuses the listener and wastes precious time.

Correct communication is that which is accurate and is aligned to rules, regulations, or job descriptions. Are the room number, patient name, and other identifiers correct? Are there two patients with similar last names? Can this task be delegated to this individual? Correct communication is not cloudy or confusing (Hansten and Jackson, 2009, pp. 287–288; Hansten, 2021, p. 318).

Complete communication leaves no room for doubt on the part of supervisor or delegatees. Staff members often say, "I would do whatever the nurses want if they would just tell me what they want me to do and how to do it." Incomplete communication wins the top prize for creating team strife and substandard work. Assuming that staff "know" what to do and how to do it, along with what information to report and when, creates havoc, rework, and frustration for patients and staff alike. Each staff member should have in mind a clear map or plan for the day, what to do and why, and what and when to report to the team leader. Parameters for reporting and the results that should be expected are often left in the team leader's brain rather than being discussed and spelled out in sufficient detail. Nurses are accountable for clear, concise, correct, and complete initial and ongoing direction.

Right Supervision and Evaluation

After prioritization, assignment, and delegation have been considered, determined, and communicated, the nurse remains accountable for the total care of the patients throughout the tour of duty. Recall that the definition of **supervision** includes not only initial direction but also that "supervision is the active process of directing, guiding, and influencing the outcome of an individual's performance of a task." Similarly, NCSBN defines supervision as "the provision of guidance or direction, oversight, evaluation, and follow-up by the licensed nurse for the accomplishment of a delegated nursing task by assistive personnel" (ANA et al., 2014, p. 23). Nurses may not actually perform each task of care, but they must oversee the ongoing progress and results obtained, reviewing staff performance. Evaluation of the care provided, and adequate documentation of the tasks and outcomes, must be included in this last of the five rights. On a typical unit in an acute care facility, assisted living, or long-term care setting, the RN can ensure optimal performance as the RN begins the shift by holding a short "second report" meeting with AP, outlining the day's plan and the plan for each patient, and giving initial direction at that time. Subsequent short team update or "checkpoint" meetings should be held before and after breaks and meals and before the end of the shift (Hansten, 2005, 2008a, 2008b, 2019). During each short update, feedback is often offered and plans are altered. The last checkpoint presents all team members with an opportunity to give feedback to one another using the step-by-step feedback process (Hansten, 2008a, pp. 79–84; Hansten, 2021 pp. 301–302). This step is often called the "debriefing" checkpoint or huddle, in which the team's processes are also examined. In ambulatory care settings, this checkpoint may be toward the end of each patient's visit or the end of the shift; in home health care, these conversations are often conducted on a weekly basis. Questions such as "What would you recommend I do differently if we worked together tomorrow on the same group of patients? What can we do better as a team to help us navigate the patients toward their preferred results?" will help the team function more effectively in the future.

1. **The team member's input should be solicited first.** "I noted that the vital signs for the first four patients aren't yet on the electronic record. Do you know what's been done?" rather than "WHY haven't those vital signs been recorded yet?" At the end of the shift, the questions might be global, as in "How did we do today?" "What would you do differently if we had it to do over?" "What should I do differently tomorrow?"

2. **Credit should be given for all that has been accomplished.** "Oh, so you have the vital signs done, but they aren't recorded? Great, I'm so glad they are done so I can find out about Ms. Johnson's temperature before I call Dr. Smith." "You did a fantastic job with cleaning Mr. Hu after his incontinence episodes; his family is very appreciative of our respect for his dignity."

3. **Observations or concerns should be offered.** "The vital signs are routinely recorded on the electronic medical record (EMR) before patients are sent for surgery and procedures and before the doctor's round so that we can see the big picture of patients' progress before they leave the unit and to make sure they are stable for their procedures." Or, "I think I should have assigned another RN to Ms. A. I had no idea that your mother recently died of breast cancer."

4. **The delegatee should be asked for ideas on how to resolve the issue.** "What are your thoughts on how you could order your work to get the vital signs on the EMR before 8:30 AM?" Or, "What would you like to do with your work plan for tomorrow? Should we change Ms. A's team?"

5. **A course of action and plan for the future should be agreed upon.** "That sounds great. Practice use of the handheld computers today before you leave, and that should resolve the issue. When we work together tomorrow, let me know whether that resolves the time issue for recording; if not, we will go to another plan." Or, "If you still feel that you want to stay with this assignment tomorrow after you've slept on it, we will keep it as is. If not, please let me know first thing tomorrow morning when you awaken so we can change all the assignments before the staff arrive."

PRACTICE BASED ON RESEARCH EVIDENCE

Rationale for Maximizing Nursing Leadership Skills at the Point of Care

If the skills presented in this book are used to save lives by providing care prioritized to attend to the most unstable patients first, optimally delegated to be delivered by the right personnel, and assigned using appropriate language with the most motivational and conscientious supervisory follow-up, then clinical outcomes should be optimal and work satisfaction should flourish. Solid correlational research evidence has been lacking related to "the best use of personnel to multiply the RN's ability to remain vigilant over patients' progress and avoid failures to rescue, but common sense would advise that better delegation and supervision skills would prevent errors and omissions as well as unobserved patient decline" (Hansten, 2008b, 2019).

In an era of value-based health care reimbursement based on clinical results with linkages for care along the continuum from site to site, a nurse's accountability has irrevocably moved beyond task orientation to leadership practices that ensure better outcomes for patients, families, and populations. The necessity of efficiency and effectiveness in health care means that nurses must delegate and supervise appropriately so that all tasks that can be safely assigned to AP are completed flawlessly. Patient safety experts have linked interpersonal communication errors and teamwork communication gaps as major sources of medical errors while The Joint Commission associated these as root causes of 70% or more of serious reportable events (Grant, 2016, p. 11). Severe events that harm patients (sentinel events) can occur through inadequate hand-offs between caregivers and along the health care continuum as patients are transferred (The Joint Commission, 2017).

Nurses are accountable for processes as well as outcomes measures so that insurers will reimburse health care organizations. If hospital-acquired conditions occur, such as pressure injuries, falls with injury, and some infections, reimbursement for the care of that condition will be negatively impacted.

- Nurses have been reported to spend more than half their time on tasks other than patient care, including searching for team members and internal communications (Voalte, 2013). Shift report at the bedside, along with better initial direction and a plan for supervision during the day, all ultimately decrease the time wasted when nurses must attempt to connect with team members when delegation and assignment processes do not include the five rights. At one facility in the Midwest, shift hand-offs were reduced to 10–15 minutes per shift per RN as a result of a planned approach to initial direction and care planning, which thus saved each RN 30–45 minutes per day (Hansten, 2008a, p. 34). Better use of nursing and AP time can result in more time to care for patients, giving nurses the opportunity to teach patients self-care or to maintain functional status.

- When nurses did not appropriately implement the five rights of delegation and supervision with AP, errors occurred that potentially could have been avoided with better nurse leadership behaviors. Early research about the impact of supervision on errors showed that about 14% of task errors or care omissions related to teamwork were due to lack of RN direction or communication, and approximately 12% of the issues stemmed from lack of supervision or follow-up (Standing et al., 2001). Lack of communication among staff members has been an international issue leading to care that is not completed appropriately (Diab & Ebrahim, 2019). Errors can result in uncompensated conditions or readmissions; unhappy patients and providers; disgruntled health care purchasers; and a disloyal, anxious patient community (Hansten, 2019).

- Teamwork and job satisfaction have been found to be negatively correlated with over-delegation and a hierarchical relationship between nurses and AP (Kalisch, 2015, pp. 266–67), but offering feedback effectively has been shown to improve team thinking and performance (Mizne, 2018 at https://www.15five.com/blog/7-employee-engagement-trends-2018/). Workplace injuries, expensive employee turnover, and patient safety have been linked with employee morale. Daily or weekly feedback has been requested by a majority of teams and this could be achieved by excellent delegation, assignment and supervision shift routines (McNee, 2017, https://www.mcknights.com/blogs/guest-columns/nurse-morale-and-its-impact-on-ltc/). Best practices for deployment of personnel include a connection to patient outcomes, which can occur during initial direction and debriefing supervision checkpoints (Hansten, 2021 in Zerwehk and Garneau).

- Unplanned readmissions to acute care within 30 days of discharge are linked to potential penalties and reduced reimbursements. Inadequate nurse initial direction and supervision of AP can lead to missed mobilization, hydration, and nutrition of patients, thereby discharging deconditioned patients and can be traced to ED visits and subsequent readmissions. Reimbursement bundling for specific care pathways such as total joint replacements or acute exacerbation of chronic obstructive pulmonary disease (COPD) requires that team communication and nurse supervision of coworkers along the full continuum must be seamless from ambulatory care to acute care, rehabilitation, and home settings (Kalisch, 2015; Hansten, 2019).

- As public quality transparency and competition for best value becomes the norm, ineffective delegation has been a significant source of missed care, such as lack of care planning, lack of turning or ambulation, delayed or missed nutrition, and lack of hygiene (Bittner et al., 2011; Kalisch, 2015, pp. 266–270). These care omissions can be contributing factors for the occurrence of unreimbursed "never events" (events that should never occur) such as pressure injuries and pneumonia, as well as prolonged lengths of stay. Other nurse-sensitive quality indicators such as catheter-associated urinary tract infections (CAUTIs) could be correlated to omitted perineal hygiene and inattention to discontinuation of catheters. Useful models that link delegation with care omissions and ensuing care hazards, such as thrombosis, pressure injuries, constipation and infection, combined with a Swiss Cheese Safety Model showing defensive steps against health care–acquired conditions and errors through excellence in nurse leadership can be accessed in the August 2014 *Nurse Leader* at https://doi.org/10.1016/j.mnl.2013.10.007 (Hansten, 2014a, 2020b).

- In perioperative nursing, omissions such as lack of warming, oral care, head elevation, and deep breathing can lead to postoperative pneumonia and lack of optimal healing (Ralph & Viljoen, 2018). Many of these interventions could be delegated or assigned.

Evidence does indicate that appropriate nursing judgment in prioritization, delegation, and supervision can save time and improve communication and thereby improve care, patient safety, clinical outcomes, and job satisfaction, potentially saving patient-days and absenteeism and recruitment costs. Patient satisfaction, staff satisfaction, and clinical results decline when nursing care is poor. Potential reimbursement is lost, patients and families suffer, and the health of our communities decays when nurses do not assume the leadership necessary to work effectively with all team members (Bittner et al., 2011; Kalisch, 2015; Hansten, 2019).

PRINCIPLES FOR IMPLEMENTATION OF PRIORITIZATION, DELEGATION, AND ASSIGNMENT

Return to our goalposts of the four Ps (purpose, picture, plan, and part) as a framework as you answer the questions in this workbook and further develop your own expertise and recall the following principles:

- The nurse should always start with the patient's and family's preferred outcomes in mind. The nurse should be first clear about the patient's purpose for accessing care and their picture for a successful outcome.
- The nurse should refer to the applicable state nursing practice statute and rules as well as the organization's job descriptions for current information about roles and responsibilities of RNs, LPNs/LVNs, and AP. (These are the roles or the parts that people play.)
- Student nurses, novices, float nurses, and other infrequent workers also require variable levels of supervision, guidance, or support (The workers' abilities and roles become a piece of the plan.) (NCSBN, 2016b).
- The nurse is accountable for nursing judgment decisions and for ongoing supervision of any care that is delegated or assigned.
- The nurse cannot delegate the nursing process (in particular the assessment, planning, and evaluation phases)

or clinical judgment to a non-nurse. Some interventions or data-gathering activities may be delegated based on the circumstances.

- The nurse must know as much as practical about the patients and their conditions, as well as the skills and competency of team members, to prioritize, delegate, and assign. Decisions must be specifically individualized to the patient, the delegatees, and the situation.
- In a clinical situation, everything is fluid and shifting. No priority, assignment, or delegation is written indelibly and cannot be altered. The nurse in charge of a unit, a team, or one patient is accountable to choose the best course to achieve the patient's and family's preferred results.

Best wishes in completing this workbook! The authors invite you to use the questions as an exercise in assembling the pieces to the puzzle that will become a picture of health-promoting practice.

REFERENCES

Alfaro-LeFevre, R. (2017). *Critical thinking, clinical reasoning, and clinical judgment: A practical approach* (6th ed.). St Louis: Saunders.

American Nurses Association & National Council of State Boards of Nursing. (2019). *National guidelines for nursing delegation* https://www.nursingworld.org/practice-policy/nursing-excellence/official-position-statements/id/joint-statement-on-delegation-by-ANA-and-NCSBN/. (File available to members only at https://www.nursingworld.org/globalassets/practiceand policy/nursing-excellence/ana-position-statements-secure/ana--ncsbn-joint-statement-on-delegation.pdf.)

American Nurses Association, Duffy, M., & McCoy, S. F. (2014). *Delegation and YOU: When to delegate and to whom.* Silver Springs, MD: ANA.

Bittner, N., Gravlin, G., Hansten, R., et al. (2011). Unraveling care omissions. *Journal of Nursing Administration, 41*(12), 510–512.

Brous, E. (2014). Lessons learned from litigation: The case of Bernard Travaglini. *American Journal of Nursing, 114*(5), 68–70.

Carder, P. C., & O'Keeffe, J. (2016). State regulation of medication administration by unlicensed assistive personnel in residential care and adult day services settings. *Research Gerontological Nursing, 7*, 1–14.

Diab, G., & Ebrahim, R. (2019). Factors leading to missed nursing care among nurses at selected hospitals. *American Journal of Nursing Research, 7*(2), 136–147.

Dyck, M., & Novotny, N. (2018). Exploring reported practice habits of registered nurses and licensed practical nurses at Illinois nursing homes. *Journal of Nursing Regulation, 9*(2), 18–30.

Grant, V. (2016). Sharpening your legal IQ: Safeguarding your license. *Viewpoint, 38*(3), 10–12.

Hansten, R. (2005). Relationship and results-oriented healthcare: Evaluate the basics. *Journal of Nursing Administration, 35*(12), 522–524.

Hansten, R. (2008a). *Relationship and results oriented healthcare™ planning and implementation manual.* Port Ludlow, WA: Hansten Healthcare PLLC.

Hansten, R. (2008b). Why nurses still must learn to delegate. *Nurse Leader, 6*(5), 19–26.

Hansten, R. (2011). *Leadership at the point of care: Nursing delegation.* http://www.MyFreeCE.com.

Hansten, R. (2014a). Coach as chief correlator of tasks to results through delegation skill and teamwork development. *Nurse Leader, 12*(4), 69–73.

Hansten, R. (2014b). *The master coach manual for the relationship & results oriented healthcare program.* Port Ludlow, WA: Hansten Healthcare PLLC.

Hansten, R. (2019). *Another look at RN leadership skill level and patient outcomes.* LinkedIn Pulse. https://www.linkedin.com/pulse/another-look-rn-leadership-skill-level-patient-hansten-rn-mba-phd.

Hansten, R. (2020a). *Delegation/supervision/assignment during a pandemic.* LinkedIn Pulse. https://www.linkedin.com/pulse/delegationassignmentsupervision-pandemic-ruth-hansten-rn-mba-phd/.

Hansten, R. (2020b). Delegation, assignment, and supervision. In P. K. Vana, & J. Tazbir (Eds.), *Nursing leadership and management* (4th ed.). Hoboken, NJ: Wiley.

Hansten, R. (2021). Delegation in the clinical setting. In J. Zerwekh, & A. Garneau (Eds.), *Nursing today: Transitions and trends* (10th ed.). St Louis: Elsevier.

Hansten, R., & Jackson, M. (2009). *Clinical delegation skills: A handbook for professional practice* (4th ed.). Sudbury, MA: Jones & Bartlett.

Interprofessional Education Collaborative. (2016). *Core competencies for interprofessional collaborative practice: 2016 Update.* Washington, DC: Interprofessional Education Collaborative. https://ipecollaborative.org.

Kalisch, B. (2015). *Errors of omission: How missed nursing care imperils patents.* Silver Springs, MD: ANA.

Maningo, M. J., & Panthofer, N. (2018). Appropriate delegation in an ambulatory care setting. *AAACN Viewpoint, 40*(1), 1–2.

McMullen, T. L., Resnick, B., Chin-Hansen, J., et al. (2015). Certified nurse aide scope of practice: State-by-state differences in allowable delegated activities. *Journal of American Medical Directors Association, 6*(1), 20–24.

Mizne, D. (2018). *7 Fascinating employee engagement trends for 2018*, 1–11. https://www.15five.com/blog/7-employee-engagement-trends-2018/.

McNee, B. (2017). *Nurse morale and its impact on LTC.* McKnights Long-Term Care News, 1–2. https://www.mcknights.com/blogs/guest-columns/nurse-morale-and-its-impact-on-ltc/.

Mueller, C., Vogelsmeier, A., Anderson, R., et al. (2018). Interchangeability of licensed nurses in nursing homes: Perspective of directors of nursing. *The End to End Journal, 1*, 1–27.

National Council of State Boards of Nursing. (1995). Delegation: Concepts and decision-making process. *Issues, 16*(4), 1–4.

National Council of State Boards of Nursing. (2016a). Medical Assistant-Certified Model Curriculum. https://www.ncsbn.org/07_Final_MAC.pdf.

National Council of State Boards of Nursing. (2016b). National guidelines for nursing delegation. *Journal of Nursing Regulation, 7*(1), 5–14. https://www.ncsbn.org/NCSBN_Delegation_Guidelines.pdf.

National Council of State Boards of Nursing. (2019a). *Participating states in the nurse licensure compact implementation.* https://www.ncsbn.org/compacts.htm.

National Council of State Boards of Nursing. (2019b). 2018 LPN/VN practice analysis: Linking the NCLEX-PN examination to practice. *NCSBN Research Brief, 75.* https://www.ncsbn.org/13443.htm.

QSEN Institute. (2019). *QSEN competencies.* http://qsen.org/competencies/graduate-ksas/.

Ralph, N., & Viljoen, B. (2018). Fundamentals of missed care: Implications for the perioperative environment. *ACORN Journal of Perioperative Nursing, 31*(3), 3–4.

Revised Code of Washington. (2012). *Registered nurse—Activities allowed—Delegation of tasks.* Title 18, Chapter 18.79, Section 18.79.260). http://apps.leg.wa.gov/RCW/default.aspx?cite=18.79.260.

Silvestri, L., & Silvestri, A. (2018). *Saunders 2018-2019 strategies for test success* (p. 66). St Louis: Elsevier.

Standing, T., Anthony, M., & Hertz, J. (2001). Nurses' narratives of outcomes after delegation to unlicensed assistive personnel. *Outcomes Management of Nursing Practice, 5*(1), 18–23.

The Joint Commission. (2017). Inadequate hand-off communication. *Sentinel Event Alert, 58.*

Texas Board of Nursing. (2019). *Frequently asked questions: Delegation*, 1–7. http://www.bon.texas.gov/faq_delegation.asp#t6.

Voalte. (2013). *Special report: Top 10 clinical communication trends*, 1–16. https://www.voalte.com/press-releases/new-survey-finds-hospital-nurses-spend-half-shift-tasks-patient-care.

Washington State Administrative. (2019). *Definitions.* https://app.leg.wa.gov/wac/default.aspx?cite=246-840-010. 2019.

Washington State Department of Health Nursing Care Quality Assurance Commission. (2019). Registered nurse and licensed practical nurse scope of practice. *Advisory opinion*, 1–12. https://www.doh.wa.gov/Portals/1/Documents/6000/NCAO13.pdf.

RECOMMENDED RESOURCES

Alfaro-LeFevre, R. (2017). In *Critical thinking, clinical reasoning, and clinical judgment: A practical approach* (6th ed.). St Louis: Saunders.

Hansten, R. (2008). *Relationship and results oriented healthcare™ planning and implementation manual.* Port Ludlow, WA: Hansten Healthcare PLLC.

Hansten, R. (2014). *The master coach manual for the relationship & results oriented healthcare program.* Port Ludlow, WA: Hansten Healthcare PLLC.

Hansten, R., & Jackson, M. (2009). *Clinical delegation skills: A handbook for professional practice* (4th ed.). Sudbury, MA: Jones & Bartlett.

Hansten, R. (2014). Coach as chief correlator of tasks to results through delegation skill and teamwork development. *Nurse Leader, 12*(4), 69–73.

Hansten Healthcare PLLC website, http://www.Hansten.com or http://www.RROHC.com. Check for new delegation/supervision resources, online delegation, and assignment education modules at http://learning.Hansten.com/.

Kalisch, B. (2006). Missed nursing care. *Journal of Nursing Care Quality, 21*(4), 306–313.

National Council of State Boards of Nursing website. http://www.ncsbn.org. Contains links to state boards and abundant resources relating to delegation and supervision. Also download the ANA and NCSBN Joint Statement on Delegation. The decision trees and step-by-step process through the five rights are exceptionally clear and a great review to prepare for the NCLEX at https://www.ncsbn.org/NCSBN_Delegation_Guidelines.pdf and https://www.ncsbn.org/Delegation_joint_statement_NCSBN-ANA.pdf.

Introduction PART 1

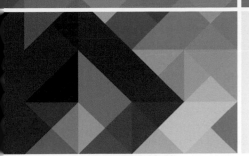

CHAPTER 1

Fundamentals of Nursing

Questions

1. A newly hired nurse experienced harsh criticism from the preceptor during orientation. Upon completing orientation, the charge nurse assigned her the most difficult and complex patients. What would the new nurse do **first**?
   1. Use assertive communication to discuss the assignments with the charge nurse
   2. Talk to the nurse manager about the behavior of the charge nurse and preceptor
   3. Make a formal written complaint and submit it to the human resources department
   4. Review the facility's policies on horizontal violence (e.g., bullying and harassment)

2. Which assistive personnel (AP) needs a reminder on providing denture care?
   1. AP-A places a towel in the sink, then fills the sink with 1 inch of tepid water
   2. AP-B puts on gloves and grasps the front teeth to remove the upper denture
   3. AP-C brushes all denture surfaces with a brush using a commercial paste
   4. AP-D rinses the dentures with hot water and stores them in a clean dry cup

3. Which specimen collection method is the **most** important to modify if a patient has a low platelet count?
   1. Blood serum sample for blood typing
   2. Stool sample for ova and parasites
   3. Midstream urine sample for urinalysis
   4. Expectorated sputum sample for culture

4. Before the end of the shift, the nurse is rounding on assigned patients and performing a quick head-to-toe assessment. Which patient has the **priority** finding?
   1. Patient with kidney stones has a score of 7/10 on pain scale
   2. Opioid-naïve patient has slow, shallow respirations
   3. Postsurgical patient has pale, clammy skin
   4. Elderly patient is more confused compared to baseline

5. Which guidelines are included as good body mechanics for lifting and moving? **Select all that apply.**
   1. Bend forward from the waist to pick up objects
   2. Use thigh, arm, or leg muscles rather than the back muscles
   3. Elevate the bed to work at a height that minimizes bending
   4. Keep the trunk straight; do not twist when lifting
   5. Use a wide base of support; feet apart at shoulder width
   6. Push objects away rather than pulling them toward

6. Which incident would involve the state board of nursing in fulfilling its **primary** purpose?
   1. Older, experienced nurse receives less pay than a recently hired new graduate nurse
   2. Nurse experiences sexual harassment from a supervisor and health care providers
   3. Nurse is practicing with an expired license and fails to assess a patient's cast forearm
   4. Several nurses are fired by hospital administration for trying to start a nurses' union

7. Which documentation entry needs to be flagged so that the general guidelines for documentation can be reviewed with the nurse who made the entry?
   1. 1330: Dr. Smith reviewed and explained surgical procedure; consent form signed and witnessed. Nurse A LPN/LVN
   2. 1400: Registered nurse assesses patient's pain at 7/10 on the pain scale and administers morphine as needed (PRN). Nurse B LPN/LVN
   3. 1545: Sacral wound irrigated with 100 mL sterile normal saline. Pink tissue and small amount of serous drainage noted. Nurse C LPN/LVN
   4. 1730: Liquid nutritional supplement refused; "I don't like the taste." Other flavors offered, but declined. Nurse D LPN/LVN

8. Which nurse is **most** likely to be held liable for nursing malpractice?
   1. Nurse A assigns too many patients to AP; some do not get a shower
   2. Nurse B fails to report worsening condition and the patient sustains permanent damage
   3. Nurse C leaves before shift report; no patient is harmed but oncoming nurses are upset
   4. Nurse D is demeaning and uses condescending language and the patient gets angry

9. The nurse is supervising the nursing student who is performing a procedure. Which action by the nursing student requires correction?
   1. Checks agency policy and procedure manual before beginning the procedure
   2. Checks the order, collects equipment, and performs hand hygiene
   3. Provides privacy, raises the bed to working height, and ensures that wheels are locked
   4. Identifies self, starts procedure, and explains each step as it is performed

10. Which patient would benefit the **most** from a therapeutic oatmeal bath?
    1. Has itching and irritation secondary to dermatitis
    2. Has an open wound in the lower extremity
    3. Has a fever and needs cooling measures
    4. Has discomfort secondary to rectal surgery

11. The nurse is using the PQRST mnemonic device for pain assessment. Which question would the nurse ask to assess the "S" portion of the mnemonic?
    1. Is the pain in a single location or does it radiate to other parts of your body?
    2. On a scale of 1–10, 1 as the least and 10 as the worst, which number best describes your pain?
    3. When did the pain start and approximately how long did each episode last?
    4. Do you have any ideas or thoughts about what could be causing the pain?

12. The nurse needs data to determine if the patient has a pulse deficit. Which task would be **best** to delegate to the AP?
    1. Begin counting the radial pulse for a full minute, when signaled
    2. Take a radial pulse, then listen to the apical pulse for a full minute
    3. Check and report pulse deficit when taking routine vital signs
    4. Check the radial pulse for a full minute on each wrist

13. In which situation has the nurse made the **greatest** error in delegation and instruction to the AP regarding the movement or transfer of a patient?
    1. Tells AP to put the ambulatory patient in a wheelchair and push him to the dining room
    2. Asks AP to use a drawsheet and pull the patient from the bed to a stretcher
    3. Tells the AP to logroll and reposition a patient with a recent spinal cord injury
    4. Asks the AP to remind a quadriplegic patient to do range-of-motion (ROM) exercises

14. During bed-making, which nursing student requires a reminder from the supervising nurse?
    1. Student A raises the bed to working height and uses a wide base of support
    2. Student B changes linen on one side of the bed before moving to the other side
    3. Student C carries soiled linens away from the body and puts them in a linen hamper
    4. Student D takes unused and unsoiled linens back to the central linen cart

15. Four patients need vital signs, assessment, and care after undergoing various diagnostic procedures. Which patient can be safely assigned to the AP for assistance and taking vital signs?
    1. Patient had a thoracentesis that was performed at bedside
    2. Patient had a pelvic exam and a Papanicolaou smear
    3. Patient had a lumbar puncture performed 1 hour ago
    4. Patient returns from the x-ray department after having an arteriogram

16. Which of the displayed heart rhythms would the nurse identify as tachycardia?

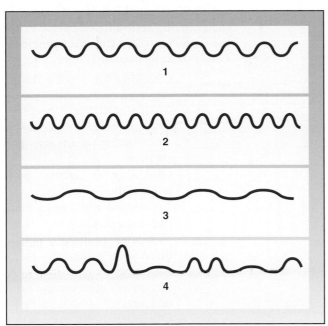

(Figure from Williams P deWit's (2021) *Fundamental Concepts and Skills for Nursing* (6th ed.), Elsevier.)

17. The nurse instructs the AP to collect stool specimens from several patients. Which patient's specimen must be **immediately** taken to the laboratory after the AP collects it?
    1. Patient has diarrhea and stool culture is needed to rule out *Clostridium difficile* infection
    2. Patient reports dark-colored stool for several days with subjective feelings of fatigue
    3. Patient has diarrhea and mucus stools after drinking water from a mountain stream
    4. Patient reports pain and small amounts of bright red blood during defecation

18. Which instruction would the nurse give to the AP regarding the use of the temporal artery thermometer?
    1. If the patient has been eating or drinking, wait for 15—30 minutes before taking the temperature
    2. Switch the thermometer to the temporal artery setting and use the red probe
    3. Slide probe across forehead; keep button depressed, lift probe, and touch on the neck just behind the earlobe
    4. Place the patient in the Sims' position and wipe the skin to remove perspiration

19. Drop and Drag

Scenario: The patient reports stomach pain. "A dull ache, right here in the middle (points to midepigastric area) that wakes me in the middle of the night, and it bothers me when I don't eat on a regular schedule. It started about 2 or 3 months ago. When it starts to hurt, I eat a couple of crackers or take an over-the-counter antacid and then I feel better. It's usually mild, but when I am very worried or stressed out, I feel stomach acid churning and at that point the pain is moderate. Occasionally, I get nauseated, but I never actually vomit."

The nurse will use the guidelines for documenting a sign or a symptom. The guidelines include six categories:
A. Location in the body
B. Quality
C. Quantity
D. Chronology
E. Setting
F. Aggravating or alleviating factors
G. Associated manifestations

Six categories for documentation guidelines are listed in the left column. Match the documentation samples below with one of the categories. Write the correct letter in the space provided. Note that all responses are used only once.

1. _____ Discomfort described as a dull ache
2. _____ Symptoms relieved by eating crackers or taking over-the-counter antacids
3. _____ Wakes in the middle of the night with dull ache
4. _____ Occasional nausea, but no vomiting
5. _____ Onset about 2–3 months ago
6. _____ Points to midepigastric area, "right here in the middle"
7. _____ Discomfort described as "usually mild" but moderate during stress

 Answer Key for this chapter begins on p. 15

20. Drop and Drag

Scenario: The nurse uses knowledge of anatomy and physiology to locate the pulse points for assessment and intervention.

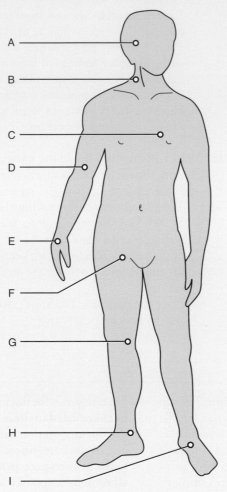

A
B
C
D
E
F
G
H
I

(Figure from Williams P: deWit's (2018) *Fundamental Concepts and Skills for Nursing* (6th ed.) , Elsevier.)

Refer to the figure in the left-hand column and select the best pulse site for each nursing action listed below. Write the correct letter in the space provided. Letters may be used only once.

_____ 1. Checking for a pulse during one-man cardiopulmonary resuscitation (CPR)

_____ 2. Taking a routine blood pressure

_____ 3. Auscultating heart rate and rhythm

_____ 4. Obtaining an arterial body temperature

_____ 5. Locating dorsalis pedis pulse was unsuccessful

_____ 6. Checking perfusion in the distal lower extremities

_____ 7. Assessing femoral artery insertion site after cardiac catherization

_____ 8. Obtaining pulse rate during routine vital signs

_____ 9. Assessing lower extremity for peripheral artery disease; Doppler device may be needed

Answers

1. **Ans: 1** The first action would be to talk directly to the charge nurse about the assignments. This could be difficult for a new nurse, but assertive communication can be carefully planned and then delivered with a calm and nonconfrontive tone of voice. The other options may also be considered if the nurse continues to experience harassment or bullying from other members of the health care team. **Focus:** Prioritization; **QSEN:** TC; **Concept:** Communication, Professional Identity; **Cognitive Level:** Applying; **IPEC:** IC

2. **Ans: 4** AP-D needs a reminder. Hot water may warp or soften dentures, so tepid water is used for cleaning and rinsing. Cleaned dentures are stored in a clean labeled cup with cool water. The other APs are performing correctly. **Focus:** Prioritization, Supervision; **QSEN:** N/A; **Concept:** Clinical Judgment; **Cognitive Level:** Applying; **IPEC:** IC

3. **Ans: 1** Platelets are important for blood clotting and a low platelet count can cause excessive bleeding. To prevent untoward bleeding, the collection method for drawing blood would include using a small gauge needle and holding firm pressure on the puncture site for at least 5 minutes and thereafter rechecking the site for continued bleeding or oozing. For stool, urine, or sputum, the collection method would not be affected by a low platelet count; however, the nurse would observe each specimen for frank blood. **Focus:** Prioritization; **QSEN:** S; **Concept:** Perfusion; **Cognitive Level:** Analyzing

4. **Ans: 2** The nurse uses the ABCs (airway, breathing, circulation) to prioritize and the patient with slow shallow respirations could be having respiratory depression secondary to opioids. The nurse would assess responsiveness, check the pulse oximeter reading, reposition as necessary, and obtain a prescription for naloxone as needed. The other patients have problems that require additional assessment. The patient with pain and kidney stones needs a pain assessment and the nurse must note the time of the last dose of pain medication and assess urinary output. For the post-surgical patient, pain and the surgical site must be assessed. Vitals signs should also be obtained since hemorrhage is a concern. Pale, clammy skin also occurs with hypoglycemia, so the nurse would obtain a blood glucose reading as needed. Increased confusion in elderly patients could be caused by many things, such as medication side effects, infection, anxiety, unfamiliar environment, decreased cerebral perfusion, or oxygen deficit. The nurse must assess confusion, take vital signs and a pulse oximeter reading, and check blood glucose. Findings are reported and recorded. **Focus:** Prioritization; **QSEN:** S; **Concept:** Gas Exchange; **Cognitive Level:** Analyzing

5. **Ans: 2, 3, 4, 5** The goal is to decrease stress and strain on the back muscles. Use large muscles, such as the thighs, arms, and legs, rather than relying on the back muscles. Working at a comfortable height that minimizes bending; squatting, rather than bending; keeping the back straight; and maintaining a wide base of support are actions that preserve the back muscles. Using the Leg muscles and shifting body weight allows the object to be pulled, whereas pushing objects utilizes the upper and lower back and the arms. **Focus:** Prioritization; **QSEN:** S; **Concept:** Safety; **Cognitive Level:** Applying

6. **Ans: 3** The primary purpose of the state board of nursing is to protect the public and promote safe practice by ensuring that nurses are licensed, competent, and acting within the scope of practice. The board of nursing does not regulate or oversee agency/facility policies and practices. For salary or sexual harassment issues, nurses can seek resolution within the agency or facility. Professional nursing organizations can offer additional assistance in and advice on salary, harassment, hiring/firing, nurses' unions, and other workplace issues. **Focus:** Prioritization; **QSEN:** S; **Concept:** Health Policy; **Cognitive Level:** Analyzing; **IPEC:** V/E

7. **Ans: 2** Documentation should be done by the health team member who performs the action. (Note to student: during emergency situations, for example, during cardiac arrest, one nurse may be designated as the recorder to document the actions of the resuscitation team. Follow agency policies for emergency situations.) When the actions of team members, such as health care providers and therapists, are documented, name and title should be included. Objective data is included after performing a task or giving care. When a patient declines a treatment, use direct quotes and include actions that were taken. **Focus:** Prioritization **QSEN:** I; **Concept:** Technology and Informatics; **Cognitive Level:** Analyzing; **Test Taking Tip:** As you are reading and studying, notice that textbooks and journal articles highlight and summarize important guidelines in boxes, tables, or bullet lists.

8. **Ans: 2** All of these nurses have failed to give high-quality nursing care; however, a malpractice claim includes four elements: duty, breach of duty, causation, and damage. Nurse B had a duty to the patient, failed

PART 2 Common Health Scenarios

to fulfill that duty, and this breach resulted in permanent damage. The other nurses would be referred to the nurse manager for discussion, problem-solving, and counseling so that quality of care is achieved and maintained. **Focus:** Prioritization **QSEN:** EBP; **Concept:** Health Care Law; **Cognitive Level:** Analyzing

9. **Ans: 4**   Student has skipped the critical element of identifying the patient using two identifiers before beginning the procedure. The other actions are correct. **Focus:** Prioritization, Supervision; **QSEN:** S; **Concept:** Safety; **Cognitive Level:** Applying; **Test Taking Tip:** An important step that is emphasized in fundamentals textbooks is identifying the patient before proceeding with care. Safety measures and actions that reduce error are likely to be tested during NCLEX.

10. **Ans: 1**   Oatmeal or starch baths are soothing for irritated skin; also skin is patted dry rather than rubbed; this decreases itching and scratching. Open wounds must be kept clean and are treated with medicated soaks. The health care provider may order cooling sponge baths with tepid water for patients with fever. Sitz bath is a comfort measure that is offered after vaginal or rectal surgery or childbirth. **Focus:** Prioritization; **QSEN:** N/A; **Concept:** Inflammation; **Cognitive Level:** Applying

11. **Ans: 2**   In the PQRST mnemonic, P stands for precipitating events (cause of pain); Q is the quality of pain (patient's own words, such as throbbing, burning, dull); R is for radiation of pain (location of pain with radiation or spreading to other body parts); S is for severity (scales are often used to rate severity; verbal rating includes mild, moderate, severe); and T is for timing (onset, duration, episodic) **Focus:** Prioritization; **QSEN:** EBP; **Concept:** Pain; **Cognitive Level:** Applying

12. **Ans: 1**   A pulse deficit is noted when there is a discrepancy between the apical pulse and the radial pulse. Two members of the health care team must work together. Upon signal, one counts the apical pulse and the other counts the radial pulse for a full minute; then the radial pulse is subtracted from the apical pulse. If the nurse took a radial pulse and suspected an irregularity, then listening to the apical pulse would be a correct action, but this action should not be delegated to the AP. Likewise, it would be inappropriate to ask the AP to check for a pulse deficit during routine vital signs because the nurse is responsible to assess for irregular heart rhythms. Checking the radial pulse on each wrist is done when there is a possible perfusion problem in one or both arms. **Focus:** Prioritization, Supervision; **QSEN:** TC; **Concept:** Perfusion; **Cognitive Level:** Analyzing; **IPEC:** R/R

13. **Ans: 3**   All of these instructions could use improvement; however, the AP should not independently logroll or reposition a patient with a recent spinal cord injury. Improper technique could cause damage to the spinal cord and permanent paralysis. The AP can assist the nurse; logrolling requires two to three team members (depending on the size of the patient) and the patient's body must be kept in a straight alignment. Ambulatory patients should be assisted to walk to the dining area rather than being pushed in a wheelchair. Pulling a patient can cause shearing forces, which contributes to pressure injuries; a sliding board and two to three helpers would be preferable. Quadriplegic patients require passive ROM exercises; reminders are insufficient, and most patients with quadriplegia will require total assistance with ROM. **Focus:** Prioritization; **QSEN:** S; **Concept:** Safety, Immobility; **Cognitive Level:** Analyzing

14. **Ans: 4**   Student-D needs a reminder. Linen that is taken into a patient's room should not be returned to the central cart. Even if it is unused and appears clean it is considered contaminated for use for other patients. The other students are performing correctly. **Focus:** Prioritization, Supervision; **QSEN:** EBP; **Concept:** Infection; **Cognitive Level:** Applying; **IPEC:** IC

15. **Ans: 2**   To correctly assign and delegate this task, the nurse must know the possible postprocedure complications and take responsibility to evaluate vital signs in the context of the assessment findings. A pelvic exam and a Papanicolaou smear are noninvasive. A Pap smear involves scraping some cells from the cervix. The AP can be assigned to take vital signs and assist the patient in wiping the perineal area after the examination. Postprocedural care for a thoracentesis, a lumbar puncture, and an arteriogram requires concurrent critical thinking about the patient's condition, assessment findings, vital signs, teaching, and other interventions. For example, complications of a thoracentesis include impaired breathing, decreased oxygenation, and bleeding; the patient may need pain medication or reassurance. For a lumbar puncture, the patient is instructed to lie flat, report a headache (which is a common side effect), and drink as much fluid as possible. Puncture site must be observed for leakage and signs of infection. For an arteriogram, bleeding at the insertion site must be observed; depending on the health care provider's orders, the site may be immobilized. The tissue distal to the insertion site must also be assessed for perfusion. **Focus:** Prioritization; **QSEN:** S; **Concept:** Clinical Judgement; **Cognitive Level:** Analyzing; **Test Taking Tip:** In addition to knowing which tasks the APs can perform, the nurse must use clinical judgment related to the patient's condition. When the patient is unstable or if there is a possibility for complications, the AP is not the right

person, even if the task is simple and within the AP's scope of practice.

16. **Ans: 2**   Tachycardia is a rapid or fast heartbeat. In a normal rhythm, the heartbeat is regular and the pauses between beats are even. Bradycardia is a slow heartbeat. An irregular heartbeat is characterized by erratic pauses between beats and an uneven rate. **Focus:** Prioritization; **QSEN:** N/A; **Concept:** Perfusion; **Cognitive Level:** Applying

17. **Ans: 3**   Ideally, all specimens are transported to the laboratory as soon as possible; however, the onset of diarrhea and change in stools after drinking contaminated water indicate testing for ova and parasites and the specimen must be fresh (within 2 hours). Stool specimens for *Clostridium difficile* are usable up to 24 hours if they are refrigerated. Stool for culture and dark stool for hemoccult are less time sensitive. Reports of pain and bright red blood during defecation suggest that the patient has a hemorrhoid; however, stool cytology may also be ordered if cancer is suspected. **Focus:** Prioritization; **QSEN:** N/A; **Concept:** Elimination; **Cognitive Level:** Analyzing

18. **Ans: 3**   A temporal artery thermometer is considered the most accurate way to measure temperature. The probe is usually slid across the forehead above the brow. If perspiration is present, the temperature can be measured by touching the neck, just behind the earlobe. Oral temperatures are affected if the patient has been eating or drinking. For taking the rectal temperature, the red probe is used; some electronic thermometers have a setting for rectal or oral. Sims' position is comfortable for the patient when rectal temperature is taken. Skin is wiped for axillary or temporal artery measurement, but for rectal temperatures, the skin is wiped afterward to remove any excessive lubricant that was used on the probe. **Focus:** Prioritization; **QSEN:** N/A; **Concept:** Thermoregulation; **Cognitive Level:** Applying

19. **Nextgen Ans: 1B, 2F, 3E, 4G, 5D, 6A, 7C**   Using the guidelines, the nurse would include what the patient says in the documentation. The nurse also asks focused questions to elicit additional information, such as asking about the radiation of pain (Location), asking for additional descriptors (Quality), using a pain scale to quantify the discomfort (Quantity), and asking about the duration of episodes (Chronology). Questions about place, such as the work environment (Setting), or dietary habits and types of food (Aggravating factors) would be appropriate when gastroesophageal reflux disease is suspected. Based on the patient's report, the nurse would consider asking additional questions about other gastrointestinal symptoms, such as a change in bowel pattern, blood or dark-colored stool, or change in eating habits (Associated manifestations). The nurse would also perform and document a physical assessment. **Focus:** Prioritization; **QSEN:** I; **Concept:** Technology and Informatics; **Cognitive Level:** Analyzing; **Cognitive Skill:** Recognize Cues

20. **Nextgen Ans:**

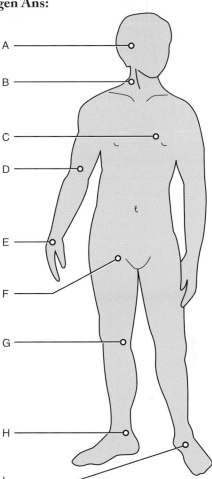

(Figure from Williams P. deWit's (2018) *Fundamental Concepts and Skills for Nursing* (6th ed.) Elsevier.)

1B Carotid, 2D Brachial, 3C Apical, 4A Temporal, 5H Posterior tibial, 6I Dorsalis pedis, 7F Femoral, 8E Radial, 9G Popliteal   During one-man CPR, the rescuer is close to the carotid artery. The carotid pulse is easier to palpate compared to peripheral pulses when cardiac output is decreased. The brachial artery is the common site to take blood pressures; it is easy to locate and access in most patients. The apical pulse is the best site to auscultate heart sounds. Temporal arterial thermometers are designed to give accurate body temperatures. Ideally, the skin is clean and dry. Press the button and slide the probe across the forehead. If perspiration is present, an accurate temperature can be obtained by touching on the neck just behind the earlobe. When the dorsalis pedis pulse is not palpable, the nurse moves up the leg and checks the posterior tibial. Dorsalis pedis is the main arterial supply for the foot and is usually readily located; however, the posterior tibial artery does provide some oxygenated blood to the foot. If no pulses are felt, the nurse would continue up the leg until a palpable pulse is obtained. The presence or absence of pulses at each site should be recorded and reported. The femoral artery is a common insertion site for cardiac catheterization. Postprocedure care includes examination of the site for bleeding or hematoma formation and perfusion distal to the insertion site. The radial pulse is the most common site to take a routine pulse. It is easily palpated and readily accessible. The popliteal pulse is checked if the patient has peripheral artery disease. It can also be used for blood pressure measurement if there is a problem with the upper extremities. The popliteal pulse can be difficult to locate because of the tissue behind the knee. A Doppler device may be used to locate any pulse that is difficult to palpate. The use of the Doppler is recorded and reported to the health care provider. **Focus:** Prioritization; **QSEN:** EBP; **Concept:** Perfusion; **Cognitive Level:** Analyzing; **Cognitive Skill:** Recognize Cues

QSEN Key: PCC, Patient-Centered Care; **TC,** Teamwork & Collaboration; **EBP,** Evidence-Based Practice; **QI,** Quality Improvement; **S,** Safety; **I,** Informatics. **IPEC Key:** Domain 1 Values/Ethics (**V/E**); Domain 2 Roles/Responsibilities (**R/R**); Domain 3 Interprofessional Communication (**IC**); Domain 4 Teams/Teamwork (**T/T**)

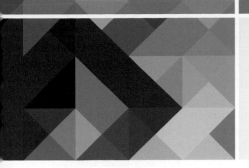

CHAPTER 2

Respiratory Problems

Questions

1. A 74-year-old patient with chronic obstructive pulmonary disease (COPD) displays difficulty breathing and increased coughing productive of yellow-green sputum. Vital signs are temperature 37.7°C (100°F), pulse 88 irregular, respiration rate 24, blood pressure 140/88, O_2 sat 92% on 1 L of oxygen. What is the **priority** nursing action?
   1. Report the findings to the health care provider (HCP).
   2. Ask the respiratory therapist to deliver an as-needed (PRN) breathing treatment.
   3. Increase oxygen as needed until the O_2 sat is 98%.
   4. Administer acetaminophen 650 mg by mouth for fever.

2. A patient who returned from a bronchoscopy several hours ago develops difficulty breathing and chest pain and is coughing up blood. Which interventions should the nurse perform first?
   1. Place the patient in a semi-Fowler's position.
   2. Apply electrocardiogram electrodes.
   3. Apply oxygen as ordered.
   4. Immediately report the findings to the registered nurse (RN).

3. For a patient with a tracheostomy, which duties can the nurse safely delegate to assistive personnel (AP)? **Select all that apply**.
   1. Holding the tracheostomy tube when the nurse is changing the ties and tube holder.
   2. Instructing the patient on how to cough effectively to remove secretions.
   3. Gathering tracheostomy sterile supply kits prior to the dressing change.
   4. Checking tracheostomy cuff pressure with a manometer.
   5. Assisting the nurse in delivering oxygen before and during sterile suctioning.
   6. Auscultating the lungs before and after suctioning the tracheostomy tube.

4. A student nurse is assisting the nurse with a hypertensive patient who suddenly develops epistaxis (nosebleed). The student nurse has been pinching the nostrils with the patient's head in a retrograde position for 5 minutes, but the bleeding continues. What is the **priority** nursing action?
   1. Apply ice to the bridge of the nose.
   2. Instruct the student nurse to continue the intervention and remain with the patient for at least 10 more minutes.
   3. Tell the student nurse to place the patient's head in a forward position while pinching the nostrils.
   4. Recheck the blood pressure and notify the HCP immediately.

5. The nurse is caring for a patient with COPD who has chest tightness, rapid, labored breathing, and a productive cough. Vital signs are: T 100°F (37.7°C), P 98, R 28, BP 158/88, O_2 sat is 70% room air. He is unable to speak more than five words at a time. Which intervention should the nurse institute immediately?
   1. Suction secretions from the patient's oropharynx.
   2. Notify the rapid response team.
   3. Apply electrocardiogram electrodes.
   4. Administer 100% oxygen via a nonbreather mask.

6. A student nurse is assigned to a patient with pneumonia. Which statement made by the student nurse regarding how to obtain a sputum specimen should the nurse correct?
   1. "I will obtain the specimen right after my patient receives his nebulizer treatment."
   2. "I will ask the patient to take several deep breaths, cough, and spit in the cup."
   3. "I will use a sterile specimen cup."
   4. "I will make sure that the mouth care has been given before the procedure."

7. The nurse is assisting the critical care RN in the intensive care unit (ICU) with a mechanically ventilated patient. Which intervention by the nurse is a priority to prevent ventilator-acquired pneumonia (VAP)?
   1. Suctioning the endotracheal tube every 2 hours.
   2. Administration of prophylactic antibiotics.
   3. Oral care with chlorhexidine every 2 hours.
   4. Positioning the patient in a prone position.

8. The nurse is caring for a patient with a right pneumonectomy. Which AP statement would prompt the nurse to intervene?
   1. "I have positioned the patient with his head at a 45-degree angle."
   2. "The chest tube is draining small amounts of blood."
   3. "I placed the patient on his side so he could look out the window."
   4. "The patient is resting with the head of the bed at a 30-degree angle."

9. The nurse has received reports on four patients. Which patient should the nurse make rounds on **first**?
   1. A 77-year-old male admitted with a pelvic fracture who is short of breath, anxious, and restless and was medicated for pain 15 minutes ago. T 99°F (37.2°C), P 100, R 24, BP 90/72, O$_2$ sat 92% room air.
   2. A 57-year-old female 1 day status–post–knee replacement patient who refused her albuterol breathing medications. T 100 °F (37.7°C), P 74, R 24, BP 104/72, O$_2$ sat 91% room air.
   3. A 35-year-old female with asthmatic bronchitis coughing up yellow-green sputum who is on antibiotics. T 101.4°F (38.5°C), P 92, R 24, O$_2$ sat 96% on 2 L oxygen.
   4. A 68-year-old male with emphysema who is dyspneic and is in atrial fibrillation. T 99°F (37.2°C), P 88, R 22, BP 140/90, O$_2$ sat 90% on 2 L oxygen.

10. The charge nurse has delegated reading the labs of a patient with COPD to a float nurse. The patient has the following arterial blood gases (ABG): pH 7.35, (PaCO$_2$) 48 mmHg, (PaCO$_2$) 80 mmHg, (HCO$_3$) 28 mEq/L. The float nurse is unsure if he should take any further action based on the ABGs. Which course of action should the charge nurse suggest?
   1. Suction the patient.
   2. Increase oxygen to 3 L/minute.
   3. Notify respiratory therapy for a PRN breathing treatment.
   4. Continue to monitor the patient.

11. The nurse has delegated all the personal care of her patients to the AP. Which of the following situations would warrant the nurse to give additional guidance to the AP?
    1. A patient with COPD who is reclining in a chair at a 120-degree angle.
    2. A patient with tuberculosis (TB) in a negative-pressure room with the door closed.
    3. A patient on a clear liquid diet who is eating a popsicle.
    4. A patient with viral pneumonia being transported to x-ray with a surgical mask on.

12. The nurse is caring for a postoperative patient with a tonsillectomy. Vital signs upon return to the unit were T 37°C (98.7°F), P 76, R 20, BP 134/72, O$_2$ sat 98% on 2 L of oxygen and have remained stable for the past hour. Which postoperative duty should not be delegated to the AP?
    1. Check vital signs every 30 minutes for 2 hours.
    2. Position the patient in a semi-Fowler's position.
    3. Assess the patient for frequent swallowing.
    4. Place an ice pack around the neck.

13. A patient is being treated for a community-acquired pneumonia with levofloxacin. Which statement made by the patient would cause the nurse to notify the HCP immediately?
    1. "I have to eat before taking this drug, so it doesn't cause nausea."
    2. "I must have hurt my knee because I have a pain under my kneecap, and it hurts to walk."
    3. "I've been on this drug for almost 2 days and I still don't feel well."
    4. "I don't take the drug with dairy products."

14. The nurse is assigned a patient with COPD and hypertension. The patient's wife asks the nurse what could have caused her husband's illness. Which risk factors are significant when the nurse considers the etiology of COPD in this patient? **Select all that apply**.
    1. Smoking
    2. Working as a firefighter
    3. Living in a dry desert climate
    4. Overweight
    5. Age over 50 years old
    6. Low-protein diet

15. The nurse and an AP are assigned to a patient on mechanical ventilation. Which action should the nurse delegate to the AP?
    1. Assessing the need to suction the endotracheal tube.
    2. Assisting the respiratory therapist with obtaining an ABG.
    3. Evaluating the response to medication.
    4. Cleansing and reapplying a transparent dressing to a stage 1 pressure injury.

16. A patient with TB is ready for discharge. Which statement made by the patient indicates that the nurse must reinforce the discharge instructions?
    1. "I will cover my nose and mouth when I cough or sneeze."
    2. "I will continue to take all the medications as prescribed for 6 months."
    3. "I will only drink two beers a day."
    4. "I will make sure that my family members are tested for TB."

17. The nurse is assisting an RN with a patient who is on mechanical ventilation. The patient's ABGs are as follows: pH 7.35, (PaO_2) 75 mmHg, ($PaCO_2$) 60 mmHg, (HCO_3) 28 mEq/L. Which order given by the HCP will correct the respiratory acidosis?
    1. Increase the FiO_2 on the ventilator to 40%.
    2. Insert a nasogastric tube.
    3. Increase the respiratory rate on the ventilator from 8 to 12 a minute.
    4. Draw samples for a complete blood count (CBC) and electrolyte levels.

18. _____

Case Study: The nurse is caring for a patient in an assisted living center. He presents with a dry, irritated throat, nasal congestion, sneezing, and a nonproductive cough. Vital signs are T 37.2°C (99°F), P 87, R 16, BP 132/74, O_2 sat 96% on room air.

Question: Which interventions by the nurse are important to carry out with this patient? **Select all that apply:**

1. Administer acetaminophen 650 mg by mouth for a fever of 37.2°C (99°F).
2. Tell the patient that she should avoid going outside during allergy season.
3. Instruct the patient how to properly wash her hands.
4. Tell the patient it is okay to use decongestant nose drops for 3 days.
5. Ask the provider for an order for a throat culture and antibiotic therapy.
6. Request that the patient not eat in the dining hall with other residents for several days.
7. Instruct the patient to increase fluids such as citrus juices.

19. Drag and Drop _____

Scenario: The nurse is caring for a 25-year-old patient with chest trauma following a motor vehicle crash. A thoracostomy (chest) tube was inserted into the left pleural cavity 2 days ago to alleviate a hemothorax. Vital signs are stable, and the patient is alert and oriented.
1. _____Temporarily clamp the tube to assess for an air leak.
2. _____Mark the amount of drainage in the water seal collection every 8 hours.
3. _____ Monitor and chart the amount and character of the drainage.
4. _____Instruct the patient to cough and deep-breathe.
5. _____Replace the water seal drainage system as necessary.
6. _____Monitor the patient for crepitus.
7. _____Assist the patient in changing positions to enable drainage and ventilation.
8. _____Assist the patient with bathing.
9. _____Assess complaints of new-onset left chest discomfort.

Question: Select the appropriate staff for each action and place the correct letter in the space next to each action. (Letters may be used more than once.)
A. Supervising RN
B. LPN/LVN
C. AP

 Answer Key for this chapter begins on p. 23

20. Drag and Drop

Scenario: The nurse is reinforcing patient teaching for a patient on how to use a peak flowmeter.

Instructions: Place the steps in the correct order for how to use the peak flowmeter. Write the letter from the left column next to the number on the left column to indicate the correct order.

Steps that are included in the procedure:		Correct order of steps:
A. The patient records the value and resets the pointer		1. _____
B. Rest for a few breaths		2. _____
C. The nurse instructs the patient to set the pointer to zero		3. _____
D. Take a deep breath while standing		4. _____
E. Make a firm seal with lips around the mouthpiece and then blow fast and hard		5. _____
F. Rest, repeat the process for a total of three readings		6. _____

Common Health Scenarios   PART 2

Answers

1. **Ans: 1** The patient's fever and yellow-green sputum indicate a possible respiratory infection. The HCP should be notified for assessment, diagnosis, and treatment. A respiratory treatment may be given but is not the priority and could delay treatment of an infection. An O_2 sat of 92% is adequate, so increasing oxygen is not necessary and could have a negative effect on a COPD patient by interfering with the mechanism to breathe. Fever stimulates the production of white blood cells to fight infection and generally should not be treated unless it is 38.8°C (102°F) or the patient is uncomfortable. **Focus**: Prioritization; **QSEN**: EBP **Concept**: Infection/Gas Exchange; **Cognitive Level:** Analyzing

2. **Ans: 1** The first thing the nurse should do is protect the airway by placing the patient in a semi-Fowler's position. Although applying oxygen and electrodes is reasonable, airway is the priority action and should be done first. The RN must be notified, but only after the nurse has made sure the patient has a patent airway. **Focus**: Prioritization; **QSEN**: EBP; **Concept**: Gas Exchange; **Cognitive Level**: Analyzing

3. **Ans: 1, 3, 5** The AP can assist the nurse with holding the tracheostomy tube to ensure the tube stays in place while the tube holder and ties are being replaced. The AP may also assist the nurse in delivering oxygen so the nurse can remain sterile during the suctioning procedure, and the AP can be delegated to gather the supply kit prior to the dressing change. Instruction on coughing, checking cuff pressures, and auscultating lungs need to be done by the nurse. **Focus**: Delegation; **QSEN**: S/T/C; **IPEC**: T/T; **Concept**: Care Coordination; **Cognitive Level**: Analyzing

4. **Ans: 3** The priority is airway. If the patient's head is in a retrograde position, bleeding can enter the throat and cause an airway obstruction or aspiration. Ice can be applied to the nose but is not the priority. Immediately notifying the HCP is not necessary unless the bleeding continues and cannot be stopped. **Focus**: Prioritization; **QSEN**: T/C; **IPEC**: R/R; **Concept**: Gas Exchange; **Cognitive Level**: Analyzing

5. **Ans: 4** For this patient, who is exhibiting signs of respiratory distress, 100% oxygen is needed. If hypoxia is not treated for more than 4 to 6 minutes, sudden cardiopulmonary arrest and irreversible damage to the brain can occur. There is no indication that there is an airway obstruction as the patient can still speak, so suctioning the oropharynx is not warranted and would waste time. The rapid response team should be notified immediately after oxygen is applied. EKG electrodes can be applied while waiting for the rapid response team to arrive. **Focus**: Prioritization; **QSEN**: EBP; **Concept**: Gas Exchange; **Cognitive Level**: Analyzing

6. **Ans: 2** Sputum needs to be coughed up from the respiratory tract. The patient should be told to forcefully cough and expectorate into the sterile specimen cup. Because saliva will be mixed in with the sputum, the patient's mouth should be clean and rinsed with water prior. The best sputum specimen is taken first thing in the morning before breakfast. **Focus**: Assignment, Supervision; **QSEN**: T/C; **IPEC**: R/R; **Concept**: Patient Education; **Cognitive Level**: Applying

7. **Ans: 3** Chlorhexidine oral care at least four times a day is proven to reduce VAP and is part of the ventilator bundle. Suctioning the endotracheal tube should be done only as needed to remove secretions. Frequent suctioning increases secretions and can cause trauma to the respiratory tract. Probiotics and not antibiotics are used prophylactically to decrease infection. Positioning the patient in a prone position improves oxygenation but does not prevent VAP. **Focus**: Priority; **QSEN**: EBP; **Concept**: Gas Exchange/Infection; **Cognitive Level**: Analyzing

8. **Ans: 3** The patient with a pneumonectomy should not be placed in a lateral position. The mediastinum can shift because there is no longer lung tissue in place. This can compress the remaining lung. **Focus**: Prioritization; **QSEN**: EBP/S; **Concept**: Gas Exchange; **Cognitive Level**: Analyzing

9. **Ans: 1** This patient is at a high risk for a fat embolus from his pelvic fracture. Early symptoms of a fat embolus include shortness of breath, feelings of apprehension, and restlessness. This patient should be assessed first, so either the rapid response team or the HCP are to be notified immediately. The head of the bed should be elevated, and oxygen should be administered. **Focus**: Prioritization; **QSEN**: S; **Concept**: Gas Exchange; **Cognitive Level**: Analyzing

10. **Ans: 4** Normal ABG values are pH 7.35–7.45, (PaO_2) 75–100 mmHg, ($PaCO_2$) 35–45 mmHg, (HCO_3) 22–26 mEq/L. A patient with COPD normally retains carbon dioxide, so it is expected that their $PaCO_2$ would be higher (48 mmHg) and their pH would be more toward the acidic side (pH 7.35). The patient's bicarbonate is higher (alkaline) to compensate for the pH from dropping below 7.35. **Focus**: Delegation; **QSEN**: T/C; **IPEC**: R/R; **Concept**: Acid Base Balance; **Cognitive Level**: Analyzing. **Test Taking Tip**: Knowing or memorizing normal range laboratory values allows you to quickly evaluate the data in the question and apply it to the patient's condition.

PART 2 Common Health Scenarios

11. **Ans: 1** A patient with COPD should be placed sitting in a Fowler's position, leaning forward to help with breathing. The elbows may be placed either on the patient's knees or with their arms folded and placed on a nightstand with a couple of pillows on top. The door to a negative-pressure room should be closed, popsicles are considered a clear liquid, and a patient with pneumonia should wear a surgical mask to minimize droplet exposure to the staff. **Focus:** Delegation; **QSEN:** PCC; **Concept:** Gas Exchange; **Cognitive Level:** Analyzing

12. **Ans: 3** A patient who is swallowing frequently could indicate excessive bleeding. The nurse should examine the patient for frequent swallowing as it could represent a bleeding emergency. **Focus:** Delegation; **QSEN:** T/C; **IPEC:** R/R; **Concept:** Perfusion; **Cognitive Level:** Analyzing

13. **Ans: 2** Levofloxacin is a quinolone and can cause tendon ruptures and serious nerve damage. The HCP should be notified immediately so the drug can be stopped and replaced with a different antibiotic and thus further damage to the tendons can be avoided. Levofloxacin should be taken 2 hours before or 2 hours after a meal. The nurse can counsel the patient that if nausea occurs, it is best to take the drug with a full glass of water. Antibiotics can take up to 3 days before the patient begins to feel better. Levofloxacin should not be taken with dairy products. **Focus:** Prioritization; **QSEN:** EBP; **Concept:** Clinical Judgement; **Cognitive Level:** Analyzing

14. **Ans: 1, 2, 3** Smoking is the cause of around 90% of COPD risk. Persons who live in dust-filled environments or have occupations that have exposure to dust, fly ash, soot, smoke, aerosols, and fumes are also considered at high risk for developing COPD. **Focus:** Priority **QSEN:** PCC; **Concept:** Patient Education; **Cognitive Level:** Applying

15. **Ans: 2** The AP can assist the respiratory therapist as needed but cannot assess the need for suctioning or evaluate a medication response. These are nursing actions. Cleansing and reapplying a dressing should be done by the nurse so she can note any changes in the pressure injury. **Focus:** Delegation; **QSEN:** T/C; **IPEC:** R/R; **Concept:** Care Coordination; **Cognitive Level:** Analyzing

16. **Ans: 3** Patients should not drink alcohol because it increases the risk for liver damage while they are on TB medications. The patient should cover their nose and mouth when sneezing and coughing and put the tissue directly in the trash. TB medications are prescribed for 6 months and anyone that was in close contact with the patient should receive a TB test. **Focus:** Prioritization; **QSEN:** EBP; **Concept:** Adherence; **Cognitive Level:** Applying

17. **Ans: 3** Increasing the respiratory rate from 8 to 12 times a minute will drive the CO_2 out of the lungs, decreasing the $PaCO_2$. Increasing the FiO_2 will not decrease the $PaCO_2$ but will increase the PaO_2. Inserting a nasogastric tube and ordering a CBC and electrolyte level will not decrease respiratory acidosis. **Focus:** Prioritization; **QSEN:** EBP; **Concept:** Acid Base Balance; **Cognitive Level:** Analyzing

18. **Ans: 3, 4, 6, 7** The patient is exhibiting symptoms of the common cold as evidenced by a low-grade fever, which would not be present if she had allergic symptoms. Acetaminophen does not need to be administered for a low-grade fever but may be advisable for discomfort that may accompany the cold. Correct handwashing for 20 seconds is advisable to prevent further infection or spread of the cold. Decongestant nose drops will help the congestion but can have a rebound effect after 3 days. A throat culture and antibiotics do not need to be requested at this time as there is no indication of a bacterial throat infection. It is advisable to keep away from others because a cold is contagious for 3 days after symptoms appear. Increasing fluids is advisable, particularly citrus juices that have vitamin C. **Focus:** Prioritization; **QSEN:** EBP; **Concept:** Clinical Judgement; **Cognitive Level:** Analyzing; **Cognitive Skill:** Prioritize hypothesis. **Test Taking Tip:** Know the signs/symptoms of common disorders; this helps you to quickly identify nursing concerns and to prioritize actions.

19. **Ans: 1.A, 2.B, 3.B, 4.B, 5.A, 6.B, 7.C, 8.C, 9.A** Clamping of the chest tube to assess for air leaks must be done by the supervising RN. The LPN/LVN should monitor, chart, and mark the amount of drainage on the drainage system and instruct the patient in coughing and deep breathing, as well as monitoring the patient for crepitus to assure accuracy. An AP can assist with position changes and bathing. The supervising RN must replace the water seal drainage system if it becomes full or cracked. The RN should assess any new complaints of chest discomfort. **Focus:** Delegation; **QSEN:** T/C; **IPEC:** T/T; **Concept:** Collaboration; **Cognitive Level:** Analyzing; **Cognitive Skill:** Take Action

20. **Ans: 1.C, 2.D, 3.E, 4.B, 5.A, 6.F Focus:** Priority; **QSEN:** EBP; **Concept:** Patient Education; **Cognitive Level:** Application; **Cognitive Skill:** Take Action

QSEN Key: PCC, Patient-Centered Care; **TC,** Teamwork & Collaboration; **EBP,** Evidence-Based Practice; **QI,** Quality Improvement; **S,** Safety; **I,** Informatics

IPEC Key: Domain 1 Values/Ethics (**V/E**); Domain 2 Roles/Responsibilities (**R/R**); Domain 3 Interprofessional Communication (**IC**); Domain 4 Teams/Teamwork (**T/T**)

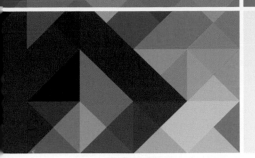

CHAPTER 3
Cardiovascular Problems

1. The nurse is assigned a patient with right-sided heart failure. Morning vital signs are T 37°C (98.6°F), P 110, R 26, O_2 sat 90%, BP 140/74. Which additional finding would require the nurse to notify the registered nurse (RN) or health care provider (HCP)?
   1. Hourly urine output of 15 mL/hour.
   2. 2+ pedal edema.
   3. S_2 heart sounds.
   4. Vesicular breath sounds.

2. For a patient with mild heart failure, which newly prescribed medication prescription prompts the nurse to observe for worsening signs of heart failure?
   1. Lisinopril 10 mg every day.
   2. Hydrochlorothiazide 25 mg every day.
   3. Synthroid 25 mcg every day.
   4. Loratadine 10 mg every day.

3. Which statement made by the nurse will give the clearest direction to the assistive personnel (AP) about assignments?
   1. "The patient needs to be walked down the hall today."
   2. "Place the patient in the chair for at least 1 hour today."
   3. "Please bathe and dress the patient by 10 a.m. for transfer."
   4. "Put a suture tray in the room for the surgeon."

4. The nurse is supervising a graduate nurse on a skilled nursing unit. A resident with a history of angina is complaining of chest pain after receiving news that his brother died. Vital signs are T 98.6°F (37°C), P 105 irregular, R 22, O_2 sat 94%, BP 110/64. He was given one nitroglycerine sublingual tablet 1 minute ago and the graduate nurse is preparing to administer 325 mg of aspirin. Which statement made by the graduate nurse is an indication for the supervising nurse to intervene?
   1. "The aspirin will prevent further blood clot formation."
   2. "You will need to chew this tablet."
   3. "The aspirin will improve blood flow to the heart."
   4. "The aspirin will help relieve the chest pain."

5. The nurse is assigned four patients. Which patient should the nurse round on **first**?
   1. A 55-year-old patient with Dressler syndrome who had cardiac surgery 2 weeks ago. T 37.7°C (100°F), P 84, R 22, O_2 sat 94%, BP 140/82.
   2. An 85-year-old patient with mitral valve stenosis and new-onset atrial fibrillation who is on coumadin. T 37°C (98.6°F), P 110 irregular, R 26, O_2 sat 90%, BP 140/74.
   3. A 65-year-old patient who had a permanent pacemaker inserted 1 day ago who has dementia and is agitated and flailing his arms. T 37°C (98.6°F), P 72, R 22, O_2 sat 96%, BP 130/72.
   4. A 77-year-old patient with pneumonia who is on antibiotics. T 37.7°C (100°F), P 90, R 22, O_2 sat 90%, BP 140/72.

6. The nurse is making assignments for the medical surgical care unit. Which patient should the nurse assign to an AP who has floated from the maternity unit?
   1. A post–coronary artery bypass graft (CABG) patient who is stable and needs support to cough and deep breathe.
   2. A patient with a new tracheostomy who is coughing up copious amount of sputum.
   3. A patient with coronary artery disease (CAD) who will be coming back to the unit after a cardiac catheterization.
   4. A patient recently diagnosed with angina.

7. The nurse is taking care of a patient with CAD who states, "All of a sudden it's hard to breathe and my left arm feels numb and it hurts." Vital signs are T 37.2°C (99°F), P 100 regular, R 26, O_2 sat 95%, BP 88/72. Which action will the nurse take **first**?
   1. Notify the rapid response team (RRT).
   2. Apply oxygen at 2 L/minute via nasal cannula.
   3. Administer nitroglycerine 1/150 sublingual tablet.
   4. Perform a 12-lead electrocardiogram (EKG).

Common Health Scenarios
PART 2

8. The nurse is assigned to a patient with stable angina who is scheduled for a cardiac catheterization arteriogram the next morning. Which actions will the nurse be prepared to take? **Select all that apply.**
   1. Hold metformin for 3 days.
   2. Keep the patient nothing by mouth (NPO).
   3. Assure the patient has signed a consent form.
   4. Review renal function, PT, PTT, and INR for abnormal values.
   5. Increase fluids after the arteriogram.
   6. Insert a urinary catheter to prevent bladder distention.

9. A patient with a history of CAD tells the nurse that he is nervous about his heartbeat being irregular sometimes. Which nursing intervention is the **priority**?
   1. Ask the patient about his daily intake of caffeinated beverages.
   2. Ask the RN if the patient should be put on telemetry.
   3. Offer the patient a PRN antianxiety medication.
   4. Update the nursing care plan to indicate the patient has an intermittent irregular heart rate.

10. The nurse is caring for a postoperative patient who underwent surgery for placement of a porcine valve. Which instructions should the nurse give to the AP regarding the postop care of the patient? **Select all that apply.**
    1. Use a soft toothbrush when providing oral care twice a day.
    2. Chart intake and output.
    3. Observe for and report obvious blood on the surface of the dressing.
    4. Report any complaints of chest pain or discomfort.
    5. Apply oxygen via nasal cannula at 2 L/minute.
    6. Remind the patient to cough and deep breath every 2 hours.

11. The nurse is auscultating apical heart sounds on a patient with heart failure. Place an X over the area where the nurse should place the diaphragm of the stethoscope to best listen for S_3 and S_4 sounds.

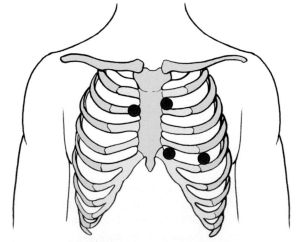

Figure from Stromberg, H. (2021) *deWit's Medical-Surgical Nursing* (4th ed.), Elsevier.

12. The nurse is caring for several patients on the cardiac unit. Which patient should the nurse see **first** on morning rounds?
    1. A 66-year-old patient, admitted to the unit during the night, who has abnormal CK-MB and troponin I levels.
    2. An 18-year-old patient with endocarditis who is on vancomycin and is complaining of night sweats.
    3. A 66-year-old patient who is 1 week post–cardiac bypass and received an opioid 1 hour ago for complaints of chest discomfort.
    4. A 77-year-old patient with peripheral artery disease (PAD) who is complaining of leg cramping.

13. The nurse is caring for a newly admitted patient from the emergency department with acute substernal chest pain. Which actions can the nurse assign to an AP?
    1. Questioning the patient about his medication history.
    2. Obtaining a capillary blood glucose level.
    3. Applying electrodes for cardiac monitoring.
    4. Notifying the primary HCP of the patient's admission.

14. The telemetry technician on the cardiac stepdown unit has notified the nurse that a patient's heart rate has decreased from a rate of 72 to a rate of 56, indicating bradycardia. What is the **first** action the nurse will take?
    1. Notify the RRT.
    2. Check vital signs, level of consciousness, and oxygen saturation.
    3. Alert the supervising RN.
    4. Perform a 12-lead EKG.

15. A 76-year-old patient with a history of congestive heart failure (CHF) and CAD is complaining of muscle cramping, drowsiness, and confusion. Vital signs are T 98.6°F (37°C), P 64, R 16, O_2 sat 95%, BP 100/74. Which medication will the nurse hold?
    1. Carvedilol 12.5 mg by mouth twice a day.
    2. Ibuprofen 400 mg by mouth every 8 hours with food.
    3. Bumetanide 0.5 mg by mouth every morning.
    4. Lisinopril 10 mg every day.

16. The nurse is assigned a patient with hypertension and type 2 diabetes who is prescribed atenolol 50 mg by mouth every day. Which signs and symptoms should the nurse be particularly alert about and concerned for?
    1. Nausea, sweating, and shakiness.
    2. Difficult breathing.
    3. Increased thirst and increased urination.
    4. Weakness and fatigue.

17. Which positioning instruction should the nurse give to the AP regarding the care of a patient with PAD who is having moderately severe pain and numbness in her lower extremities?
    1. Place the patient in bed and raise the foot of the bed above the level of the heart.
    2. Place the patient in a reclining chair with the legs positioned at a 180-degree angle.
    3. Place the patient in a chair with the legs hanging down at a 90-degree angle.
    4. Place the patient in bed in a supine position with a pillow under her knees.

18. Which medication should the nurse question when prescribed for a patient who is taking a daily aspirin for stroke prevention?
    1. Metoprolol succinate 50 mg by mouth every day.
    2. Atorvastatin 20 mg by mouth every day.
    3. Clopidogrel 75 mg by mouth every day.
    4. Naproxen 250 mg by mouth twice a day.

19. Matrix. The nurse is caring for a 62-year-old patient who is having dysrhythmias after a myocardial infarction (MI) 1 week ago. Vital signs are stable, and the patient is alert and oriented. For each potential HCP order, place an X in the box to indicate whether it is essential, nonessential, or contraindicated.

Potential Order	Essential	Nonessential	Contraindicated
24-hour telemetry			
Monitor vital signs every 2 hours			
Insert a urinary catheter			
Insert an intravenous (IV) catheter saline lock			
Place the patient on intake and output			
Monitor and chart daily weights			
Strict bed rest			
Administer morphine sulfate 10 mg IV for complaints of chest pain			
Dietary Approaches to Stop Hypertension diet			

20. **Complete the sentences below by choosing the most probable option for the omitted information that corresponds with the same numbered list of options provided.**

    Pulmonary edema is caused by ___1___ sided heart failure. Nursing priority interventions for acute pulmonary edema includes placing the patient in a ___2___, administering oxygen to keep the oxygen saturation between ___3___. Administration of ___4___ is given for diuresis. ___5___ is the best indicator of fluid increase.

Options for 1	Options for 2	Options for 3	Options for 4	Options for 5
Right	Semi fowlers position	89%–90%	Furosemide	Weight gain
Left	Tri-pod position	98%–100%	Morphine Sulfate	Lung auscultation
	Reverse Trendelenburg position	93%–95%	Fluconazole	Chest x-ray
	High fowlers			

    Answer Key for this chapter begins on p. 28

Answers

1. **Ans: 1**   Decreased urine output in right-sided heart failure indicates poor perfusion to the kidneys. Urine output should be at least 30 mL/hour. 2+ pedal edema would be considered a normal finding in right-sided heart failure and an S_2 heart sound and vesicular breath sounds are both normal findings. **Focus**: Prioritization; **QSEN**: EBP; **Concept**: Perfusion; **Cognitive Level**: Analyzing

2. **Ans: 3**   Synthroid is a thyroid hormone replacement medication. Thyroid hormone regulates cellular metabolism by converting oxygen and calories into energy and may worsen heart failure by increasing the metabolic and oxygen demands of the heart. **Focus**: Prioritization; **QSEN**: EBP/S; **Concept**: Cellular Regulation; **Cognitive Level**: Analyzing. **Test Taking Tip**: It is likely that you have cared for patients who were prescribed at least one of the medications in this question. A good way to study pharmacology is to pay attention to medications that are commonly prescribed.

3. **Ans: 3**   The direction is clear and specific on what needs to be done, why it needs to be done, and what time it needs to be done at. It is not clear how far the patient should be walked in number 1. In number 2 "at least" an hour is not specific enough. Number 4 is not specific as to when the surgeon needs the suture tray. **Focus**: Assignment, Supervision; **QSEN**: T/C; **Concept**: Communication; **Cognitive Level**: Analyzing

4. **Ans: 4**   Aspirin prevents platelets from sticking together and forming a clot. Blood flow to the heart is improved when blood can flow freely through the coronary arteries and can help prevent MI. Although aspirin is used to decrease fever and pain from inflammation, this is not the reason aspirin is given to a patient with angina who may be having an MI. Chewing the aspirin allows for faster absorption in the event of an MI when time is of the essence. **Focus**: Prioritization, Supervision; **QSEN**: EBP, T/C; **IPEC**: IC; **Concept**: Perfusion; **Cognitive Level**: Analyzing

5. **Ans: 3**   Moving your arms for normal daily motion is acceptable after a permanent pacemaker. However, flailing your arms or engaging in activities such as tennis or swimming that accentuates arm movement can dislodge the leads and lead to life-threatening dysrhythmias and cardiac instability. **Focus**: Prioritization; **QSEN**: EBP; **Concept**: Clinical Judgement; **Cognitive Level**: Analyzing

6. **Ans: 1**   Patients 2, 3, and 4 have conditions that warrant an experienced AP care for them. The experienced AP will be more comfortable, practiced, and knowledgeable about airway, breathing, and circulation issues in less stable patients on the unit. The AP from the maternity unit should be familiar with the coughing and deep breathing techniques. **Focus**: Assignment; **QSEN**: T/C; **IPEC**: R/R; **Concept**: Care Coordination; **Cognitive Level**: Analyzing

7. **Ans: 1**   The patient's O_2 sat is 95%, which is adequate, so the nurse should stay with the patient and alert the RRT first. Nitroglycerine might lower the BP even further and administration should be left to the RRT. A 12-lead EKG could be performed while waiting for the RRT. **Focus**: Prioritization; **QSEN**: EBP; **Concept**: Perfusion; **Cognitive Level**: Analyzing

8. **Ans: 1, 2, 3, 4, 5**   Metformin is held before procedures requiring contrast to prevent lactic acidosis should kidney function become impaired. Patients are kept NPO to avoid aspiration. When the HCP explains the procedure, the permit is usually signed. The nurse must assure the consent form has been signed prior to the procedure. Renal function, PT, PTT, and INR should be done prior to the procedure for a baseline so that the procedure can be canceled in the case of abnormalities. Fluid should be increased after any procedure that utilizes dye, so avoid kidney disfunction. Although the dye used in the arteriogram can act as a diuretic and cause bladder distention, it is not necessary to insert a urinary catheter. **Focus**: Prioritization; **QSEN**: EBP; **Concept**; Perfusion; **Cognitive Level**: Analyzing

9. **Ans. 1**   Caffeine can cause nervousness, increased BP, and a rapid and/or irregular heartbeat. Collecting data to report to the RN is the first phase of the nursing process, making this the priority intervention. Asking the RN about placing the patient on telemetry is a good idea but would be part of the planning process and requires an HCP order. Offering a PRN antianxiety drug would likely not relieve the irregular heart rate but, if done, it would be part of the implementation process. Updating the nursing care plan would be part of the evaluation process. **Focus**: Prioritization; **QSEN**: PCC; **Concept**: Care Coordination; **Cognitive Level**: Analyzing

10. **Ans: 1, 2, 3, 4, 6**   The AP is allowed to observe for any postop complications and report back to the nurse. Oxygen is a medication and the AP is not allowed to administer medications. **Focus**: Delegation; **QSEN**: PCC; **Concept**: Care Coordination; **Cognitive Level**: Analyzing

11. **Ans:**   Mitral area (5th intercostal space at the midclavicular line). **Focus**: Prioritization; **QSEN**: N/A; **Concept**: Perfusion; **Cognitive Level**: Applying

12. **Ans: 1** CK-MB and troponin levels are specific for myocardial muscle damage and rise within 6 hours after an MI. This patient should be seen first, and the provider notified of the abnormal lab results. Night sweats are normal for a person with endocarditis as it is an infectious process. The patient is on antibiotics, so this does not represent a priority. The patient who received an opioid an hour ago should be evaluated for relief of chest pain, but it is nonemergent. Leg cramping is a normal finding in a patient with PAD. **Focus**: Prioritization; **QSEN**: S; **Concept**: Clinical Judgement; **Cognitive Level**: Analyzing

13. **Ans: 3** The AP may assist the nurse with the admission assessment by applying EKG electrodes. Asking about medication history, collecting and measuring specimens such as capillary blood glucose, and notifying the HCP of an admission are actions that need to be completed by the nurse for continuity of quality care. **Focus**: Assignment; **QSEN**: PCC; **Concept**: Care Coordination, S; **Cognitive Level**: Analyzing

14. **Ans: 2** Bradycardia occurs frequently in athletes, elderly people, and those on certain medications. It does not need to be treated unless the patient is symptomatic. The first action is to gather information by measuring vital signs. If the BP is low or there is a change in consciousness, poor perfusion is indicated. If the respirations are abnormal or the oxygen saturation is low, hypoxia is indicated. The RRT should be notified for symptomatic bradycardia. **Focus**: Prioritization; **QSEN**: S; **Concept**: Perfusion; **Cognitive Level**: Analyzing

15. **Ans: 3** Bumetanide is a potent potassium wasting diuretic. The patient is having symptoms of hypokalemia, as evidenced by symptoms of muscle cramping, drowsiness, and confusion. The bumetanide should be held temporarily until the HCP can be notified and new orders are given. Hypokalemia can cause lethal dysrhythmias. **Focus**: Prioritization; **QSEN**: S; **Concept**: Fluid and Electrolytes; **Cognitive Level**: Analyzing

16. **Ans: 3** Increased thirst and urination are signs of hyperglycemia. Atenolol is a beta-blocker that can raise blood sugar in diabetic patients and mask symptoms of hypoglycemia such as nausea, sweating, and shakiness. At therapeutic doses, atenolol does not affect the beta-2 receptors in the lungs to affect breathing. Weakness and fatigue are signs of hypokalemia. **Focus**: Prioritization; **QSEN**: S, PCC; **Concept**: Glucose regulation; **Cognitive Level**: Analyzing

17. **Ans: 3** PAD affects the arteries of the lower extremities. By placing the legs in a downward position, more blood flow is delivered to the lower extremities, relieving pain and numbness. Additionally, foot and leg exercises as tolerated will help encourage venous return. Positioning with the foot of the bed raised above the heart level or placing a pillow under the knees will further impede arterial blood flow and worsen the symptoms. **Focus**: Assignment/Supervision; **QSEN**: PCC, T/C; **Concept**: Perfusion; **IPEC**: T/T; **Cognitive Level**: Applying

18. **Ans: 4** Nonsteroidal antiinflammatory drugs (NSAIDs), such as naproxen and ibuprofen, should not be used in conjunction with aspirin. NSAIDs can interfere with aspirin's effect of decreasing platelet aggregation; which is necessary for continued cardioprotection. **Focus**: Prioritization; **QSEN**: S; **Concept**: Perfusion; **Cognitive Level**: Analyzing

19. **Ans:**

Potential Order	Essential	Nonessential	Contraindicated
24-hour telemetry	X		
Monitor vital signs every 2 hours		X	
Insert a urinary catheter			X
Insert an intravenous (IV) catheter saline lock	X		
Place the patient on intake and output	X		
Monitor and chart daily weights	X		
Activity: bed rest		X	
Administer morphine sulfate 10 mg IV for complaints of chest pain			X
DASH diet	X		

Monitoring vital signs every 2 hours for a stable post-MI patient is not essential. Waking the patient every 2 hours can stress the heart and prevent healing. Every 4 to 8 hours is appropriate while the patient is on telemetry. Insertion of a urinary catheter is contraindicated due to the increased risk for infection. Strict bed rest for a stable post-MI patient is not necessary. Patients with uncomplicated MI are usually out of bed within 2 days. Morphine sulfate 10 mg IV is contraindicated and should be administered in small increments to relieve chest pain so that the blood pressure remains stable. DASH stands for a diet approach to stop hypertension. The DASH diet encourages eating foods low in sodium and rich in potassium, magnesium, and calcium. **Focus**:   Prioritization; **QSEN**: PCC; **Concept**: Perfusion; **Cognitive Level**: Analyzing; **Cognitive Skill**: Take Action

20. **Ans: b, d, f, h, k, o, n**   Pulmonary edema is caused by <u>left sided</u> heart failure. Nursing priority interventions for acute pulmonary edema includes placing the patient in a <u>high fowlers</u>, administering oxygen to keep the oxygen saturation between <u>93%-95%</u>. Administration of <u>furosemide</u> is given for diuresis. <u>Weight gain</u> is the best indicator of fluid increase. **Focus**: Prioritization; **QSEN**: EBP; **Concept**: Perfusion; **Cognitive Level**: Analyzing

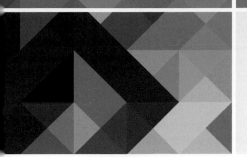

CHAPTER 4
Changes in Level of Consciousness

Questions

1. A patient with a history of chronic alcohol abuse displays short-term memory loss, long-term memory gaps, and confabulation. The health care provider (HCP) prescribes medication to prevent progression to Wernicke encephalopathy. Which medication prescription does the nurse anticipate?
   1. Parenteral dose of lorazepam followed by oral doses of lorazepam.
   2. Intramuscular (IM) dose of thiamine followed by oral doses of thiamine.
   3. Oral doses or monthly IM doses of naltrexone.
   4. Oral doses of methadone with dosage adjustments as needed.

2. The nurse tells the assistive personnel (AP) to check on a patient who had a hypoglycemic reaction. The AP reports back that the patient is asleep. One hour later, the patient is discovered unresponsive and despite resuscitation efforts, the patient dies. Which member of the health care team is **most** likely to be held liable in a malpractice suit?
   1. AP who reported to the nurse that the patient was asleep.
   2. Clinical educator who checked off AP's skills proficiency.
   3. Nurse who instructed the AP to check on the patient.
   4. Supervising registered nurse (RN) who was available by phone.

3. In change of shift report, the oncoming nurse hears that the older patient was confused and lethargic during the afternoon and early evening and then finally fell asleep and is now sleeping soundly. Which question is the **most** important to ask the off-going nurse?
   1. Did you notify the HCP about the confusion?
   2. When was the last time you tried to arouse the patient?
   3. Were vital signs and pulse oximeter readings within normal limits?
   4. How does the patient usually behave in the afternoon and evening?

4. The patient's wife tells the nurse that her husband frequently has difficulty concentrating and is unexpectedly groggy and lethargic in the middle of the day. Which question would the nurse ask **first** to assist the HCP in diagnosing obstructive sleep apnea (OSA)?
   1. "Does he ever have trouble recognizing you?"
   2. "Have you heard him snoring at night?"
   3. "Does he drink alcohol in the evening?"
   4. "Has he ever had problems with his heart?"

5. An older patient has nausea and copious vomiting for several days and now appears weak, confused, and disoriented to time. Which fluid and electrolyte imbalances are **most** likely to be causing these symptoms?
   1. Normal fluid volume with hypernatremia.
   2. Decreased fluid volume with hyponatremia.
   3. Normal fluid volume with hyperkalemia.
   4. Increased fluid volume with hypokalemia.

6. A family member tells that nurse that the patient was feeling fairly good "after we turned up his oxygen, but now he's too groggy to talk, so we'll leave and let him sleep." Which action would the nurse perform **first**?
   1. Instruct the family that oxygen should not be changed without a doctor's order.
   2. Arouse the patient, readjust the oxygen level, and monitor level of consciousness.
   3. Notify the charge nurse, document patient status, and write an incident report.
   4. Ask the AP to check the vital signs and make the patient comfortable.

7. For an overdose of opioid medication, an intravenous (IV) bolus of naloxone was administered by the emergency medical system personnel; the patient who was stuporous with respiratory depression aroused suddenly and was then transported to the hospital. What is the **most** important posttreatment assessment that the nurse would make?
   1. Continuously monitor for nausea and vomiting.
   2. Observe for anxiety, paranoia, or hypervigilance.
   3. Monitor for increasing lethargy or slow breathing.
   4. Monitor for fever, chills, and excessive sweating.

Common Health Scenarios PART 2

8. In which disorder is the patient **most** likely to display an acute onset or unexpected change of mental status and a decreased level of consciousness (LOC)?
   1. Paranoid schizophrenia.
   2. Major depression.
   3. Alzheimer disease.
   4. Delirium.

9. Which instruction would the nurse give to AP about caring for a patient who has altered mental status during the postictal phase of a grand mal seizure?
   1. Stay with the patient until he is alert and able to recall events.
   2. Assist the patient to a side-lying position and encourage rest.
   3. Arouse the patient every 15–20 minutes and give sips of fluid.
   4. Observe, report, and document the return to baseline behavior.

10. Which patient with an altered mental status is **most** likely to be prescribed lactulose?
    1. Patient is in a diabetic coma.
    2. Patient has hepatic encephalopathy.
    3. Patient has residual stroke symptoms.
    4. Patient sustained traumatic brain injury.

11. The patient has a Glasgow Coma Scale (GCS) score of 8. Which instruction would the nurse give to the AP?
    1. Encourage the patient to independently do as much self-care as possible.

2. Remind the patient to use the call bell whenever assistance is needed.
3. Identify yourself and explain everything that you are doing as you do it.
4. Raise the head of the bed before feeding the patient or giving fluids.

12. A patient who drank an excessive amount of alcohol is stuporous, difficult to arouse, and hypothermic. Breathing is irregular and skin is cool and bluish. The medical diagnosis is alcohol poisoning. What is the **priority** nursing concern?
    1. Cognition.
    2. Oxygenation.
    3. Perfusion.
    4. Thermoregulation.

13. A neighbor calls the nurse and describes having sudden unilateral weakness, confusion, and loss of balance that resolved spontaneously after 2 hours. Which response is the **best**?
    1. "When did you first notice the symptoms?"
    2. "You probably had a transient ischemic attack (TIA)."
    3. "You need to seek immediate medical attention."
    4. "Are you having a headache or blurred vision?"

14. The nurse is assessing a patient who is unresponsive to verbal stimuli. Which pupil abnormality is the **most** serious and could be caused by severe pressure in the midbrain or hypoxia associated with cardiopulmonary arrest?

Assessment Data	Appearance
1. Unilateral fixed, dilated pupil, unreactive to light	
2. Bilateral dilated, fixed pupils do not react to light	
3. Bilateral small, fixed pupils do not react to light	
4. Unequal pupil size, both react to light	

(Figures from Stromberg H. (2021) *deWit's Medical-Surgical Nursing* (4th ed), Elsevier.)

15. In caring for an unconscious patient, which instruction would the nurse give to the AP about positioning the patient?
1. Put the patient in a lateral recumbent position.
2. Place the patient prone with head turned to the side.
3. Place the patient supine; align head and neck.
4. Put the patient in a high Fowler's with siderails up.

16. In caring for a patient who has risk for increased intracranial pressure (ICP), which medication would the nurse query?
1. Labetalol.
2. Acetaminophen.
3. Morphine sulfate.
4. Mannitol.

17. A patient who has schizophrenia is at risk for water intoxication and displays lethargy, confusion, and a change in baseline mental status. Which laboratory result is the nurse likely to check **first** before calling the HCP?
1. Sodium level.
2. Glucose level.
3. White blood cell count.
4. Blood urea nitrogen level.

18. A patient is newly diagnosed and admitted for schizophrenia. The nurse notices that every day at around 10:00 a.m., the patient is drowsy and falls asleep in the dayroom. Which action would the nurse use **first**?
1. Encourage the patient to go to bed earlier.
2. Report observations to the RN.
3. Check the side effects of new prescription medications.
4. Assess for ingestion or inhalation of illicit substances.

19. The nurse is assessing the central pain response in a patient who is not responding to voice commands. Which response indicates retention of the **highest** level of function?
1. Frowns and moves arms and legs in a random fashion.
2. Extends and stiffens legs; arms are adducted; wrists are flexed on the chest.
3. Extends and stiffens legs, toes, and arms; head and neck arch backward.
4. Attempts to push nurse's hand away and tries to move away from stimuli.

20. Enhanced Multiple Response

> **Scenario:** The nurse and AP are assigned to care for a patient who has been unresponsive for several weeks after a drug overdose. The patient is breathing and displays purposeful withdrawal from painful stimuli and occasional incomprehensible sounds.

The patient requires total assistance for activities of daily living (ADLs). Which tasks could be delegated or assigned to the AP? **Select all that apply.**
Instructions: Place an X in the space provided or highlight each task that could be delegated or assigned to the AP. Select all that apply.
1. _____ Take and record vital signs every 4 hours
2. _____ Thoroughly clean and dry perineal area after episodes of incontinence
3. _____ Talk to patient and explain actions as care is given
4. _____ Give tube feedings and report problems
5. _____ Carefully check skin and document findings
6. _____ Perform mouth care every 2 hours with sponge swabs
7. _____ Perform passive range-of-motion exercises
8. _____ Assess respiratory effort and listen to breath sounds
9. _____ Reposition patient at least every 2 hours

PART 2 Common Health Scenarios

 Answer Key for this chapter begins on p. 34

Answers

PART 2

Common Health Scenarios

1. **Ans: 2** The patient is displaying signs and symptoms of Korsakoff syndrome, which is brought on by a thiamine deficiency. An IM dose of thiamine followed by oral doses of thiamine is used to prevent progression to Wernicke encephalopathy. Wernicke encephalopathy (sudden onset of symptoms, such as confusion, nystagmus, and unsteady gait) is a reversible medical emergency that is treated with IV administration of thiamine for rapid effect. Benzodiazepines (e.g., lorazepam) are used for alcohol withdrawal syndrome. The IV route is preferred for seizures or delirium tremens. Oral naltrexone is used for opioid use disorder and alcohol use disorder. A monthly injection of naltrexone may be given to select patients who do not require hospitalization and are able to abstain from alcohol. Oral methadone is used for opioid use disorder. **Focus:** Prioritization; **QSEN:** EBP; **Concept:** Addiction, Cognition; **Cognitive Level:** Applying

2. **Ans: 3** The nurse who instructed the AP to check on the patient failed to follow up on the AP's report and assess for symptoms of insulin shock. There was a duty to the patient, a breach of duty, and a harmful outcome. The AP is not expected to recognize the difference between normal sleep and insulin shock. When patients have conditions that affect (or potentially affect) mental status, the nurse must assess to differentiate small changes in responsiveness. The AP and supervising RN could be interviewed during an investigation of this sentinel event (as defined by the Joint Commission, a sentinel event is a patient safety occurrence that results in harm or death). The clinical educator could be asked to remediate the nurse and AP who were involved or to educate the staff about the prevention of future events. **Focus:** Prioritization; **QSEN:** EBP; **Concept:** Health Care Law; **Cognitive Level:** Analyzing

3. **Ans: 4** Knowledge of the patient's baseline behavior is essential for prioritizing nursing actions. For example, if the patient is prone to sundowner syndrome, the behavior described by the off-going nurse would be expected and interventions would be designed accordingly. If confusion and lethargy are unusual for the patient, then the nurse would ask other questions. For example, were there events (e.g., long visits with family) or activities (e.g., physical therapy) that could have caused stress or fatigue? Were any new medications administered? Did the patient have any other symptoms? The oncoming nurse can ask any question during shift report and would then assess arousability, vital signs, and oxygen saturation and then notify the HCP accordingly. **Focus:** Prioritization; **QSEN:** EBP; **Concept:** Cognition; **Cognitive Level:** Analyzing. **Test Taking Tip:** Knowledge of baseline behavior is essential for differentiating an acute condition, such as delirium, from a chronic condition, such as dementia. This is particularly important for older people who have risk for many conditions that can affect cognition or alter the level of consciousness

4. **Ans: 2** Snoring is a common symptom of OSA and partners are frequently the first to notice the condition. Inability to recognize familiar people occurs with advanced dementia or other severe cognitive disorders. Avoiding alcohol in the evening is a first-line recommendation in the treatment of OSA. Risk for heart problems or stroke is higher for untreated OSA. **Focus:** Prioritization; **QSEN:** EBP; **Concept:** Gas Exchange; **Cognitive Level:** Applying

5. **Ans: 2** The patient is likely to have fluid volume deficit and sodium loss because of vomiting. Fluid volume deficit is likely to accompany hypernatremia. Increasing the fluid intake to facilitate urinary excretion of potassium would be a treatment for hyperkalemia (unless the hyperkalemia is related to kidney failure). Decreased fluid volume and hypokalemia could also be caused by excessive vomiting. **Focus:** Prioritization; **QSEN:** EBP; **Concept:** Fluid and Electrolytes; **Cognitive Level:** Analyzing

6. **Ans: 2** The priority is to arouse the patient, correct the oxygen flow, and continue to monitor. The patient may be tired because of the visit; however, patients who have respiratory disorders, such as chronic obstructive pulmonary disease (COPD), need carefully controlled supplemental oxygen. Educating the family on disease processes, such as COPD, notifying the charge nurse, documenting the patient status, checking vital signs, and making the patient comfortable would be done after safety needs are met. An incident report would help the nurse manager prevent future occurrences. Even if the patient did not suffer immediate harm, temporary hypoxia and hypercapnia may have caused tissue damage that could cause long-term problems. **Focus:** Prioritization; **QSEN:** EBP; **Concept:** Gas Exchange; **Cognitive Level:** Analyzing

7. **Ans: 3** A bolus of IV naloxone can immediately reverse the effects of opioid medications; however, the effect may only last between 30 minutes and 3–4 hours and then the symptoms of overdose can reoccur. An infusion of naloxone is usually started as soon as possible. The other signs/symptoms (nausea, vomiting, feelings of anxiety and paranoia, fever, chills, and sweating) are evidence of opioid withdrawal, which can occur after naloxone administration if the patient has opioid addiction. **Focus:** Prioritization; **QSEN:** EBP; **Concept:** Gas Exchange, Addiction; **Cognitive Level:** Analyzing

8. **Ans: 4** Delirium can be caused by many things, for example, infection, drug overdose, electrolyte imbalance, or stroke. Acute onset of impaired cognitive function and decreased LOC require immediate assessment. Patients who have paranoid schizophrenia or Alzheimer's disease can have chronic cognitive dysfunction, but a sudden decreased LOC is not expected. Patients with major depression have decreased energy, but impaired cognitive function and decreased LOC are not expected. **Focus:** Prioritization; **QSEN:** EBP; **Concept:** Cognition; **Cognitive Level:** Analyzing

9. **Ans: 2** The AP can assist the patient to a side-lying position; this decreases the risk for aspiration. During the postictal phase the patient will be tired and should be encouraged to rest and sleep as needed. Even when fully alert, the patient may be unable to recall events immediately preceding or following a seizure. Arousing the patient to give fluids is not necessary. Observing and documenting return to baseline behavior is a nursing task that cannot be delegated to the AP. **Focus:** Delegation, Supervision; **QSEN:** S; **Concept:** Safety; **Cognitive Level:** Analyzing; **IPEC:** IC.

10. **Ans: 2** In hepatic encephalopathy, liver failure causes ammonia to build up and the result is acute confusion. Lactulose draws ammonia from the bloodstream into the colon. Byproducts are then expelled. **Focus:** Prioritization; **QSEN:** N/A; **Concept:** Cognition, Elimination; **Cognitive Level:** Analyzing

11. **Ans: 3** A GCS score of 8 means that the patient is in a coma. The AP would be reminded to continue to talk to the patient and explain actions, because patients in a comatose state may retain hearing. Also, communicating with the patient is always done to show respect and caring. **Focus:** Delegation, Supervision; **QSEN:** EBP; **Concept:** Intracranial Regulation, Communication; **Cognitive Level:** Analyzing; **IPEC:** IC.

12. **Ans: 2** For patients with alcohol poisoning, the priority is oxygenation, because excessive alcohol can depress respirations. Airway management is also a priority because the gag reflex may not be present. The other nursing concerns also need to be addressed after the oxygen needs are met. **Focus:** Prioritization; **QSEN:** S; **Concept:** Gas Exchange; **Cognitive Level:** Applying

13. **Ans: 3** TIA includes the signs/symptoms described by the neighbor, but the symptoms are also consistent with a stroke. The American Stroke Association recommends immediate assessment. In addition, there is about a 12% increased risk for stroke within 90 days of a TIA. Time of symptom onset is assessed by the stroke team to guide the use of thrombolytic therapy. Headache or blurred vision may accompany TIA or stroke. **Focus:** Prioritization; **QSEN:** S; **Concept:** Intracranial Regulation; **Cognitive Level:** Analyzing

14. **Ans: 2** Bilateral fixed and dilated pupils accompany severe pressure in the midbrain or hypoxia related to cardiopulmonary arrest. Nervous system disorders and drug overdose could also cause pupils to appear fixed and dilated. Unilateral dilation could be caused by damage to the oculomotor nerve or by head trauma. Small, fixed pupils are related to some drugs or damage to certain parts of the brain. Unequal and reactive pupils could be congenital or caused by ocular inflammation or adhesion of the iris, cornea, or lens. **Focus:** Prioritization; **QSEN:** S; **Concept:** Intracranial Regulation; **Cognitive Level:** Analyzing

15. **Ans: 1** The lateral recumbent position is preferred to prevent aspiration. The prone position would not be a good choice because the patient's random head movements could obstruct the breathing. Supine position increases the risk for aspiration. High Fowler's position increases the risk for shearing forces as the patient slips down in bed; injury could also occur if the patient falls or slumps against siderails. **Focus:** Delegation, Supervision; **QSEN:** S; **Concept:** Safety; **Cognitive Level:** Applying; **IPEC:** IC.

16. **Ans: 3** Morphine is an opioid, which can cause increased ICP and respiratory depression. It can interfere with the accurate assessment of mental status and level of consciousness. Morphine may be cautiously prescribed for patients with severe head trauma to decrease agitation related to pain. Antipyretics, antihypertensives, hyperosmotic medications, antiseizure medications, muscle relaxants, corticosteroids, and IV fluids may be prescribed in the treatment of ICP. **Focus:** Prioritization; **QSEN:** S; **Concept:** Safety, Intracranial Regulation; **Cognitive Level:** Analyzing

17. **Ans: 1** Excessive water consumption can cause water intoxication, and this increases the risk for hyponatremia. Patients with schizophrenia who are unable to follow instructions may need close observation to prevent frequent use of drinking fountain, taking fluids from other patients, or drinking water from the toilet. Low blood glucose could cause the symptoms, but there is no connection to water intoxication. Elevated glucose can cause thirst and the patient's inclination is to increase fluid intake, but hyperglycemia causes overall dehydration. An increase in white cell count could signal infection, which can cause change in mental status, particularly in older adults. Elevated blood urea nitrogen does occur with renal failure and the byproducts of renal failure contribute to changes in mental status. The nurse would also report other available laboratory results to the HCP. **Focus:** Prioritization; **QSEN:** EBP; **Concept:** Fluid and Electrolytes; **Cognitive Level:** Analyzing. **Test Taking Tip:** Abnormalities in any of these laboratory results could account for change of mental status. To answer this type of question, examine how the past medical history connects with the options

Common Health Scenarios
PART 2

18. **Ans: 3** The nurse notices the pattern and timing of the behavior and recognizes that morning medications are usually administered between 8 a.m. and 9 a.m. Many medications that are prescribed for mental health will initially cause drowsiness. The nurse may also assess sleep habits and the use of illicit substances and then report findings to the RN. **Focus:** Prioritization; **QSEN:** S; **Concept:** Clinical Judgment; **Cognitive Level:** Analyzing

19. **Ans: 4** The highest level of response is the purposeful movement of trying to avoid the noxious stimuli. Frowning and moving randomly is the next level. Stiff extended legs and adduction of upper extremities is decorticate posturing. Decerebrate posturing (stiffness, rigidity, and arching) is the lowest level of response and suggests severe brain damage. **Focus:** Prioritization; **QSEN:** EBP; **Concept:** Intracranial Regulation; **Cognitive Level:** Applying. **Test Taking Tip:** A way to remember decorticate posturing is that the arms and wrists are turning inward toward the *core* of the body

20. **Ans: 1, 2, 3, 6, 7, 9** The AP can be assigned many of the tasks for a patient that requires full assistance for ADLs. Vital signs, hygiene, range-of-motion exercises, and positioning are within the scope of practice of the AP. The nurse must perform the assessment tasks. Invasive procedures, such as tube feedings, are generally not delegated to the AP. All caregivers should be talking to the patient and explaining care. The nurse and AP would make every effort to work as a team to make tasks easier and safer. **Focus:** Delegation, Supervision; **QSEN:** TC; **Concept:** Care Coordination; **Cognitive Level:** Applying; **IPEC:** T/T.

QSEN Key: PCC, Patient-Centered Care; **TC,** Teamwork & Collaboration; **EBP,** Evidence-Based Practice; **QI,** Quality Improvement; **S,** Safety; **I,** Informatics.
IPEC Key: Domain 1 Values/Ethics (**V/E**); Domain 2 Roles/Responsibilities (**R/R**); Domain 3 Interprofessional Communication (**IC**); Domain 4 Teams/Teamwork (**T/T**)

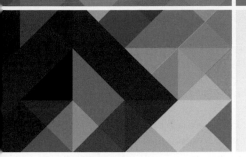

Questions

1. Which patient will the nurse watch **most** closely because of risk for a pressure injury?
   1. Patient who is ambulatory but has occasional urinary incontinence.
   2. Patient who is very thin and refuses to eat meals.
   3. Patient who can sit up in a chair three times a day with assistance.
   4. Patient who is confused but can use the bathroom with assistance.

2. Which areas of a patient's body will the nurse assess often for a patient at risk for a pressure injury when placed in the position depicted in this picture? **Select all that apply.**

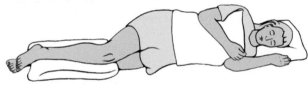

Figure from Stromberg H. (2022) *deWit's Medical-Surgical Nursing* (4th ed.), Elsevier.

   1. Scapula.
   2. Head of the fibula.
   3. Trochanter.
   4. Sacrum.
   5. Patella.
   6. Greater tuberosity of the humerus.

3. The nurse is assessing a patient's skin and finds the buttocks area is reddened with intact skin that is mottled but does not blanch. Which pressure injury staging classification does the nurse suspect?

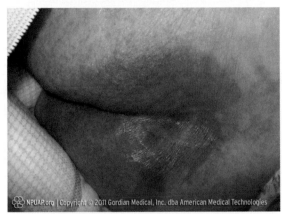

Figure from the National Pressure Ulcer Advisory Panel and European Pressure Ulcer Advisory Panel. (2009) Pressure ulcer prevention and treatment: clinical practice guideline. *National Pressure Ulcer Advisory Panel.*

   1. Stage 1.
   2. Stage 2.
   3. Stage 3.
   4. Stage 4.

4. Which actions can the nurse safely delegate to an assistive personnel (AP) when caring for a patient at risk for pressure injury? **Select all that apply.**
   1. Turn and reposition the patient every 1 to 2 hours.
   2. Check and record vital signs every 4 hours.
   3. Assess pressure points for redness and blanching.
   4. Assist the patient to the bathroom as needed.
   5. Remind the patient to sit up in a chair three times a day.
   6. Administer the patient's daily vitamin supplement.

Common Health Scenarios   PART 2

5. The AP asks the registered dietetic nutritionist (RDN) which nutritional sources will help decrease the risk for a patient to develop a pressure injury and help to heal for an existing pressure injury. What is the RDN's **best** response?
   1. Complex carbohydrates.
   2. Extra fat sources.
   3. Proteins; zinc; and vitamins A, C, and E.
   4. Simple carbohydrates and iron supplements.

6. Which patient care actions for a patient with a Stage 3 pressure injury would be **best** to assign to the Licensed Practical Nurse/Licensed Vocational Nurse (LPN/LVN)? **Select all that apply.**
   1. Repositioning the patient every 2 hours.
   2. Irrigating the patient's wound and changing the dressing.
   3. Performing the patient's admission assessment.
   4. Inserting a urinary catheter as prescribed by the health care provider (HCP).
   5. Administering as-needed (PRN) prescribed oral medication for discomfort.
   6. Providing mouth care before the patient's breakfast tray is served.

7. Which order prescribed by the HCP, for a patient with a healing Stage 3 pressure injury in the coccyx area, would the nurse be sure to question?
   1. Provide protein shakes three times a day.
   2. Normal saline wound irrigation with each dressing change.
   3. Sprinkle dextranomer beads over the wound with each dressing change.
   4. Wet to dry dressing changes three times a day.

8. Which health care team member would be **best** for the nurse to consult about for advice on the treatment of a pressure injury?
   1. HCP.
   2. Wound care nurse specialist.
   3. Infection control specialist.
   4. Surgeon.

9. Which instruction will the nurse provide an AP for providing skin care on a patient at risk for a pressure injury due to immobility and incontinence?
   1. Use an antibiotic soap with hot water to wash the skin.
   2. Vigorously scrub the skin to promote perfusion.
   3. Apply powder after cleansing the affected area.
   4. Clean the skin gently and apply a moisturizer after drying.

10. The nurse notes that a patient with a pressure injury has a Braden scale score of 11 from the charge RN. Which category of risk does this score indicate?
    1. At risk.
    2. Moderate risk.
    3. High risk.
    4. Severe risk.

11. Two APs are moving a patient at risk for pressure injury up in bed. Which action requires that the nurse intervene and provide additional instruction to the APs?
    1. APs position themselves on opposite sides of the patient.
    2. APs raise the patient's bed to a comfortable working level.
    3. APs remind the patient to cross arms across the chest.
    4. APs move the patient by pulling under the patient's arms.

12. A patient has developed a reddened area on his ankle. Which dressing type will the nurse apply?
    1. Thin film dressing.
    2. Gauze dressing with tape.
    3. Hydrocolloid dressing.
    4. Wet-to-dry dressing.

13. The HCP prescribes irrigation using 250 mL of a nontoxic solution for a patient's clean Stage 3 pressure injury with each sterile dressing change. Which solution is **best** for the nurse to use?
    1. Povidone iodine.
    2. Normal saline.
    3. Hydrogen peroxide.
    4. Sodium hypochlorite.

14. Which key elements will the nurse include when documenting the assessment of a patient's pressure injury? **Select all that apply.**
    1. Size of pressure injury.
    2. Cause of injury.
    3. Appearance of exudate.
    4. Presence of granulation tissue.
    5. Type of irrigation solution.
    6. Degree of intactness of skin.

15. Which treatment or intervention will the nurse expect the HCP to prescribe when a patient's pressure injury wound requires mechanical debridement?
    1. Application of a proteolytic enzyme.
    2. Electrical stimulation.
    3. Negative pressure wound therapy.
    4. Hyperbaric oxygen therapy.

16. The AP asks the nurse why a patient's wound is packed with gauze each time the dressing is changed. Which is the nurse's **best** response?
    1. "The wound is packed with gauze because that is part of the wound care nurse's instructions for this patient's dressing change."
    2. "The patient's wound is packed with gauze because it helps the development of granulation tissue for healing."
    3. "The wound is packed with gauze to help prevent the presence of infectious organisms."
    4. "I will ask the health care provider why we are packing the wound with gauze and let you know later."

17. The nurse notes a patient's pressure injury wound has creamy yellow exudate. What is the nurse's **first** action?
    1. Change the wound dressing.
    2. Irrigate the wound with normal saline.
    3. Notify the HCP.
    4. Carefully document the finding.

18. The nurse is assisting with the admission of a patient from a long-term care facility who has a Stage 4 pressure injury wound. Which actions or interventions will the nurse delegate to the experienced AP? **Select all that apply.**
    1. Help move the patient from the stretcher to the bed.
    2. Orient the patient to unit policies.
    3. Take the patient's temperature.
    4. Assist the patient in changing into a hospital gown.
    5. Assess the patient's wound.
    6. Check the patient's oxygen saturation.

19. Nextgen (Enhanced Hot Spot)

Case Study: The nurse is providing care for a 79-year-old patient who has dementia and is unable to perform self-care. He is incontinent and wears adult diapers. His medical history includes cataract surgery and hypotension. He is unable to feed himself and has a poor appetite and has lost 10 pounds over the past month. The AP checks his diaper every hour and changes it as needed. He is repositioned every 2 hours using a pull/draw sheet. The HCP is planning to insert a feeding tube.

Instructions: Underline or highlight the factors in the case study that increase the patient's risk for developing a pressure injury.

20. Nextgen (Cloze)

Scenario:
The nurse is assigned to care for patients at risk for pressure injuries.

Patients:

A. 84-year-old with an open wound deep crater on the sacrum with areas of granulation tissue when dressing was last changed. Vital signs: T 98.8°F (37.1°C), P 84 regular, R 18, BP 128/76. Alert and oriented.
B. 72-year-old with a reddened area on the right hip that does not blanch with finger pressure. Vital signs: T 99.2°F (37.3°C), P 80 regular, R 18, BP 142/80. Drowsy and napping.
C. 78-year-old with a pink wound that is moist with a ruptured blister on the left heel. Vital Signs: T 102.8°F (39.3°C), P 96 irregular, BP 108/60. Confused.
D. 66-year-old who is obese with the sacral region wound reddened, warm, and hard. Vital signs: T 97.6°F (36.4°C), P 92 regular, R 24, BP 164/92. Requesting PRN pain medication.

Instructions:
Prioritize the order in which these patients should be seen by the nurse in order to ensure safe and efficient patient care.

Place the letter of the patients from the column on the left in the correct order they should be assessed below.

1. _____

2. _____

3. _____

4. _____

Answer Key for this chapter begins on p. 40

PART 2 Common Health Scenarios

Answers

1. **Ans: 2**   Patients who are poorly nourished are at risk for pressure injuries. Other risk factors include lack of mobility, exposure of skin to excessive moisture (e.g., urinary or fecal incontinence), and aging skin. **Focus:** Prioritization; **QSEN:** PCC; **Concept:** Perfusion, Tissue Integrity, Nutrition; **Cognitive Level:** Analyzing. **Test Taking Tip:** Be alert to keywords in questions such as **most** and **best** when choosing the correct answer. These words indicate that although more than one answer may be correct, one of the responses is better or more important than the rest.

2. **Ans: 2, 3, 6**   When a patient is placed in a position, the areas where the bones press the skin and the skin is pressed against the bed are at risk for pressure injury. Areas of the body at risk when a patient is in a side-lying position include ears, greater tuberosity of the humerus (shoulder), trochanter (hip), head of the fibula (knee), and lateral malleolus (ankle). Scapula and sacrum are at risk with supine positioning. Patellae are at risk with prone positioning. **Focus:** Prioritization; **QSEN:** PCC; **Concept:** Perfusion, Tissue Integrity; **Cognitive Level:** Applying

3. **Ans: 1**   The appearance of a stage 1 pressure injury includes that the skin is intact but is reddened, color may be pink or mottled, and the skin does not blanch. **Focus:** Prioritization; **QSEN:** PCC; **Concept:** Perfusion, Tissue integrity; **Cognitive Level:** Applying

4. **Ans: 1, 2, 4, 5**   The AP's scope of practice includes basic patient care and assistance with activities of daily living (ADLs), as well as checking and recording vital signs and reminding or encouraging patients about information already taught by the nurse. The nurse is responsible for assessing patients and administering medications. **Focus:** Delegation; **QSEN:** PCC, S; **Concept:** Safety; **Cognitive Level:** Applying; **IPEC:** R/R

5. **Ans: 3**   Research has demonstrated that increasing calories, proteins, zinc, and vitamins (A, C, and E) reduce the risk for pressure injury and promote the healing of existing pressure injuries. **Focus:** Prioritization; **QSEN:** PCC, TC, EBP; **Concept:** Tissue integrity; **Cognitive Level:** Analyzing; **IPEC:** R/R, IC

6. **Ans: 2, 4, 5**   Administering oral drugs, changing wound dressings, and inserting urinary catheters are all within the scope of practice for an LPN/LVN. The RN would do a patient's initial admission assessment. Although an LPN/LVN could certainly reposition and provide mouth care for a patient, these actions would be better delegated to an AP. **Focus:** Assignment; **QSEN:** PCC, TC; **Concept:** Health

care quality; **Cognitive Level:** Applying; **IPEC:** R/R. **Test Taking Tip:** It is essential to be familiar with scopes of practice when assigning or delegating tasks to members of the patient care team.

7. **Ans: 4**   Wet-to-dry dressings are not recommended for healing pressure injuries because this can damage new granulation tissue when the dressing is removed. All of the other prescribed actions are appropriate for care of a healing pressure injury in the coccyx region. **Focus:** Prioritization; **QSEN:** PCC, EBP; **Concept:** Tissue integrity; **Cognitive Level:** Analyzing

8. **Ans: 2**   A wound care nurse specialist has training and knowledge about care of wounds, including cleaning and dressing materials. They will assess a patient's wound, then provide advice for the best methods to promote healing and follow the patient's progress. **Focus:** Prioritization; **QSEN:** PCC, TC; **Concept:** Tissue integrity; **Cognitive Level:** Analyzing; **IPEC:** IC

9. **Ans: 4**   The AP is taught to clean the skin as soon as possible after soiling occurs and at routine intervals, then moisturize the skin. Skin should be washed gently with clean, warm water and mild soap. The AP should not scrub, but use only the amount of pressure necessary to clean the skin. Skin should be patted dry. **Focus:** Delegation, Supervision; **QSEN:** PCC; **Concept:** Tissue integrity; **Cognitive Level:** Applying; **IPEC:** IC

10. **Ans: 3**   Braden scale risk categories are at risk (15–18), moderate risk (13–14), high risk (10–12), and severe risk (9). **Focus:** Prioritization; **QSEN:** EBP; **Concept:** Tissue integrity; **Cognitive Level:** Applying. **Test Taking Tip:** Become familiar with commonly used scales and assessment tools. This allows you to quickly answer questions and to readily detect problems in the clinical setting

11. **Ans: 4**   A patient at risk for pressure injury has thin, easily injured skin. Pulling the patient up in bed causes shearing, which can result in skin tears. The nurse would instruct the APs to place a draw (pull) sheet under the patient and use that for moving them up higher in the bed. This prevents shearing and skin injury. All of the other actions are appropriate to repositioning the patient. **Focus:** Prioritization; **QSEN:** PCC, S; **Concept:** Tissue integrity; **Cognitive Level:** Analyzing

12. **Ans: 1**   A reddened area suggests a stage 1 pressure injury. The application of a thin film dressing (e.g., Tegaderm) protects the injury from shearing forces and keeps it moist. **Focus:** Prioritization; **QSEN:** PCC, EBP; **Concept:** Tissue integrity; **Cognitive Level:** Analyzing

PART 2 Common Health Scenarios

13. **Ans: 2** Normal saline is isotonic and the most commonly used wound irrigation solution due to safety (lowest toxicity). Povidone iodine is a broad-spectrum antimicrobial solution. Hydrogen peroxide is a commonly used wound antiseptic. Sodium hypochlorite (e.g., Dakin's solution) is used in pressure ulcers with necrotic tissue to help control infection. **Focus:** Prioritization; **QSEN:** PCC; **Concept:** Tissue integrity; **Cognitive Level:** Analyzing

14. **Ans: 1, 3, 4, 6** The nurse documents the appearance of the pressure injury wound after assessment. Size, presence and appearance or exudate, presence and amount of granulation tissue (indicates healing is occurring), and whether the skin is intact or the wound has a crater are all important findings to include in the documentation. Cause of injury and type of irrigation are important but are not part of the pressure injury assessment. **Focus:** Prioritization; **QSEN:** PCC; **Concept:** Tissue integrity; **Cognitive Level:** Applying

15. **Ans: 1** Mechanical debridement is accomplished by the use of whirlpool baths, wet-to-dry saline dressings, sprinkling dextranomer beads over the wound, and proteolytic enzymes or other chemicals that break down dead tissue and absorb exudate. **Focus:** Prioritization; **QSEN:** PCC; **Concept:** Tissue integrity; **Cognitive Level:** Analyzing; **IPEC:** IC

16. **Ans: 2** A patient's pressure injury wound with a crater is packed with gauze because it facilitates the formation of granulation tissue (e.g., connective tissue with multiple small vessels) and healing by second intention to debride the wound. Responses 1 and 3 are not accurate. Response 4 does not respond to the AP's question. **Focus:** Prioritization; **QSEN:** EBP; **Concept:** Tissue integrity; **Cognitive Level:** Analyzing; **IPEC:** IC

17. **Ans: 3** A wound exudate that is creamy yellow indicates infection, most likely with staphylococcus. The priority action is to notify the HCP of the infection so that changes in the health care plan can be implemented to treat the infection. The changes may include dressing changes and irrigation, but the HCP must be notified first. Careful documentation is essential but is not the highest priority at this time. **Focus:** Prioritization; **QSEN:** PCC, S; **Concept:** Tissue Integrity, Infection, Clinical Judgment; **Cognitive Level:** Analyzing

18. **Ans: 1, 3, 4, 6** The nurse delegates care that is within the AP's scope of practice, such as repositioning, checking vital signs, and assisting with changing to a hospital gown. An experienced AP would also know how to check oxygen saturation using a pulse oximeter. The nurse is responsible for ensuring that the AP knows this skill. Assessing and orienting are more complex skills that should be completed by nurses. **Focus:** Delegation, Supervision; **QSEN:** PCC, TC; **Concept:** Leadership; **Cognitive Level:** Applying; **IPEC:** R/R, IC

19. **Ans:** Pressure injury risk factors include immobility, inactivity, moisture, malnutrition, advanced age, altered sensory perception, and decreased mental awareness, as well as friction and shear. Contributing factors include dehydration, obesity, and edema. **Focus:** Prioritization; **QSEN:** PCC, EBP; **Concept:** Perfusion, Tissue Integrity; **Cognitive Level:** Analyzing

Case Study: The nurse is providing care for a 79-year-old patient who has dementia and is unable to perform self-care. He is incontinent and wears adult diapers. His medical history includes cataract surgery and hypotension. He is unable to feed himself and has a poor appetite and has lost 10 pounds over the past month. The AP check his diaper every hour and changes it as needed. He is repositioned every 2 hours using a pull/draw sheet. The HCP is planning to insert a feeding tube.

Instructions: Underline or highlight the factors in the case study that increase the patient's risk for developing a pressure injury.

20. **Ans: Nextgen**

Scenario: The nurse is assigned to care for patients at risk for pressure injuries.

Patients:

Instructions:

Prioritize the in the order in which these patients should be seen by the nurse in order to ensure safe and efficient patient care.

Place the letter of the patients from the column on the left in the correct order they should be assessed below.

A. 84-year-old with an open wound deep crater on the sacrum with areas of granulation tissue when dressing was last changed. Vital signs: T 98.8°F (37.1°C), P 84 regular, R 18, BP 128/76. Alert and oriented, watching TV.

B. 72-year-old with a new reddened area on the right hip that does not blanch with finger pressure. Vital signs: T 99.2°F (37.3°C), P 80 regular, R 18, BP 142/80. Drowsy and napping.

C. 78-year-old with a pink wound that is moist with a ruptured blister on the left heel. Vital Signs: T 102.8°F (39.3°C), P 110 irregular, BP 108/60. Confused.

D. 66-year-old who is obese with the sacral region wound reddened, warm, and hard. Vital signs: T 97.6°F (36.4°C), P 92 regular, R 24, BP 164/92. Requesting PRN pain medication.

1.____C_____
2.____B_____
3.____D_____
4.____A_____

Patient C has an elevated temperature, increased heart rate, and is confused, which may indicate an infection, and so should be assessed first so the HCP can be notified and appropriate interventions started. Patient B has a new reddened area and a slightly elevated temperature that needs to be assessed next. Patient D's pain level needs to be assessed and they should be given pain medication. Patient A has a healing pressure wound, for which the dressing has been changed, and is in no discomfort at this time. **Focus:** Prioritization; **QSEN:** PCC; **Concept:** Clinical judgment; Tissue Integrity; **Cognitive Level:** Analyzing

QSEN Key: PCC, Patient-Centered Care; **TC,** Teamwork & Collaboration; **EBP,** Evidence-Based Practice; **QI,** Quality Improvement; **S,** Safety; **I,** Informatics.

IPEC Key: Domain 1 Values/Ethics (**V/E**); Domain 2 Roles/Responsibilities (**R/R**); Domain 3 Interprofessional Communication (**IC**); Domain 4 Teams/Teamwork (**T/T**).

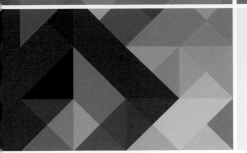

CHAPTER 6
Patients With Dementia

Questions

1. Which instruction is the **best** to give to assistive personnel (AP) for a patient with mild Alzheimer's disease (AD)?
   1. Check to see if the patient remembered to comb her hair.
   2. Coach the patient step by step to don and button her blouse.
   3. Select clothes for the day and dress the patient before breakfast.
   4. Brush the patient's teeth and ensure that no toothpaste is swallowed.

2. Which medication prescribed for dementia must be administered in the evening?
   1. Donepezil.
   2. Sertraline.
   3. Risperidone.
   4. Zolpidem.

3. A patient with mild AD is living at home with his spouse. Which task is **most** appropriate for the home health LPN/LVN to perform in the care of this patient?
   1. Identify a family member or friend who could monitor financial issues.
   2. Teach the patient and spouse how to use and organize medications in a pill box.
   3. Assess the initial home health needs and the family's use of community resources.
   4. Initiate the discussion of nutritional therapies that may preserve cognitive function.

4. Which class of prescribed medication would the nurse question because there is a **greater** risk for death for patients with AD?
   1. Cholinesterase inhibitors.
   2. Selective serotonin reuptake inhibitors.
   3. Antipsychotics.
   4. Benzodiazepines.

5. The nurse has been caring for a person with dementia for several weeks. Today, as the nurse approaches the person, he appears fearful and anxious. Which action would the nurse take **first**?
   1. Slowly back away and come back later to check on the person.
   2. Call the person by name, reintroduce self, and give reassurance.
   3. Check the immediate environment for disturbing stimuli.
   4. Assess the person for symptoms of medication side effects.

6. Which person is displaying an **early** sign of AD?
   1. Person A cannot remember where she left her reading glasses.
   2. Person B cannot remember her eldest daughter's first name.
   3. Person C shows less interest in work and socializing.
   4. Person D has weight loss and requires verbal coaching to eat meals.

7. A family member has been caring for an older relative with dementia for a long time. Which action related to caregiver burnout could be delegated to the home health aide?
   1. Observe the quality of interaction and caring between the caregiver and person who has dementia.
   2. Inform family members that the home health agency is holding a seminar for family caregivers next month.
   3. Suggest strategies that can help the primary caregiver to maintain own health and emotional well-being.
   4. Role model care and attention toward the person with dementia to decrease caregiver guilt and burnout.

8. Which nursing concern represents a **priority** for a patient with dementia who is displaying agitation?
   1. Cognition.
   2. Communication.
   3. Safety.
   4. Anxiety.

9. Which instruction would the nurse give to the AP for a patient with sundowner syndrome?
   1. Help the patient to do complex tasks, such as filling out a menu in the morning.
   2. Help the patient to perform bedtime rituals and get into bed before sundown.
   3. Encourage the patient to take a nap between lunchtime and dinnertime.
   4. Assist the patient with attending a fun and interactive social event after dinner.

10. A team leader at a long-term care center must assign a nurse to care for a resident with severe AD. Which nursing ability would be the **most** important to consider in making this assignment?
    1. Expertise in delegation skills.
    2. Proficiency in psychomotor skills.
    3. Good time management skills.
    4. Excellent communication skills.

11. The nurse is preparing to apply a rivastigmine patch at the prescribed time. The nurse notices that there is a rivastigmine patch on the right side of the patient's chest and another rivastigmine patch on the left side of the chest. What would the nurse do **first**?
    1. Notify the registered nurse (RN) about the potential for medication overdose.
    2. Check the medication administration record to verify the time of application.
    3. Remove both patches, clean the skin and assess for medication side effects.
    4. Call poison control for advice about possible rivastigmine overdose.

12. A patient with dementia displays a catastrophic reaction while visiting with family members. Which action would the nurse take **first**?
    1. Speak calmly, listen to the patient's concerns, and redirect with reassurance.
    2. Call the health care provider (HCP) and report the sudden behavior change.
    3. Direct several staff members to escort the patient to another room.

    4. Ask the family to leave and come back on a day when the patient is calm.

13. Which instruction would the nurse give to the home health aide for a patient who has confusion related to Korsakoff syndrome?
    1. Encourage the family to take the saltshaker off of the table.
    2. Remind the family to store alcoholic beverages in a locked cabinet.
    3. Supervise smoking and limit the patient to two cigarettes per day.
    4. Offer the patient food and snacks that do not contain refined sugar.

14. A patient with moderate AD has a history of chronic back pain, but today the patient cannot accurately describe the location of the pain or rate the intensity. Which action would the nurse take **first**?
    1. Closely assess for grimacing, guarding, or difficulties with movement.
    2. Call a family member and ask how they usually manage the pain medication.
    3. Note the time of the last dose of analgesic and give according to the prescribed schedule.
    4. Hold the as-needed (PRN) dose and document that pain assessment was not possible.

15. Which AP needs additional supervision related to caring for a resident who has dementia and is displaying agitated behavior?
    1. AP-A uses a calm and quiet tone of voice to reassure the resident.
    2. AP-B removes potentially hazardous objects from the environment.
    3. AP-C tries to physically hold the resident until agitation subsides.
    4. AP-D redirects the resident to a pleasant non-threatening activity.

16. The nurse is gathering data about risk factors that a patient might have for AD. Which questions would the nurse ask? **Select all that apply.**
    1. Do you have a family history of Down syndrome?
    2. Do you have a personal history of high cholesterol?
    3. How old are you?
    4. Do you have a family history of cancer?
    5. Have you ever sustained a head injury?
    6. Do you have a personal history of high blood pressure?

17. For a patient with dementia who is prone to confabulation, which instruction would be the **best** to give to the AP?
    1. "Don't believe anything the patient says, he will try to trick you to get his own way."
    2. "Gently correct the patient if you notice errors or falsehoods in what he is saying."
    3. "Ask the patient to give specific details related to the topic to stimulate his memory."
    4. "Accept what the patient is saying because it is his way of filling conversational gaps."

18. A patient with advanced AD has weight loss, decreased fluid intake, a low cholesterol level, and physical inactivity. Which prescription related to the patient's nutritional status would the nurse question?
    1. Daily calorie counts.
    2. Feeding tube.
    3. Thickened liquid supplements.
    4. Weekly weights.

19. Enhanced Multiple Response. _____

Scenario: Residents who live in a long-term care center can have varying degrees of dementia. Some need reminders to perform activities of daily living (ADLs). Some can function with step-by-step coaching. Others will require modified, partial, or total assistance to achieve tasks. The nurse works in a facility where the nurse-to-resident ratio is 1:30, whereas the ratio of AP to residents is 1:10; therefore the nurse must delegate or assign much of the bedside care and interaction to the APs. With appropriate supervision from the LPN/LVN, which tasks related to reality orientation for residents with dementia can be delegated or assigned to APs? **Select all that apply.**

Instructions: Place an X in the space provided or highlight each task that can be delegated or assigned to the APs.

1. _____Lead a reality orientation group for residents and interested family members.
2. _____Position a clock with large numbers in a resident's room in clear view.
3. _____For residents with global amnesia, repeat orientation to person, place, and time.
4. _____Provide care and mental stimulation according to the resident's wishes.
5. _____Keep environmental lighting low and dim to minimize confusion.
6. _____Ask one simple question at a time and allow adequate time for a response.
7. _____Engage residents in conversational topics at a normal pace as care is performed.
8. _____Look directly at the residents when speaking.
9. _____Place seasonally appropriate decorations in the day area.

Answer Key for this chapter begins on p. 47

PART 2 Common Health Scenarios

20. Enhanced Multiple Response.

Scenario: The nurse works for a home health agency and is assigned to be part of the team that will care for a new patient. The patient is an elderly gentleman who has AD. He lives at home with his wife, who is the primary caregiver. The wife reluctantly agreed to home health care after being convinced by her daughter. The patient's symptoms are progressing slowly from mild to moderate and there has been a recent change in his medications. Which tasks are **best** performed by the LPN/LVN? **Select all that apply.**

Instructions: Place an X in the space provided or highlight the tasks that are best performed by the LPN/LVN.

1. _____Monitor abilities to perform ADLs.
2. _____Encourage family members to express concerns.
3. _____Assist the patient with bathing and showering on scheduled days.
4. _____Assist with the planning of a consistent daily routine.
5. _____Observe the home environment for safety hazards during every visit.
6. _____Perform initial assessment to establish baseline behaviors and abilities in ADLs.
7. _____Instruct home health aide on ways to increase patient independence.
8. _____Administer medications and document and report efficacy and side effects.
9. _____Evaluate family members' response to support group and other resources.
10. _____Listen to and acknowledge the patient's expression of feelings.

Answer

1. **Ans: 1** Patients with mild AD can be forgetful and may need reminders, but most would have the motor and cognitive abilities to independently complete ADLs. For people with moderate AD, coaching tasks step by step is helpful. People in the severe stage need total assistance in decision-making, dressing, hygiene, eating, and toileting. **Focus:** Prioritization, Supervision; **QSEN:** PCC; **Concept:** Cognition; **Cognitive Level:** Analyzing; **IPEC:** IC

2. **Ans: 4** Any of these medications may cause drowsiness; however, zolpidem is prescribed short-term for insomnia. Donepezil is prescribed to help improve memory and cognition. Sertraline is an antidepressant, which may cause drowsiness but may also worsen insomnia. Risperidone may be prescribed to patients with dementia for agitation or aggression. **Focus:** Prioritization; **QSEN:** EBP; **Concept:** Sleep; **Cognitive Level:** Applying; **Test Taking Tip:** Pharmacology is a complicated and important area of study. Recognizing the purpose of commonly prescribed medications is a good place to start.

3. **Ans: 2** The LPN/LVN is well trained in medication administration. Organizing medication in a pill box helps to decrease confusion, particularly if the person needs to take several medications at different times during the day. Identifying family members or friends to take over finances should be done by the RN or a social worker. The initial health assessment and the use of resources should be done by the RN. Discussion of nutritional therapies should be initiated by the HCP or a registered dietician. **Focus:** Assignment; **QSEN:** TC; **Concept:** Care Coordination; **Cognitive Level:** Analyzing

4. **Ans: 3** Antipsychotic medications are associated with risk for death in older adult patients. The US Food and Drug Administration recommends that antipsychotic medications not be used for dementia-related psychosis, but they are prescribed for agitation and aggression for patients with AD. Patients with AD have low levels of acetylcholine; cholinesterase inhibitors counteract the breakdown of this neurotransmitter. Selective serotonin reuptake inhibitors are prescribed for depression. Benzodiazepines are prescribed with caution; the nurse would monitor for cognitive changes and initiate fall precautions. **Focus:** Prioritization; **QSEN:** S; **Concept:** Safety; **Cognitive Level:** Applying

5. **Ans: 2** First, the nurse would calmly call the person by name and identify self. Persons with dementia can experience episodic paranoia and fear and be unable to recognize familiar people. Slow movements are appropriate, and the nurse would move away if the person displayed aggression; however, the nurse would not leave the person alone. Environmental stimuli should be minimized. Other factors, such as medication side effects, time of day, hallucinations, or sources of actual danger (e.g., abuse or threats of abuse), should be considered and addressed. **Focus:** Prioritization; **QSEN:** PCC; **Concept:** Cognition; **Cognitive Level:** Analyzing

6. **Ans: 3** Early signs of AD include withdrawal from social/work activities, changes in mood or personality, memory loss that disrupts daily life, difficulties with planning or problem solving, difficulties with familiar tasks, confusion regarding time and place, trouble understanding spatial relationships, difficulty finding the right words, inability to retrace steps, and poor judgment. Person A shows behavior that could be normal aging or normal for her. Person B displays a behavior associated with moderate AD, and Person D has behaviors associated with advanced disease. **Focus:** Prioritization; **QSEN:** EBP; **Concept:** Cognition; **Cognitive Level:** Analyzing. **Test Taking Tip:** NCLEX will test your ability to recognize early signs and symptoms because early recognition and intervention is typically associated with better patient outcomes.

7. **Ans: 2** The nurse can instruct the home health aide to give the date, time, and location of programs that may be of interest to family members and patients. The home health aide would not be expected to explain the benefit or subject matter of the programs. Observing family dynamics, suggesting strategies, and role modeling are nursing responsibilities that should not be delegated to the AP. **Focus:** Delegation; **QSEN:** TC; **Concept:** Care Coordination; **Cognitive Level:** Analyzing; **IPEC:** R/R

8. **Ans: 3** The priority is safety. The nurse selects the best interventions based on the knowledge of how dementia affects cognition and an awareness of the patient's baseline behavior. Using good communication skills is the first-line intervention to help the patient remain safe and decrease agitation. Identifying sources of anxiety and triggers for agitated behavior helps to prevent future incidents. **Focus:** Prioritization; **QSEN:** S; **Concept:** Safety; **Cognitive Level:** Applying

9. **Ans: 1** Complex tasks should be done in the morning. Sundowner syndrome can occur in cognitive disorders, such as delirium, dementia, or AD. Behaviors such as confusion, wandering, suspicion, agitation, or restlessness occur in the late afternoon and may continue into the night. Early bedtimes may be convenient for the staff but are not necessarily in

PART 2   Common Health Scenarios

the patient's best interest. Discouraging daytime naps and performing bedtime rituals may be helpful in establishing a regular sleep schedule. Interactive social activities in the evening hours may increase confusion. **Focus:** Delegation, Supervision; **QSEN:** PCC; **Concept:** Cognition; **Cognitive Level:** Analyzing; **IPEC:** IC

10. **Ans: 3**   All of these skills are important for quality nursing care; however, persons with severe AD require total assistance for ADLs and they require continuous assessment of body systems. Care will be time consuming; thus good time management and task organization skills are important. Some aspects of ADLs can be delegated, but the nurse must be present to assess the skin during bathing and there is a greater risk for aspiration when the person is eating or drinking. Assessment of swallow and portion size of each spoonful must be monitored to prevent pouching of food; therefore delegation of feeding to the AP may be inappropriate. Likewise, APs can perform range-of-motion exercises but are not expected to interpret moaning or grimacing as pain or baseline response. Persons with severe AD will not be able to communicate; nevertheless, all health care staff are expected to explain procedures and to display respect; however, socialization needs are of lower priority than physical needs. **Focus:** Prioritization; **QSEN:** PCC; **Concept:** Clinical Judgment; **Cognitive Level:** Analyzing

11. **Ans: 3**   Rivastigmine is used to treat dementia in AD and Parkinson disease. The presence of two patches creates a concern that the patient may have received an overdose of the medication. The nurse would remove both patches and clean the skin to prevent additional absorption, and then assess for common side effects (e.g., nausea, vomiting, abdominal pain, dizziness, diarrhea, skin irritation) and serious side effects (e.g., irregular or slow heart rate, fainting, severe abdominal pain, dark stool/emesis). Based on the assessment, the nurse would implement emergency measures as needed. The RN and HCP would be notified. The HCP may request that poison control be contacted. An incident report would include the description of the two patches and what actions were taken. **Focus:** Prioritization; **QSEN:** S; **Concept:** Safety; **Cognitive Level:** Analyzing

12. **Ans: 1**   First, the nurse would calmly assess the situation and listen to the person (the inciting incident could be very minor, but acknowledging feelings is therapeutic). Persons with dementia can often be gently redirected to reduce fear and perceived threat (e.g., offer a snack). Calling the HCP may be warranted after assessment or if the agitation persists and is unrelieved by usual measures. Taking the person to another area may be necessary for safety; however, this is best accomplished by one familiar nurse if the patient is not aggressive. Family members may wish

to leave, but the nurse should explain that catastrophic reactions are related to cognitive disorders and that seemingly minor events can trigger an exaggerated response. If the family is willing, the nurse and family could explore what occurred just before the reaction. The family may identify that certain topics are upsetting or that the conversational pace was too rapid. **Focus:** Prioritization; **QSEN:** PCC; **Concept:** Cognition; **Cognitive Level:** Analyzing

13. **Ans: 2**   Korsakoff syndrome is a chronic, irreversible condition that affects memory and cognition. It is usually associated with long-term alcohol abuse. The treatment, which may improve the symptoms, includes abstaining from alcohol and administering or giving large doses of thiamine. **Focus:** Assignment, Supervision; **QSEN:** EBP; **Concept:** Cognition; **Cognitive Level:** Analyzing; **IPEC:** IC

14. **Ans: 1**   First, the nurse would observe for nonverbal signs of pain; for example, gait, posture, and movement, can be affected by pain. Other behavioral changes such as irritability, restlessness, agitation, or withdrawal may also signal pain. Family, other team members, or the charge nurse may offer information about the patient's baseline behavior. Giving prescribed medication at the correct time is appropriate, but pain assessment must be performed first, and then efficacy or response would be noted. The decision to hold a PRN dose is based on assessment and it is the nurse's responsibility to assess the patient using alternative strategies. **Focus:** Prioritization; **QSEN:** EBP; **Concept:** Pain, Cognition; **Cognitive Level:** Analyzing. **Test Taking Tip:** A pain assessment that is directly obtained from the patient should always precede the administration of pain medication. If the patient is not able to give a subjective report, then the nurse must rely more heavily on objective data and secondary sources, such as family members and the medication administration record.

15. **Ans: 3**   The nurse would remind AP-C that physically holding onto someone could be interpreted as an attack; therefore the resident's agitation and aggression could increase. There are many steps that precede physical restraints, such as those demonstrated by the other APs: quiet reassurance, removing hazardous objects, and redirecting. In addition, health care staff should never try to independently restrain a patient without having adequate assistance. **Focus:** Prioritization, Supervision; **QSEN:** EBP; **Concept:** Safety; **Cognitive Level:** Applying; **IPEC:** IC

16. **Ans: 2, 3, 5, 6**   AD is more common after age 65. High cholesterol and hypertension, history of head injury, and ethnicity (in particular Blacks) are associated with greater risk. Persons who have Down syndrome have a higher incidence, but family history is not a risk factor. Cancer is not considered a risk factor. **Focus:** Prioritization; **QSEN:** EBP; **Concept:** Cognition; **Cognitive Level:** Applying

17. **Ans: 4** The nurse would direct the AP to accept what the person is saying. Confabulation is a form of speech that can occur in cognitive disorders. The person will make up experiences, words, or answers in order to fill in conversational gaps. The intent is not to deceive but to compensate for a failing memory. Responses and comments can be vague, generalized, or untrue, but correction is not necessary and pressing the person for details may increase anxiety and defensiveness. **Focus:** Prioritization, Supervision; **QSEN:** PCC; **Concept:** Communication; **Cognitive Level:** Applying; **IPEC:** IC

18. **Ans: 2** In cases of advanced dementia, feeding tubes are not generally recommended because there is no evidence that this intervention increases survival or improves the quality of life. In addition, feeding tube complications (e.g., aspiration, infection, tube dysfunction) can outweigh any potential benefits. Calorie counts, weekly weights, and thickened liquid nutritional supplements are part of the nutritional therapy for patients with geriatric failure to thrive (GFT). Criteria for GFT include weight loss, dehydration, low cholesterol, decreased appetite, poor nutrition, physical inactivity, depression, and immune dysfunction. **Focus:** Prioritization; **QSEN:** EBP; **Concept:** Nutrition; **Cognitive Level:** Analyzing

19. **Ans: 2, 6, 8, 9** Positioning a clock or calendar, asking one simple question at a time, looking directly at the person when speaking, and placing seasonal decorations are correct interventions that can be delegated/assigned to AP. Leading a reality group should be done by an RN because formative evaluation occurs during the activity. Repetitive reality orientation for persons with global amnesia is not effective and may increase frustration or agitation. APs should follow the care plan that is specific for each resident. The AP would report to the nurse if residents refuse care or request change. The environment should be well lit; inadequate lighting is a safety issue and decreased visual acuity contributes to confusion. Engaging residents in conversational topics at a normal pace during care is generally a good strategy. However, for persons with dementia, excessive stimuli or distraction can be confusing; thus APs may need to be instructed to focus on the task at hand and to speak slowly and give brief explanations. **Focus:** Delegation, Assignment; **QSEN:** TC; **Concept:** Care Coordination; **Cognitive Level:** Analyzing; **Cognitive Skill:** Generate Solutions; **IPEC:** T/T

20. **Ans: 1, 2, 4, 5, 7, 8, 10** The LPN/LVN can assist with planning routines and is responsible for monitoring changes, observing for safety issues, supervising APs, administering medications, and documenting and reporting medication efficacy and side effects. All team members would be expected to encourage the family's expression of concerns and the patient's feelings. The AP is assigned to assist with routine ADLs, such as bathing. An RN will perform the initial intake assessment that includes baseline abilities and behaviors. The RN is also responsible for evaluating response to interventions. **Focus:** Assignment; **QSEN:** TC; **Concept:** Care Coordination; **Cognitive Level:** Analyzing; **Cognitive Skill:** Generate Solutions; **IPEC:** T/T

QSEN Key: PCC, Patient-Centered Care; **TC,** Teamwork & Collaboration; **EBP,** Evidence-Based Practice; **QI,** Quality Improvement; **S,** Safety; **I,** Informatics.

IPEC Key: Domain 1 Values/Ethics (**V/E**); Domain 2 Roles/Responsibilities (**R/R**); Domain 3 Interprofessional Communication (**IC**); Domain 4 Teams/Teamwork (**T/T**)

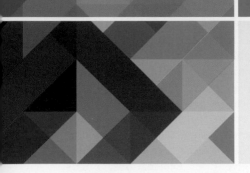

CHAPTER 7
Diabetes

Questions

1. The nurse is providing care for a patient with diabetes mellitus. Which symptoms indicate the patient has type 1 diabetes? **Select all that apply.**
   1. Weight gain.
   2. Nausea and vomiting.
   3. Extreme thirst.
   4. Numbness in the feet.
   5. Blurred vision.
   6. Frequent urination.

2. The assistive personnel (AP) asks the nurse why a patient with type 2 diabetes mellitus needs to have blood drawn to measure hemoglobin A_{1c} (HbA_{1c}) when diabetes is a problem with glucose. What is the nurse's **best** response?
   1. "When treating a patient's diabetes, it's important to know the hemoglobin level."
   2. "Hemoglobin A_{1c} levels indicate how much insulin a diabetic patient should be given each morning."
   3. "This test tells the health care provider how well the patient's body is able to make use of glucose."
   4. "HbA_{1c} is important because it indicates how well a patient's glucose has been controlled over the past 3 to 6 months."

3. What is the nurse's **best** response when a patient asks what a HbA_{1c} level of 8% means?
   1. "It means that your average blood glucose is 97 mg/dL."
   2. "It indicates that your level is considered prediabetic."
   3. "A level of 8% indicates poor glucose control."
   4. "This means that you are doing well following your diabetic diet."

4. Which action or intervention will be **best** assigned to the LPN/LVN who is caring for a patient with type 1 diabetes?
   1. Administering the patient's morning dose of subcutaneous (SC) insulin.
   2. Checking and recording morning vital signs for the patient.
   3. Setting up the patient's breakfast meal tray.
   4. Assisting the patient in ambulating to the bathroom and back.

5. Which action by the student administering a subcutaneous (SC) insulin injection requires intervention by the supervising LPN/LVN?
   1. Student puts on clean gloves.
   2. Student identifies patient using wristband.
   3. Student holds the syringe at a 45-degree angle.
   4. Student massages site after injection.

6. The nurse plans to teach a diabetic patient about foot care. Which important topics will the nurse be sure to include? **Select all that apply.**
   1. Wear clean cotton socks every day.
   2. Test the temperature of bath water before stepping into the tub.
   3. Lower your feet whenever possible to improve circulation.
   4. Wash your feet every day using hot water and soap.
   5. Never walk barefooted.
   6. Inspect your feet every day for cuts, cracks, blisters, or abrasions.
   7. Do not wear open sandals or sandals with straps between the toes.
   8. Get shoes a size larger than your feet so that they do not need to be broken in.

7. For which type 2 diabetic patient would the nurse question a prescription for oral glipizide?
   1. Patient with chronic obstructive pulmonary disease (COPD).
   2. Patient who is allergic to sulfa drugs.
   3. Patient who has renal insufficiency.
   4. Patient with flu-like symptom.s

8. The type 1 diabetic patient is prescribed a dose of regular insulin with neutral protamine hagedorn (NPH) insulin every morning. Which actions must the nurse take when administering this insulin dose? **Select all that apply.**
   1. Draw up the NPH insulin into the syringe first.
   2. Draw up the regular insulin into the syringe first.
   3. Administer the dose after breakfast.
   4. Verify that the proper dose has been drawn up with another nurse.
   5. Check the patient's fingerstick blood glucose before the dose is given.
   6. Check the patient's fingerstick blood glucose after the dose is given.

9. The AP asks the nurse why a patient's insulin dose is always given in the abdomen? What is the nurse's **best** response?
    1. "Insulin injections should be rotated between the abdomen, thighs, and arms."
    2. "The abdomen has the slowest absorption rate in the body for insulin."
    3. "Insulin should be injected by rotating sites within the abdomen to enhance absorption."
    4. "When a patient is exercising, the injection site will be changed to the thigh."

10. Which action can the nurse safely delegate to the experienced AP when caring for a patient with diabetes who develops symptoms of hypoglycemia?
    1. Administer intramuscular (IM) glucagon.
    2. Check a fingerstick glucose.
    3. Draw up insulin into a syringe.
    4. Give intravenous (IV) dextrose ($D_{50}W$).

11. A diabetic patient develops symptoms that include acetone (fruity) breath odor, deep respirations, hypotension, and abdominal rigidity. What condition does the nurse suspect?
    1. Diabetic ketoacidosis.
    2. Hypoglycemia.
    3. Hyperglycemic hyperosmolar state.
    4. Rebound hyperglycemia.

12. The AP is assisting a diabetic patient with his bath. Which **priority** instruction would the nurse be sure to provide?
    1. Check the patient's blood pressure before and after his bath.
    2. Provide the patient with a snack after his bath is completed.
    3. Assist the patient back to bed after his bath is completed.
    4. Report any breaks in the skin seen while assisting with the bath.

13. A 61-year-old patient with type 2 diabetes is NPO (nothing by mouth) after midnight for a colonoscopy in the morning. What is the **priority** assessment or intervention for this patient?
    1. Monitor the patient for signs of hypoglycemia.
    2. Prepare to administer sliding scale insulin as needed.
    3. Check fingerstick blood glucose level every 2 hours.
    4. Administer a snack if blood glucose is elevated.

14. The nurse is teaching a patient with type 2 diabetes about what to do on sick days. Which essential points will be included in the teaching plan? **Select all that apply.**
    1. Take your daily insulin as prescribed.
    2. Test your blood glucose every 4 hours.
    3. If nausea and vomiting occur, use dietary liquids with sugar.
    4. Take the prescribed dose of your oral hypoglycemic.
    5. Notify the health care provider for temperature over 100.2°F (38.8°C).
    6. Report blood glucose higher than 160 mg/dL to health care provider.

15. A 26-year-old woman who experiences diabetic symptoms during pregnancy asks the nurse if she is now diabetic. What is the nurse's **best** response?
    1. "No, once your baby is delivered the symptoms will go away."
    2. "What you have is called gestational diabetes and it occurs in less than 10% of pregnancies."
    3. "No, but 35% to 60% of women who experience gestational diabetes may develop diabetes within 5 to 10 years."
    4. "Yes, but you are a type 2 diabetic and will not need insulin to treat your condition."

16. The adult patient is admitted with symptoms of diabetes but is not overweight and has no signs of metabolic syndrome. The patient has a history of an autoimmune disease. The health care provider prescribed an oral hypoglycemic drug that did not help resolve the symptoms. What does the nurse suspect?
    1. Type 1 diabetes.
    2. Type 2 diabetes.
    3. Chemically induced diabetes.
    4. Latent autoimmune diabetes.

17. The home health nurse is visiting a diabetic patient. The patient has signs of low blood sugar (hypoglycemia) but is alert and able to swallow. What is the nurse's **best first** action?
    1. Provide 15 to 20 g of glucose or simple carbohydrate.
    2. Check the patient's fingerstick blood glucose.
    3. Ask the patient if he has taken his morning insulin.
    4. Offer a complex carbohydrate such as crackers or cheese.

18. The nurse is providing care for a patient with diabetes. Which finding would the LPN/LVN report to the supervising nurse **immediately**?
    1. Fingerstick blood glucose of 185 mg/dL.
    2. Numbness and tingling in the arches of both feet.
    3. Profuse sweating (diaphoresis).
    4. Weight gain of 1 pound over the past day.

 Answer Key for this chapter begins on p. 53

19. Nextgen (Extended Multiple Response) _____

> **Scenario:** The nurse is to administer SC regular insulin to a diabetic patient who is on sliding scale regular insulin and whose fingerstick blood glucose is 210 mg/dL. The injection site is the abdomen.

Instructions: Place an X or highlight each item that applies to the implementation of administering an SC insulin injection for this patient.

_____ Check the medication order

_____ Perform hand hygiene

_____ Identify the patient using at least three identifiers

_____ Prepare insulin by drawing up into syringe

_____ Put on sterile gloves

_____ Select site for injection and cleanse with alcohol swab using circular motion

_____ Hold syringe barrel at 30-degree angle

_____ Support skin at injection site by bunching tissue between thumb and index finger

_____ Press plunger to inject insulin using smooth motion

_____ Remove needle and activate needle guard

_____ Wipe injection site with alcohol swab to remove any blood

_____ Place needle and syringe in sharps container

 20. Nextgen (Matrix). A female client who has had type 1 diabetes mellitus for many years is having difficulty keeping her HgbA1c less than 77% with her current insulin therapy regimen and dietary modifications. She is now prescribed to take an additional insulin, high-concentration insulin glargine, subcutaneously.

Use an X for the nursing action below that is __Indicated__ (appropriate or necessary), __Contraindicated__ (could be harmful), or __Nonessential__ (makes no difference or not necessary) for the client's care with regard to administering this drug.

Nursing Action	Indicated	Contraindicated	Nonessential
Check to see when this drug was last given.			
Compare the concentration of the drug on hand with the concentration prescribed.			
If the injection is to be given close to the time another type of insulin is also to be given, carefully mix the two insulins to prevent the client from needing a second injection.			
Check the client's current blood glucose level.			
Ask the client when her most recent meal was eaten.			
After placing the needle in the SC tissue, aspirate for a blood return.			
When the injection is complete, massage the site for 30 seconds.			

Answers

1. **Ans: 2, 3, 6** Symptoms of type 1 diabetes include the three Ps, namely extreme thirst (polydipsia) and hunger (polyphagia) and frequent urination (polyuria); rapid weight loss, irritability, and weakness and fatigue; and nausea and vomiting. Weight gain, numbness in the feet, and blurred vision are symptoms of type 2 diabetes. **Focus:** Prioritization; **QSEN:** PCC; **Concept:** Glucose regulation; **Cognitive Level:** Analyzing. **Test Taking Tip:** It is very important to understand the differences between type 1 and type 2 diabetes including signs and symptoms. Treatments are different depending on the type of diabetes a patient has.

2. **Ans: 4** HbA_{1c} is drawn periodically to monitor the effectiveness of diabetic therapy and determine the degree of control over the disease process over a longer period of 3 to 6 months. This test does not measure hemoglobin, nor does it measure the amount of insulin a patient needs each morning or how well the patient's body uses glucose. **Focus:** Prioritization; **QSEN:** PCC, TC, EBP; **Concept:** Glucose Regulation, Leadership; **Cognitive Level:** Applying; **IPEC:** IC

3. **Ans: 3** Research has shown that lowering HbA_{1c} to 6.5% or less is associated with decreased risk of microvascular complications (eye, kidney, nerve) of diabetes. A high level shows poor glucose control over a period of 3 to 6 months. The nurse would remind the patient about strategies for better glucose control (e.g., diet, exercise). **Focus:** Prioritization; **QSEN:** PCC; **Concept:** Glucose Regulation, Patient Education; **Cognitive level:** Analyzing

4. **Ans: 1** While the LPN/LVN could perform all of these actions or interventions, administering SC insulin as ordered is within their scope of practice. Options 2, 3, and 4 are also within the scope of practice of an AP. **Focus:** Assignment; **QSEN:** PCC, TC; **Concept:** Clinical Judgment, Safety; **Cognitive Level:** Applying; **IPEC:** R/R

5. **Ans: 4** Options 1, 2, and 3 are correct actions when giving an SC injection. The student should not massage the site after an SC injection because this can alter the rate of absorption of the injected drug. The supervising LPN/LVN would intervene and remind the student administering the injection why massaging the site is not done. **Focus:** Supervision, Prioritization; **QSEN:** PCC, S; **Concept:** Glucose Regulation, Safety; **Cognitive Level:** Analyzing; **IPEC:** IC

6. **Ans: 1, 2, 5, 6, 7** To improve circulation, the patient would be taught to elevate, not lower, his or her feet. Feed should be washed with warm, not hot, water. Shoes should be properly fitted, not a size larger, and they should be gradually broken in. The other responses should be included when teaching about diabetic foot care. Additional important points include that after washing, feet should be dried carefully. If cream is applied for dry skin, it should not be put between toes. Toenails should be cut along the shape of the toes and filed to remove sharp edges. A podiatrist should manage any corns, calluses, and ingrown toenails. **Focus:** Prioritization; **QSEN:** PCC, S; **Concept:** Patient Education; **Cognitive Level:** Applying

7. **Ans: 2** Glipizide is a sulfonylurea drug. Sulfonylurea drugs are from the same family of drugs as sulfonamide antibiotics and must be given with caution to a patient who is allergic to sulfa drugs. **Focus:** Prioritization; **QSEN:** PCC, S; **Concept:** Clinical Judgment; **Cognitive Level:** Analyzing

8. **Ans: 2, 4, 5** If regular insulin and an intermediate-acting insulin (e.g., NPH) are to be mixed in a syringe, the regular insulin is drawn up first to prevent any contamination of the regular insulin bottle with the longer-acting insulin. Every insulin dose must be verified by another nurse as it is drawn up, every time. The patient's fingerstick blood glucose should be drawn before breakfast and before the dose is administered, not after. **Focus:** Prioritization; **QSEN:** PCC, S; **Concept:** Glucose Regulation, Safety; **Cognitive Level:** Analyzing. **Test Taking Tip:** Remember when administering regular and long-acting insulin to use the phrase "clear to cloudy." Regular insulin is clear and NPH insulin is cloudy.

9. **Ans: 3** Insulin enters the bloodstream at different rates when given in different areas of the body. The abdomen has the quickest absorption rate (most enhanced absorption), followed by the arms. The thighs and buttocks have the slowest rate of absorption. **Focus:** Prioritization; **QSEN:** PCC; **Concept:** Glucose Regulation; **Cognitive Level:** Analyzing; **IPEC:** IC. **Test Taking Tip:** Teach patients to avoid injecting insulin into an area that will soon receive extra exercise (e.g., the thigh) because exercise increases blood flow to that area and absorption will be increased.

10. **Ans: 2** An experienced AP would have been taught how to perform a fingerstick blood glucose test. The nurse would be responsible for assuring that the AP has been taught and mastered this skill. Administering IM or IV drugs must be completed by licensed nurses. A patient with hypoglycemia would not be given insulin because it would worsen the condition. The patient needs some form of glucose to correct hypoglycemia. **Focus:** Delegation, Supervision; **QSEN:** PCC, S; **Concept:** Glucose Regulation, Safety; **Cognitive Level:** Analyzing

11. **Ans: 1** Early symptoms of diabetic ketoacidosis include increased thirst (polydipsia) and urination (polyuria); acetone breath odor; dry mucous membranes and sunken eyeballs (dehydration); nausea and vomiting; deep respirations (Kussmaul breathing); abdominal pain and rigidity; and paresthesias, weakness, paralysis, and hypotension. Late symptoms include oliguria (minimal urine output) or anuria (no urine output) and stupor or coma. **Focus:** Prioritization; **QSEN:** PCC, S; **Concept:** Glucose Regulation, Safety; **Cognitive Level:** Analyzing

12. **Ans: 4** Breaks in the skin increase the patient's risk for infection and should be noted and treated as soon as possible to prevent infection. When a patient has diabetes, healing is slowed. Observing for and treating these changes can help prevent complications. **Focus:** Delegation, Supervision; **QSEN:** PCC, S; **Concept:** Communication, Safety; **Cognitive Level:** Applying; **IPEC:** IC

13. **Ans: 1** When a patient is NPO, the risk for hypoglycemia is increased and the nurse should monitor for signs of this disorder (e.g., shakiness, headache, weakness, irritability, diaphoresis, blurred vision, tachycardia, and confusion). Giving insulin will make the hypoglycemia worse. Checking fingerstick glucose is not necessary unless the patient shows signs of hypoglycemia. Administering a snack to a patient with elevated blood glucose will make their condition worse. **Focus:** Prioritization; **QSEN:** PCC, S; **Concept:** Glucose Regulation, Safety; **Cognitive Level:** Analyzing

14. **Ans: 2, 3, 4, 5** A patient with type 2 diabetes is usually prescribed an oral hypoglycemic drug not insulin. On sick days, regular insulin may be prescribed on a sliding scale basis. A blood glycose of higher than 200 mg/dL should be reported to the health care provider. Options 2, 3, 4, and 5 are appropriate actions that the nurse should teach patients for sick days. **Focus:** Prioritization; **QSEN:** PCC, S; **Concept:** Glucose Regulation, Patient Education, Safety; **Cognitive Level:** Analyzing

15. **Ans: 3** A woman who experiences gestational diabetes during pregnancy has a 35% to 60% chance of developing diabetes within 5 to 10 years. Option 1 does not inform the patient about the risks of developing diabetes. While option 2 is true, it does not answer the patient's question. Option 4 is not accurate. **Focus:** Prioritization; **QSEN:** PCC; **Concept:** Glucose Regulation, Patient Education; **Cognitive Level:** Applying

16. **Ans: 4** Patients with latent autoimmune diabetes in adults (LADA) are usually not overweight and do not have signs of metabolic syndrome. They demonstrate rapid failure of the pancreas to make insulin when treated with oral hypoglycemic drugs and are started on insulin within a year of diagnosis. **Focus:** Prioritization; **QSEN:** PCC, S; **Concept:** Glucose Regulation, Safety; **Cognitive Level:** Analyzing

17. **Ans: 1** When a patient is exhibiting signs of hypoglycemia, the first and best action for the nurse is to provide a source of glycose of a simple carbohydrate (e.g., ½ cup of juice or regular [NOT diet] soda, six to seven hard candies, three glucose tablets, a tablespoon of honey). Checking fingerstick glucose is important but not more important than giving glucose. Insulin will make hypoglycemia worse. Complex carbohydrates would be offered later, not first. **Focus:** Prioritization; **QSEN:** PCC, S; **Concept:** Glucose Regulation, Safety; **Cognitive Level:** Applying. **Test Taking Tip:** Whenever there is question about whether a patient has hypoglycemia or hyperglycemia, treatment for hypoglycemia is begun until a blood a blood glucose test can be obtained after the emergency treatment is administered. A glucose test can be obtained to prevent brain damage from extremely low cerebral glucose levels.

18. **Ans: 3** Profuse sweating is a symptom of hypoglycemia, a complication of diabetes that requires urgent treatment. A glucose level of 185 mg/dL (10.3 mmol/L) will need coverage with sliding scale insulin, but this is not urgent. Numbness and tingling are related to the chronic nature of diabetes and are not considered urgent. A weight gain of 1 pound is not urgent. **Focus:** Prioritization; **Concept:** Collaboration; **QSEN:** TC, S; **Cognitive Level:** Analyzing; **IPEC:** IC

19. Ans:

Scenario: The nurse is to administer SC regular insulin to a diabetic patient who is on sliding scale regular insulin and whose fingerstick blood glucose is 210 mg/dL. The injection site is the abdomen.

Instructions: Place an X or highlight each item that applies to the implementation of administering an SC insulin injection for this patient.

___X___ Check the medication order
___X___ Perform hand hygiene
_____ Identify the patient using at least three identifiers
___X___ Prepare insulin by drawing up into syringe
_____ Put on sterile gloves
___X___ Select site for injection and cleanse with alcohol swab using circular motion
_____ Hold syringe barrel at 30-degree angle
___X___ Support skin at injection site by bunching tissue between thumb and index finger
___X___ Press plunger to inject insulin using smooth motion
___X___ Remove needle and activate needle guard
___X___ Wipe injection site with alcohol swab to remove any blood
___X___ Place needle and syringe in sharps container

The patient would be identified using two identifiers (e.g., wrist band, state name, and birth date). The nurse wears clean gloves to give the injection. The syringe barrel would be held at a 90-degree angle to administer an SC injection in the abdomen. **Focus:** Prioritization; **QSEN:** PCC; **Concept:** Safety, Caregiving; **Cognitive Level:** Applying; **Cognitive Skills:** Generate Solutions

20. Ans:

Nursing Action	Indicated	Contraindicated	Nonessential
Check to see when this drug was last given.	X		
Compare the concentration of the drug on hand with the concentration prescribed.	X		
If the injection is to be given close to the time another type of insulin is also to be given, carefully mix the two insulins to prevent the client from needing a second injection.		X	
Check the client's current blood glucose level.	X		
Ask the client when her most recent meal was eaten.			X
After placing the needle in the SC tissue, aspirate for a blood return.		X	
When the injection is complete, massage the site for 30 seconds.		X	

Indicated: This is an ultralong-acting insulin and is only given once every 24 hours. The drug comes in two concentrations: 100 U/mL and 300 U/mL. Using the 300 U/mL concentration when the 100 U/mL is prescribed results in a medication error with an overdose three times greater than what was prescribed and can lead to severe hypoglycemia and death. Although the drug is very long acting, if the client is already hypoglycemic, the drug can worsen that condition. It is not to be given until the client's blood glucose level is at least in the normal range.

Contraindicated: Insulin glargine is not to be mixed with any other insulin (or an other drug) because of incompatibility issues and the possibility of precipitation. Aspiration is not performed when injecting any drug subcutaneously because this action can cause tissue damage. SC insulin injection sites are not massaged because this can increase the rate of drug absorption and increase the risk for hypoglycemia.

Nonessential: Because the insulin is very long acting, the timing of the most recent meal is not really relevant, although the blood glucose level is.

Focus: Prioritization; **QSEN:** PCC; **Concept:** Safety, Clinical Judgment; **Cognitive Level:** Analyzing; **Cognitive Skills:** Generate Solutions

QSEN Key: PCC, Patient-Centered Care; **TC,** Teamwork & Collaboration; **EBP,** Evidence-Based Practice; **QI,** Quality Improvement; **S,** Safety; **I,** Informatics.

IPEC Key: Domain 1 Values/Ethics (**V/E**); Domain 2 Roles/Responsibilities (**R/R**); Domain 3 Interprofessional Communication (**IC**); Domain 4 Teams/Teamwork (**T/T**).

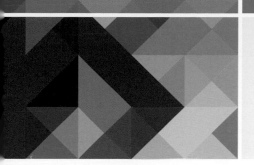

CHAPTER 8
Problems of Older Adults

Questions

1. A patient has presbycusis related to normal changes that occur with aging. Which instruction is the nurse **most** likely to give to the assistive personnel (AP)?
   1. Face the patient while speaking and maintain eye contact.
   2. Make sure eyeglasses are clean and remind patient to wear them.
   3. Ask the patient to repeat, point, or gesture to clarify intended meaning.
   4. Assist the patient with reading the menu; fine print can be difficult to see.

2. An older patient reports that his health care provider (HCP) gave him several prescriptions for constipation to use as needed (PRN) because of decreased bowel action related to aging. Which PRN medication is the nurse **most** likely to query?
   1. Docusate sodium.
   2. Methylcellulose.
   3. Senna.
   4. Loperamide hydrochloride.

3. Which statement indicates that the older person needs to be referred to their HCP for the evaluation of symptoms that exceed normal memory and cognitive changes of aging?
   1. "I have to have new information repeated a couple of times."
   2. "Multitasking is harder; I used to be able to juggle a lot of tasks."
   3. "My husband says my personality and social skills have changed."
   4. "I'd like to study a new subject, but my attention span is terrible."

4. Which AP requires a reminder and additional supervision related to the use of elderspeak?
   1. AP-A says, "Mrs. S, this is the call bell, please remember to call when you need help to go to the bathroom."
   2. AP-B says, "Mr. S, let me help you get up. Now sweetie, remember to move and stand up very slowly."
   3. AP-C says, "Mrs. S, what would you like to do first: wash your face, brush your teeth, or get dressed?"
   4. AP-D says, "Good morning, Mr. S. I am Assistant D. I am here to help you with your morning care."

5. The home health LPN/LVN notices that the older patient is taking multiple medications for his chronic health conditions: hypertension, arthritis, diabetes, depression, and pulmonary disease. Which member of the health care team would the nurse contact **first** related to the concern of polypharmacy?
   1. Each prescribing specialist.
   2. Pharmacist.
   3. Supervising registered nurse (RN).
   4. Primary HCP.

6. Based on the nurse's knowledge of genitourinary changes associated with aging, which instruction would the nurse give to the AP?
   1. Routinely check all of the older patients for urinary incontinence and assist them in cleaning up and changing clothes as needed.
   2. Older patients have increased urine production at night, so reassure them that they can call for toileting assistance at night.
   3. Urine production in older patients will exceed 2000 mL/24 h, so they need frequent assistance with toileting.
   4. Older female patients experience urinary retention related to changes in anatomical structures, so offer incontinence pads for leakage.

7. An older adult with several chronic health problems is prescribed megestrol. Which question would the nurse ask to gather data about the efficacy?
   1. Has your appetite improved?
   2. Is the urinary incontinence under control?
   3. Is the medication controlling your pain?
   4. Have the dizziness and vertigo resolved?

8. For a patient who has osteoporosis, which instruction would the nurse give to the AP to prevent the **most** serious complication?
   1. Frequently assist with toileting or other needs involving ambulation.
   2. Report complaints of back pain or discomfort with movement.
   3. Report refusal to eat foods or fluids that supply calcium and vitamin D.
   4. Encourage the patient to do range-of-motion exercises early in the morning.

9. An older adult is prescribed ferrous sulfate 200 mg three times per day for the treatment of iron deficiency anemia. Which additional medication would the nurse advocate for if the HCP fails to prescribe it?
   1. Antiemetic.
   2. Vitamin B12 injection.
   3. Antacid.
   4. Stool softener.

10. Which nursing action is the **best** example of the principle of nonmaleficence as an ethical consideration in caring for an older adult?
    1. Patient intends to smoke cigarettes despite education about the consequences, so the nurse tries to understand the patient's health goals.
    2. Patient is heavily intoxicated and belligerent; he is leaving the emergency department and intends to drive, so the nurse calls security.
    3. Patient does not have any money or health insurance, so the nurse seeks help from the RN and social worker to locate resources.
    4. Patient refuses prescribed medication and therapies, so the nurse explains the benefits of the treatment plan.

11. Which change related to aging might necessitate an age-adjusted dosage for high-protein-bound medications, such as warfarin and ibuprofen?
    1. Decreased gastric acid production.
    2. Decreased serum albumin levels.
    3. Decreased pain sensation.
    4. Increased total cholesterol levels.

12. The older female patient tells the nurse that she has been having heavy vaginal bleeding. Which question is the **priority**?
    1. When was your last normal menstrual period?
    2. Is there any chance you could be pregnant?
    3. When was your last normal Pap smear?
    4. How frequently are you changing pads for saturation?

13. For the past several months, an older female patient has been progressively lethargic, disinterested in normal activities, and having slowed thoughts processes. Which laboratory results will the nurse watch for and report to assist the HCP in differentiating major depression from an endocrine disorder?
    1. Cholesterol levels.
    2. Thyroid function tests.
    3. Blood glucose results.
    4. Coagulation studies.

14. The nurse is assigned to review hand washing as an infection control measure with a group of older adults who live in an assisted living facility. Which teaching principles will the nurse use? **Select all that apply.**
    1. Present complex information first, then review simple concepts.
    2. Assess for readiness to learn and motivation of participants.
    3. Provide written brochures at a 5th grade reading level in large print.
    4. Encourage participants to ask questions and to make comments.
    5. Extend teaching time so that all material can be covered in one session.
    6. Use a quiet and comfortable space that is well lit.

15. For an older adult with visual impairment, which instruction would the nurse give to the AP about assisting with meals?
    1. Describe the location of food on the plate using clock positions.
    2. Explain what is in each spoonful before feeding.
    3. Offer one food at a time; place it directly in front of the person.
    4. Give finger foods and serve liquids in nonspill containers.

16. An older male patient with several chronic medical problems lives alone. He sits and sleeps in a recliner and keeps the house very cold "to save money on the heating bill." What is the **best** instruction for the home health nurse to give to the AP to decrease the patient's risk for hypothermia?
    1. Locate a neighbor who would be willing to come in on a daily basis to check on him.
    2. Help the patient close off unused rooms so that only essential rooms are heated.
    3. Place quilts near the recliner; remind the patient to layer clothing and wear a hat.
    4. Check the thermostat at every visit and ensure that it is set at 70°F (21°C).

17. In the older adult, which vital sign is the **least** reliable as an indicator of health?
    1. Temperature.
    2. Pulse.
    3. Respirations.
    4. Blood pressure.

18. An older adult patient and her family are querying the fact that she has been NPO (nothing by mouth) for three days in a row for diagnostic testing. What is the **priority** nursing concern?
    1. Adherence.
    2. Fluid and electrolytes.
    3. Stress and coping.
    4. Nutrition.

19. Which factors increase the risk for HIV/AIDS among older adults? **Select all that apply.**
    1. Belief that risk is low because older adults are not interested in sex.
    2. Pregnancy is not an issue, so older adults are less likely to use condoms.
    3. Use of erectile dysfunction medications allows for prolonged sexual activity.
    4. Decreased estrogen in women causes thinning and decreased vaginal lubrication.
    5. Skin and mucous membranes are more fragile and easily torn.
    6. Primary mode of transmission in older adults is same-sex relations.

 20. Drag and Drop _____

Scenario: The nurse works in a clinic that primarily serves older adults who have a variety of chronic health problems. While assessing patients, the nurse is vigilant for evidence of elder abuse, which is divided into six categories: physical abuse, psychological or emotional abuse, sexual abuse, neglect, abandonment, and exploitation.

Which type of elder abuse is depicted in each of the patient situations?
Instructions:
Indicate which type of elder abuse listed in the left-hand column matches each patient situation. In the right-hand column, in the space provided, write in the correct letter that matches each patient situation. Note that all responses will be used and may be used more than once.

Type of Elder Abuse	Patient Situations
A. Physical abuse B. Psychological or emotional abuse C. Sexual abuse D. Neglect E. Abandonment F. Exploitation	1. _____ "I have bruises on my face, a black eye, and welts on upper arms because I fell down the stairs." 2. _____ "I give my oldest son money every week, because he can't seem to get out of debt." 3. _____ "I asked my daughter to go grocery shopping for me, but she hasn't gone for several weeks." 4. _____ "My caregiver makes fun of me when I leak urine, so I try to clean myself." 5. _____ "My lip got bruised when my caregiver was feeding me something that I don't like to eat." 6. _____ "My daughter won't talk to me; she treats me like I am not even there." 7. _____ "My husband gives me some water before he goes to work; I don't drink that much." 8 _____ "I don't like it when he does it to me, but he says that all people enjoy being touched." 9. _____ "She left me at the bus station and gave me some money for a ticket."

    Answer Key for this chapter begins on p. 60

PART 2 Common Health Scenarios

Answers

1. **Ans: 1**   Presbycusis is a gradual loss of hearing that occurs with aging. The nurse instructs the AP to face the patient and maintain eye contact while speaking; this helps the hearing impaired patient to interpret the message. For patients with visual impairment, clean lenses improve visual acuity. For patients with speech impairment, asking them to repeat, point, or use gestures can help to clarify what they are trying to express. In presbyopia, the eye loses the ability to focus on close objects, so, for example, reading becomes more difficult. **Focus:** Supervision, Assignment; **QSEN:** PCC; **Concept:** Sensory Perception; **Cognitive Level:** Analyzing; **IPEC:** IC

2. **Ans: 4**   Loperamide hydrochloride is a medication that is prescribed for diarrhea, so the nurse would assess the patient's understanding of the purpose of the drug and how to use it. The nurse would also call the HCP for clarification of PRN loperamide hydrochloride if the patient does not have any disease or disorder that causes diarrhea. The other medications are commonly prescribed for constipation: docusate sodium is a stool softener; methylcellulose is a bulk laxative; and senna is a laxative. **Focus:** Prioritization; **QSEN:** PCC; **Concept:** Elimination; **Cognitive Level:** Applying

3. **Ans: 3**   Personality changes, increased depression, and social withdrawal may be early signs of Alzheimer's disease. The other statements represent expected or normal changes associated with aging. **Focus:** Prioritization; **QSEN:** PCC; **Concept:** Cognition; **Cognitive Level:** Analyzing

4. **Ans: 2**   Although it is likely that AP-B is trying to show nurturing and patience, this AP needs a reminder about how to use clear and respectful communication. Elderspeak includes baby talk and exaggerated use of voice, pace, or tone. Another form of elderspeak is using terms of endearment, such as "honey, dear, or sweetie" that may be offensive and sound condescending. AP-C is not using elderspeak but may need a reminder that offering multiple options to patients who have cognitive impairment increases their confusion. **Focus:** Prioritization, Supervision; **QSEN:** PCC; **Concept:** Communication; **Cognitive Level:** Applying; **IPEC:** IC

5. **Ans: 3**   The nurse would consult the supervising RN for guidance. Ideally, the admission RN would have performed medication reconciliation and noticed the potential for polypharmacy during the intake assessment; contacted the primary HCP for verification of the medication list; and then documented the actions taken. If there is no documentation about the issue, the supervising RN

may follow up or instruct the nurse to follow up with the primary HCP. The primary HCP reviews the list and consults directly with any prescribing specialists for changes in medications. The pharmacist is notified whenever any changes are made in the prescriptions. **Focus:** Prioritization; **QSEN:** S; **Concept:** Safety; **Cognitive Level:** Analyzing; **IPEC:** R/R. **Test Taking Tip:** Polypharmacy is recognized as one of the major concerns for older adults. This topic is likely to be tested by NCLEX, because it is a safety issue that can be corrected by proactive nursing action.

6. **Ans: 2**   Nocturia (increased urination at night) is an expected change of aging, because the kidneys have decreased ability to concentrate the urine. One or two trips to the bathroom at night would be considered normal. Urinary incontinence is not an expected change of aging and the nurse would assess each individual for incontinence rather than instructing the AP to check and clean up every patient. Urine production of more than 2000 mL is not expected and accompanies disorders such as diabetes insipidus. Older male patients may experience urinary retention related to an enlarged prostate. Dribbling and leakage can occur. **Focus:** Prioritization, Supervision; **QSEN:** EBP; **Concept:** Elimination; **Cognitive Level:** Analyzing

7. **Ans: 1**   Megestrol can help to improve appetite. Medications such as oxybutynin are prescribed for overactive bladder, which is one cause of urinary incontinence. Opioids and nonopioid medications are commonly prescribed for pain. Medications such as meclizine are prescribed for dizziness and vertigo related to inner ear problems. **Focus:** Prioritization; **QSEN:** N/A; **Concept:** Nutrition; **Cognitive Level:** Applying

8. **Ans: 1**   For patients who have osteoporosis, risk for hip fracture sustained during a fall is the most serious complication; the bathroom is an area where falls often occur. Back pain or discomfort with movement can occur with osteoporosis and the nurse must assess these complaints. Refusing foods, fluids, or supplements that supply calcium or vitamin D could worsen the condition and cause the bone structure to become more fragile. Gentle range-of-motion exercises in the early morning would be more appropriate for patients with arthritis who experience joint stiffness after sleep; stiffness usually abates after they get up and move around. Weight-bearing exercises are recommended for patients with osteoporosis to strengthen bones. **Focus:** Prioritization; **QSEN:** S; **Concept:** Mobility; **Cognitive Level:** Applying

9. **Ans: 4** Iron supplements can cause constipation, so a stool softener is often prescribed. The nurse would also review the intake of dietary fiber and food sources that supply fiber. Iron supplements can cause nausea and cramping, but the nurse would advise taking the supplement with food rather than asking the HCP to prescribe an antiemetic medication. Vitamin B12 is a treatment for pernicious anemia. Antacids block the absorption of medications and should not be taken at the same time as iron supplements. **Focus:** Prioritization; **QSEN:** PCC; **Concept:** Elimination; **Cognitive Level:** Applying

10. **Ans: 2** Nonmaleficence is to prevent harm. If the patient is mentally impaired and his actions (e.g., driving) are a danger to self or others, the nurse would intervene to prevent harm. By attempting to understand the patient's health goals, the nurse is applying the principle of autonomy. Based on the principle of justice, the nurse helps the patient to locate resources to fund his health care needs. By explaining the benefits of the treatment plan, the nurse is applying the principle of beneficence to help the patient make informed choices and reconsider personal barriers. **Focus:** Prioritization; **QSEN:** S; **Concept:** Ethics; **Cognitive Level:** Analyzing

11. **Ans: 2** Serum albumin or prealbumin are the most common laboratory measurements of protein status. Medications that are protein bound, such as warfarin, ibuprofen, phenytoin, and furosemide, if prescribed together, can compete for binding sites and medications can be less effective. If the serum albumin level is low, medications can also be toxic. Decreased gastric acid can affect the absorption of medications. Decreased pain sensation may cause underreporting of problems, such as injury or infection. First-line interventions for high cholesterol levels are dietary and lifestyle modifications; antilipemic medications are prescribed if lifestyle modifications are insufficient. **Focus:** Prioritization; **QSEN:** S; **Concept:** Nutrition; **Cognitive Level:** Analyzing

12. **Ans: 4** Assessing blood loss and identifying active bleeding are the immediate priorities. The nurse may also ask the other questions. The date of the last menstrual period is baseline information that gives context to the current reports of vaginal bleeding. Vaginal bleeding can signal miscarriage or other problems associated with pregnancy, so pregnancy testing may be ordered. Postmenopausal vaginal bleeding could be a warning sign for cervical or uterine cancer; the date of the last normal Pap smear is obtained for baseline information. **Focus:** Prioritization; **QSEN:** S; **Concept:** Perfusion; **Cognitive Level:** Analyzing

13. **Ans: 2** Hypothyroidism can mimic the symptoms of depression, so these results would be of primary interest to the HCP. Older adults are at risk for high cholesterol levels but are typically asymptomatic with elevated levels; however, serious complications such as stroke or myocardial infarction can occur. Low blood sugar could manifest as confusion or difficulty concentrating, but effects would be acute, and the problem would have to be immediately corrected. Coagulation results would be relevant for a head injury or stroke, either of which can cause bleeding in the brain with subsequent changes in behavior or cognitive abilities. **Focus:** Prioritization; **QSEN:** N/A; **Concept:** Cellular Regulation; **Cognitive Level:** Analyzing

14. **Ans: 2, 3, 4, 6** Readiness and motivation increase success of the teaching. The Joint Commission recommends written materials, with large print at the 5th grade reading level. Written information facilitates the retention of information. By listening to questions and comments, the nurse assesses participants' understanding and teaching can be adapted accordingly. A quiet and comfortable space will decrease distractions and good lighting is essential. Simple concepts should proceed complex. Complex information should be divided into several teaching sessions rather than trying to cover all of the material in one long session. **Focus:** Prioritization; **QSEN:** PCC; **Concept:** Patient Education; **Cognitive Level:** Applying

15. **Ans: 1** Describing the location of food on the plate by using clock positions helps the person to maintain independence and dignity in self-feeding. Blindness does not prevent self-feeding. Explaining each spoonful or offering one food at a time might be useful strategies to encourage healthy eating for persons with confusion or cognitive disorders. Finger foods and nonspill containers are useful when older people have limitations in fine motor skills. **Focus:** Assignment, Supervision; **QSEN:** PCC; **Concept:** Sensory Perception; **Cognitive Level:** Applying

16. **Ans: 3** Instructing the AP to place quilts by the recliner and to layer clothes is the best intervention because it builds on the patient's existing behaviors. A social worker or nurse would be assigned to locate a neighbor or relative who would be willing to check on the patient. Closing off rooms is a possibility, but the patient might use this suggestion to save additional money by closing all rooms. Checking the thermostat at every visit is not incorrect, but the patient can readily lower the temperature as soon as the AP leaves. **Focus:** Prioritization, Supervision; **QSEN:** S; **Concept:** Thermoregulation; **Cognitive Level:** Analyzing

17. **Ans: 1** In the older adult, temperature is the least reliable indicator. Temperature may be lower than normal, possibly because of decreased metabolism or decreased physical activity. During an infection, the expected increase in temperature may not occur. Pulse rate should remain the same, but irregularities in rhythm may develop in older adults. Respiratory

rate may increase slightly due to decreased vital capacity and reserve. Systolic blood pressure may rise because of decreased elasticity in the blood vessels that can occur with aging. **Focus:** Prioritization **QSEN:** S; **Concept:** Thermoregulation; **Cognitive Level:** Applying. **Test Taking Tip:** Care of older adults and early recognition of sepsis are two topics that are likely to be tested in NCLEX. Review expected changes related to aging and know early warning signs and symptoms of disease and disorders.

18. **Ans: 2** Older adults have a higher risk for fluid and electrolyte imbalances. The nurse should observe for signs and symptoms of dehydration. Ideally, discussion with the patient and family should occur before scheduling diagnostic testing. This would increase adherence, decrease stress, and strengthen coping mechanisms. Discussion would also provide an opportunity to teach about fluid and food restrictions; questions could be addressed, and the HCP could be notified about concerns before the tests are scheduled. **Focus:** Prioritization **QSEN:** PCC; **Concept:** Fluid and Electrolytes; **Cognitive Level:** Applying

19. **Ans: 1, 2, 3, 4, 5** Factors that increase risk are a combination of physiologic changes related to aging and health beliefs. Pregnancy is not an issue, so condoms are not used for contraception. The use of erectile dysfunction medications can prolong sexual activity and therefore increases the time for exposure. Changes in mucous membranes, skin, and vaginal lubrication increase the likelihood of tearing. The belief that older adults are not interested in sex is a myth. The primary modes of transmission in older adults are opposite sex (heterosexual) relations and sharing contaminated needles among IV drug users. **Focus:** Prioritization; **QSEN:** EBP; **Concept:** Infection; **Cognitive Level:** Analyzing

20. **Ans: 1 A, 2 F, 3 D, 4 B, 5 A, 6 B, 7 D, 8 C, 9 E** The nurse must listen to reports of abuse; however, older adults may be reluctant to speak because of fear of reprisal or withdrawal of caregiver support. The nurse must analyze nonverbal behaviors, verbalized comments, physical findings, and the patient's situation to identify possible abuse. Examples of physical violence include hitting, slapping, kicking, beating, or forced feeding. Examples of psychological abuse include insults, belittling, intimidation, humiliation, or "silent treatment." Examples of sexual abuse include coerced sexual activity, forced nudity, or inappropriate photography. Examples of neglect include lack of food and fluids, poor personal hygiene, or unsafe living conditions. Caregivers or relatives abandon older adults by leaving them in hospitals, long-term care facilities, or public places such as stores or shopping centers. Older adults can be exploited for money, profit, or personal gain. **Focus:** Prioritization; **QSEN:** S; **Concept:** Interpersonal Violence; **Cognitive Level:** Analyzing; **Cognitive Skill:** Analyze Cues

QSEN Key: PCC, Patient-Centered Care; **TC,** Teamwork & Collaboration; **EBP,** Evidence-Based Practice; **QI,** Quality Improvement; **S,** Safety; **I,** Informatics.

IPEC Key: Domain 1 Values/Ethics (**V/E**); Domain 2 Roles/Responsibilities (**R/R**); Domain 3 Interprofessional Communication (**IC**); Domain 4 Teams/Teamwork (**T/T**).

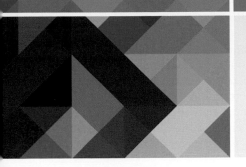

CHAPTER 9

Gastrointestinal and Nutritional Problems

Questions

1. The nurse is caring for a patient with esophageal varices. Which sign and or symptom would the nurse be **most** concerned about?
   1. Increased heart rate.
   2. Increased blood pressure.
   3. Constipation.
   4. Jaundice.

2. The nurse is feeding residents in the dining room for breakfast. Which breakfast tray should the nurse question for a resident who is Muslim?
   1. Eggs, bacon, and orange juice.
   2. Oatmeal, fruit, and coffee.
   3. French toast and a protein milkshake.
   4. Cheese and beef pastry with tea.

3. Which instructions should the nurse give a recently graduated assistive personnel (AP) regarding nutritional care of residents? **Select all that apply.**
   1. Serve patients who can feed themselves first.
   2. Hand feed the patients with advanced Parkinson disease.
   3. Open sealed packages such as utensils, sugar, and salt packets.
   4. Check each tray against the dietary order.
   5. Communicate changes of condition to the family member assisting a resident with feeding.
   6. Limit fluids for incontinent patients.

4. The nurse is administering medications on the med-surgical unit. Which patient should the nurse consult the health care provider (HCP) for before administering the ordered medication?
   1. A 37-year-old patient with irritable bowel syndrome taking methylcellulose.
   2. A 52-year-old patient with renal disease taking magnesium hydroxide.
   3. A 66-year-old patient with diverticulosis taking psyllium.
   4. A 72-year-old patient with gastroesophageal reflux disease (GERD) taking famotidine.

5. The nurse is assigned to a patient in the clinic who had a gastric bypass surgery 2 months ago. Last week the patient was cleared to start eating a regular solid food diet. Which symptoms would lead the nurse to suspect the patient has dumping syndrome?
   1. Abdominal pain and fever.
   2. Vomiting and hypotension.
   3. Nausea and diarrhea.
   4. Cramping and constipation.

6. The HCP ordered a colonoscopy for a patient to be completed the next day. Which nursing actions can the nurse safely assign to the AP?
   1. Administer the bowel prep.
   2. Provide clear liquids to the patient.
   3. Witness the signed consent for the procedure.
   4. Explain the procedure to the patient.

7. A new nurse is assigned to a patient with cirrhosis of the liver. She asks the supervising nurse if she should hold the lactulose because the patient is having six to eight diarrhea stools a day. Which statement made by the supervising nurse is correct?
   1. "Lactulose does not cause diarrhea."
   2. "Nurses should never hold ordered medications."
   3. "We can call the HCP to discontinue the lactulose."
   4. "The lactulose is necessary to decrease ammonia levels."

8. The nurse is admitting a patient from the emergency department (ED) with acute pancreatitis. Vital signs are: T 38.3°C (101°F), pulse 100 regular, R 22, BP 110/80, O_2 Sat 95% on 2 L oxygen via nasal cannula. He reports 8/10 abdominal pain. He was given 2 mg (intravenous) IV morphine 40 minutes ago in the ED. Which action should the nurse accomplish **first**?
   1. Keep the patient NPO (nothing by mouth).
   2. Place a nasogastric (NG) tube and confirm with x-ray.
   3. Administer acetaminophen 650 mg suppository for temperature of 101°F.
   4. Request the registered nurse (RN) administer 4 mg morphine sulfate via IV.

9. A patient is being admitted to the med-surgical unit from the postanesthesia care unit (PACU) following a laparoscopic cholecystectomy. Which postoperative duties can the nurse safely delegate to the AP? **Select all that apply.**
   1. Place the patient in a semi-Fowler's position.
   2. Measure vital signs every 15 minutes for 1 hour.
   3. Note the color and consistency of T-tube drainage.
   4. Empty and record the amount of T-tube drainage.
   5. Note the condition of the abdominal dressing.
   6. Question the patient regarding pain level.

10. A patient in the ED with abdominal pain is being examined for a possible appendicitis. Which action by the ED technician should the nurse question?
    1. Recording the amount of urine in the urinal.
    2. Assisting the HCP at the bedside.
    3. Accompanying the patient to radiology.
    4. Placing a heat pack on the patient's abdomen.

11. The nurse is giving preoperative care to a patient who is being prepared for a continent ileostomy. Which intervention can be assigned to the AP?
    1. Administering a saline enema.
    2. Administering bisacodyl 10 mg by mouth.
    3. Witnessing the preoperative permit.
    4. Instructing the patient on how to cough and deep breathe.

12. A patient who underwent a colectomy was admitted to the med-surgical unit. Vital signs on admission to the unit were: T 36°C (98.7°F), pulse 90 regular, R 20, BP 126/76, O_2 Sat 96% on 2 L oxygen by nasal cannula. Which observation made by the nurse 1 hour later would warrant notifying the HCP?
    1. BP 120/72, P 96, R 16, O_2 Sat 93% on room air.
    2. Urine output of 90 mL over the last hour.
    3. Complaints of abdominal pain 6/10.
    4. Firm abdomen with increased size.

13. The nurse making a home visit is reviewing medications for a colorectal cancer patient who was discharged home with an ileostomy. Which medication would warrant a call to the HCP for clarification?
    1. Famotidine 10 mg by mouth at bedtime.
    2. Morphine sulfate extended-release tablets 15 mg by mouth every morning.
    3. Vitamin B complex 1 mL sublingual twice a day.
    4. Simethicone 60 mg after meals and at bedtime.

14. The nurse has assigned obtaining intake and output measurements to the AP. Which situation would warrant the nurse to reeducate the AP?
    1. The AP recorded 8 ounces of water as 240 mL of intake.

    2. The AP donned gloves prior to emptying a urine leg bag.
    3. The AP held a graduated container of urine at eye level to obtain an output measurement.
    4. The AP recorded 5 teaspoons of ice chips as 25 mL.

15. The nurse caring for a patient with a NG tube is checking for proper placement prior to administering medications. Which data would necessitate a call to the HCP?
    1. A gastric pH of 7.
    2. Aspiration of green stomach contents.
    3. Inability to aspirate stomach contents.
    4. X-ray confirmation of placement in the stomach.

16. The nurse is making assignments for an AP on the med-surgical unit. Which nursing tasks can safely be delegated to the AP? **Select all that apply.**
    1. Application of warm, moist compresses to an infiltrated IV site.
    2. Transferring a patient with a gastroscopy tube from the bed to a chair.
    3. Administering an enema to a patient who is constipated.
    4. Administering a tube feeding to a patient with a duodenal feeding tube.
    5. Discontinuing a urinary catheter in a patient who has a fever.
    6. Performing oral care on a patient with a non-rebreather oxygen face mask.

17. The AP assigned to six patients tells the nurse that the vital signs on the other patients will not be completed on time because of near-constant cleaning of a bedridden patient with continuous diarrhea. Which statement by the nurse to the AP indicates a collaborative approach to teamwork?
    1. "I will call staffing to send someone to help."
    2. "I will call the HCP to get an order for an antidiarrheal medication."
    3. "I will come help you, let me gather some skin care supplies."
    4. "I can take the vital signs for you before I go to lunch."

18. The nurse is assigned to a patient with diverticulitis, irritable bowel syndrome-c, and GERD. The patient has received the first dose of dicyclomine 20 mg by mouth. Which symptom or symptoms relief will the nurse evaluate to determine if the medication was effective?
    1. Heartburn
    2. Diarrhea
    3. Nausea and vomiting
    4. Stomach and intestinal cramping

19. Extended Multiple Response.

The nurse is interviewing a new patient at the bariatric clinic. Vital signs are T 37°C (98.6°F), pulse 88 regular, R 20, BP 150/88, O2 Sat 98% on room air, BMI 30. She has a history of type 2 diabetes and hypertension, for which she takes metformin and lisinopril. She is here today to discuss weight loss options.

Which questions are applicable for the nurse to ask when gathering data related to factors that cause obesity? Highlight or circle numbers of the correct responses.
1. Can you tell me about your diet?
2. Do you engage in exercise?
3. What type of work do you do?
4. Do you snore or wake up suddenly in the night?
5. Do you feel fatigued or have an increased sensitivity to cold?
6. Do you have a family history of obesity?
7. Do you have back or joint pain?
8. Do you often feel overwhelmed or stressed?

20. Matrix.

The nurse in the ED is assigned a 38-year-old patient whose symptoms include nausea, vomiting, diarrhea, and abdominal discomfort for the last 3 days after attending a weekend music festival. Vital signs are T 37.7°C (100°F), pulse 110 regular, R 20, BP 90/70, O$_2$ Sat 96% on room air, skin turgor is poor. She states that she is no longer nauseated and has not vomited for 24 hours but the diarrhea continues. She reports a headache. The patient is allergic to penicillin. For each HCP order, place an X in the box to indicate whether it is indicated, nonessential, or contraindicated.

Nursing Action	Indicated	Nonessential	Contraindicated
Nothing by mouth (NPO)			
Give small amounts of electrolyte solution			
Ibuprofen 800 mg by mouth for headache			
Oxygen at 2 L per minutes via nasal cannula			
0.9% normal saline IV 250 mL/h			
Stool for culture and sensitivity			
Complete blood count (CBC)			
Amoxicillin 500 mg by mouth three times a day			
Famotidine 10 mg by mouth once a day			

PART 2 Common Health Scenarios

Answer Key for this chapter begins on p. 66

Answers

1. **Ans: 3** Coughing, vomiting, and straining for defecation causes the portal hypertension to rise suddenly and can cause bleeding and or rupture of the varices. Esophageal varices are swollen veins in the esophagus near the stomach most often caused by serious liver disease, which causes a back-up of circulation from the portal system (portal hypertension). An increased heart rate does not represent an increased danger for esophageal bleeding or rupture. Jaundice and increased blood pressure would be a normal finding in someone with portal hypertension from liver disease. **Focus:** Prioritization; **QSEN:** PCC, EBP; **Concept:** Safety, Perfusion; **Cognitive Level:** Analyzing

2. **Ans: 1** Pork may not be consumed by Muslims according to the Quran. Pork is forbidden to eat as it is considered to be impure and unhealthy. **Focus:** Prioritization; **QSEN:** PCC; **Concept:** Culture; **Cognitive Level:** Analyzing

3. **Ans: 1, 3, 4** Patients with advanced Parkinson disease have impaired swallowing. These patients should be fed by the nurse or an AP with extra training and experience to prevent aspiration. Questions or communication regarding patient condition should always be directed to the nurse or HCP. Fluids should never be limited in incontinent patients unless there is a specific HCP order to do so. Older adults have less body water and can quickly become dehydrated. **Focus:** Assignment, Supervision; **QSEN:** S, PCC; **Concept:** Nutrition; **Cognitive Level:** Analyzing

4. **Ans: 2** Medications containing magnesium should be used with caution in patients who have renal disease. The kidneys in patients with renal disease have a decreased ability to excrete excess magnesium, which can lead to magnesium toxicity. **Focus:** Prioritization; **QSEN:** S; **Concept:** Safety, Fluid and Electrolytes; **Cognitive Level:** Analyzing

5. **Ans: 3** Dumping syndrome occurs when food moves into the small intestine too quickly. Exhaustion, nausea, sweating, and diarrhea occur after eating. Eating six small meals slowly and without fluids at mealtime can prevent dumping syndrome. Abdominal pain, fever, vomiting, and hypotension would indicate leaking of stomach contents into the abdomen and typically would occur early in the postoperative period. Cramping and constipation are associated with irritable bowel syndrome. **Focus:** Prioritization; **QSEN:** PCC; **Concept:** Nutrition, Elimination; **Cognitive Level:** Analyzing

6. **Ans: 2** Providing clear liquids is within the AP's scope of practice. The nurse must administer the bowel prep as it is a medication; explanation of the procedure and witnessing the signed consent must be done by either the nurse or the HCP. **Focus:** Assignment; **QSEN:** T/C; **Concept:** Elimination; **Cognitive Level:** Applying; **IPEC:** T/T

7. **Ans: 4** Ammonia is a neurotoxin that can cause hepatic encephalopathy in a patient with liver disease. Lactulose prevents ammonia from diffusing from the colon into the blood and also draws the ammonia from the blood into the colon, decreasing ammonia levels. **Focus:** Assignment, Supervision; **QSEN:** PCC; **Concept:** Elimination; **Cognitive Level:** Analyzing

8. **Ans: 4** Pain control is the priority nursing action. NPO status, placing an NG tube, and administering acetaminophen can be accomplished after the RN administers morphine for pain relief. **Focus:** Prioritization; **QSEN:** PCC; **Concept:** Pain; **Cognitive Level:** Analyzing; **IPEC:** R/R, T/T

9. **Ans: 1, 2, 4** Positioning, measuring vital signs, and emptying and recording drainage are all duties that an AP is trained to accomplish in a safe manner. The nurse must evaluate any dressings or drainage as well as question the patient regarding his condition. **Focus:** Delegation; **QSEN:** PCC: **Concept:** PCC, Safety; **Cognitive Level:** Analyzing; **IPEC:** R/R.

10. **Ans: 4** Heat should not be used to relieve abdominal pain caused by appendicitis because it can cause vasodilation and bring excess blood to the appendix causing a rupture. An ice pack can be used to decrease abdominal inflammation in order to minimize pain. **Focus:** Supervision; **QSEN:** S; **Concept:** PCC, Safety; **Cognitive Level:** Analyzing; **IPEC:** IC

11. **Ans: 1** Only the nurse can administer medications, witness the preoperative permit, and give preoperative instructions. Enemas can be administered by the AP as long as they are not medicated. The AP can encourage the patient to cough and deep breathe but instruction must be done by the nurse. **Focus:** Assignment; **QSEN:** S; **Concept:** Safety; **Cognitive Level:** Analyzing

12. **Ans: 4** A firm abdomen that is increasing is a sign that internal bleeding could be occurring and the HCP should be notified immediately. The change in vital signs is not significant enough to notify the HCP but warrants close monitoring for continued changes. The oxygen saturation level is still within normal limits on 2 L of oxygen and could be raised by coughing and deep breathing. Urine output less than 30 mL an hour indicates decreased perfusion to the kidneys. It is not unusual for a postoperative patient to have pain and postoperative orders will include medications for pain relief. **Focus:** Prioritization; **QSEN:** PCC, S; **Concept:** Clinical Judgement; **Cognitive Level:** Analyzing

13. **Ans: 2** Patients with an ileostomy do not have enough time for extended-release or enteric-coated medication to absorb. The nurse should question the HCP regarding the extended-release morphine. Morphine can be given in dissolvable tablets or sublingual formulations as needed for pain relief. The other medications are not time released. **Focus:** Prioritization; **QSEN:** S, PCC; **Concept:** Pain; **Cognitive Level:** Analyzing

14. **Ans: 3** The proper way to measure fluid output in a graduated container is to place the container on a flat surface to read the measurement at eye level. Holding the container up to eye level can result in the wrong measurement due to the unevenness of fluid in the container. **Focus:** Assignment, Supervision; **QSEN:** S, T/C; **Concept:** Elimination; **Cognitive Level:** Analyzing; **IPEC:** R/R

15. **Ans: 1** Gastric pH is 1–4. If the pH value is over 6 it could indicate the NG tube is in the trachea or bronchus and the HCP should be notified. Green, colorless, or yellow aspirate are all normal colors of gastric aspirate. Inability to aspirate stomach contents can be a normal finding. X-ray confirmation is the gold standard for the confirmation of NG tube placement. **Focus:** Prioritization; **QSEN:** PCC, S; **Concept:** Nutrition, Safety; **Cognitive Level:** Analyzing

16. **Ans: 1, 2, 3, 5, 6** The AP can safely perform all these nursing tasks. APs are not allowed to administer a tube feeding to a patient unless this function is specifically allowed by state and agency policy. Nutritional support is a nursing responsibility. **Focus:** Delegation; **QSEN:** S, T/C; **Concept:** Care Coordination; **Cognitive Level:** Analyzing; **IPEC:** R/R

17. **Ans: 3** Taking care of this patient is not only time consuming but fatiguing. The task is easier with two people, and working together shows respect and consideration for the AP. The nurse needs to look at the patient's skin to assess for breakdown and this is a good time to complete that assessment. Calling for staffing or taking vital signs does not show the same support for the AP and calling the HCP for medication does not solve the immediate problem. **Focus:** Assignment, Supervision; **QSEN:** T/C; **Concept:** Collaboration, Care Coordination; **Cognitive Level:** Analyzing; **IPEC:** R/R, T/T

18. **Ans: 4** Dicyclomine slows intestinal movement. Relaxing the muscles in the stomach and gut relieves the stomach and intestinal cramping. **Focus:** Prioritization; **QSEN:** PCC, S; **Concept:** Pain **Cognitive Level:** Analyzing

19. **Ans: 1, 2, 3, 5, 6, 8** The causes of obesity are a high-calorie, high-fat diet, lack of exercise, sedentary work or lifestyle, and a possible genetic predisposition. Hypothyroidism, which leaves a patient sensitive to cold as well as fatigued, is also a possible cause of obesity. Overeating occurs with some people when they are stressed. Snoring or waking up in the night is a sign of obstructive sleep apnea and is not a cause but rather a complication of obesity. Back pain and joint pain are also complications of obesity as the joints become stressed from the extra weight. **Focus:** Prioritization; **QSEN:** PCC, EBP; **Concept:** Nutrition; **Cognitive Level:** Analyzing

20. **Ans:**

Nursing Action	Indicated	Nonessential	Contraindicated
Nothing by mouth (NPO)			X
Give small amounts of electrolyte solution	X		
Ibuprofen 800 mg by mouth for headache			X
Oxygen at 2 L per minutes via nasal cannula		X	
0.9% normal saline IV 250 mL/h	X		
Stool for culture and sensitivity	X		
Complete blood count (CBC)	X		
Amoxicillin 500 mg by mouth three times a day			X
Famotidine 10 mg by mouth	X		

The patient has not vomited for 24 hours, so it is no longer necessary to keep NPO status. Instead, small amounts of an electrolyte solution such as Pedialyte can be offered, so the patient does not become dehydrated. Ibuprofen is contraindicated due to the negative effects that NSAIDs have on the stomach. Oxygen saturation is within normal limits, so oxygen is not needed. An IV for hydration is indicated as the patient displays signs of dehydration as evidenced by the increased pulse rate, lowered blood pressure, and poor skin turgor. A CBC is indicated to check for an elevated white count and a stool sample should be sent for culture and sensitivity to examine for a causative agent and appropriate treatment. Amoxicillin is contraindicated because the patient is allergic to penicillin. Famotidine is indicated to decrease the hydrochloric acid. **Focus:** Prioritization; **QSEN:** PCC, EBP; **Concept:** Infection, Fluid and Electrolytes; **Cognitive Level:** Analyzing

QSEN Key: PCC, Patient-Centered Care; **TC,** Teamwork & Collaboration; **EBP,** Evidence-Based Practice; **QI,** Quality Improvement; **S,** Safety; **I,** Informatics.

IPEC Key: Domain 1 Values/Ethics (**V/E**); Domain 2 Roles/Responsibilities (**R/R**); Domain 3 Interprofessional Communication (**IC**); Domain 4 Teams/Teamwork (**T/T**).

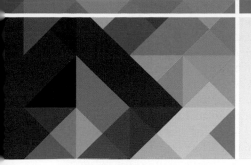

CHAPTER 10

Infection Control and Safety

Questions

1. Under nursing supervision, which actions related to the use of safety devices (restraints) can be delegated or assigned to assistive personnel (AP)? **Select all that apply.**
   1. Place familiar items, such as family pictures, near the bedside.
   2. Explain the reason for the device to the patient and family.
   3. Assess skin and perform neurocirculation checks every 30 minutes.
   4. Assist with toileting every 2 hours, or as scheduled.
   5. Assess and document behaviors related to the need for devices.
   6. Use a half-bow or safety knot to secure the device to the bed frame.

2. Which condition related to substance abuse can be fatal if the nurse fails to note and report **early** signs and symptoms?
   1. Delirium tremens.
   2. Korsakoff syndrome.
   3. Tolerance to opioids.
   4. Liver failure.

3. The nurse finds the patient lying on the floor. He is cyanotic and drooling. There is no apparent rise and fall of the chest. What does the nurse do **first**?
   1. Apply oxygen.
   2. Insert an oral airway.
   3. Check responsiveness.
   4. Initiate rescue breathing.

4. The nursing student knows to wear nonlatex gloves when caring for a patient who has a latex allergy. In which situation is the supervising nurse **most** likely to check the student's equipment before allowing the student to proceed?
   1. Gathers supplies to secure the catheter leg bag.
   2. Obtains clean linens and a clean laundry bag.
   3. Assists with preparing items on the food tray.
   4. Collects personal items to help with oral hygiene.

5. Which AP needs a reminder about actions that increase risk for falls in confused or disabled patients?
   1. AP-A checks to see if there is a notation on patients' doors for fall risk.
   2. AP-B maintains toileting and hygiene schedules throughout the shift.
   3. AP-C assists patients with getting into bed, turning out lights, and closing the doors.
   4. AP-D explains use of the call bell and reminds patients to call for help.

6. Which instruction would the nurse give to the AP about caring for a patient who has a radiation implant?
   1. Wear a dosimeter badge to protect against radiation when performing patient care.
   2. Organize supplies and care to limit time spent in close proximity to the patient.
   3. Place a lead shield over the patient's body before starting to give care.
   4. Reply to call bells by peeking around the partially opened door to see the patient.

7. A family member brings a personal handheld hairdryer to the hospital so that the patient can wash, dry, and style her hair in the preferred style. To maintain electrical safety, which action would the nurse take **first**?
   1. Inspect the hairdryer to see if the cords are frayed and to see if it functions properly.
   2. Ask the family member to bring a copy of the manufacturer's instructions.
   3. Check to see if the appliance has a three-pronged grounded electrical plug.
   4. Contact maintenance personnel to inspect the appliance for safety before usage.

8. A small fire starts in the kitchen of a long-term care facility. Which task would the nurse delegate to AP **first**?
   1. Direct ambulatory residents out of the dining area.
   2. Use the fire extinguisher to put out the fire.
   3. Check bedrooms and assist those who are bedridden.
   4. Ensure that exit doors are open and barrier doors are closed.

9. Based on the figure below, which action would the nurse take **first** to correct the problem and safely apply the principles of body mechanics?

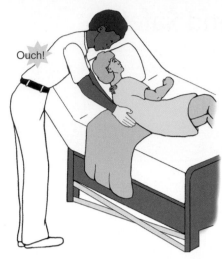

(Figure from Williams P. (2021) *deWit's Fundamental Concepts and Skills for Nursing* (6th ed.) Elsevier.)
1. Widen stance and bend or flex the knees.
2. Raise the bed to a comfortable working height.
3. Ask the patient to help by rolling forward if able.
4. Keep trunk straight and avoid using back muscles.

10. The family of an older adult is upset because a 3-year-old grandchild may have ingested some of the patient's pills. The child seems okay, but the home health nurse immediately calls poison control. Which information must the nurse include? **Select all that apply.**
1. Child's age and weight.
2. Purpose of medication.
3. Suspected number of pills ingested.
4. Name of medication.
5. Time of ingestion.
6. Symptoms/signs or complaints.

11. Which actions increase the risk for blood-borne infection related to sharps injuries? **Select all that apply.**
1. Recapping used needles by carefully placing the sheath over the needle.
2. Overloading or improperly using sharps containers.
3. Leaving contaminated sharps on trays or bedside tables.
4. Drawing blood from a confused patient with inadequate help.
5. Changing needles after drawing medication and before injecting the patient.
6. Using a plastic soda bottle to store used needles in the home setting.

12. Which task related to reducing health care–associated infections would be assigned or delegated to the AP?
1. Perform hand hygiene and change gloves between procedures that involve the perineal area or fecal matter.
2. Use an aseptic technique for cleansing the skin before an invasive procedure, such as catheter insertion.
3. Assess intravenous sites for signs of infection at least once per shift and before every use.
4. Ensure that urinary catheters are used for patients who need them and removed as soon as possible.

13. Which instruction must the nurse give to the AP about caring for a patient who has a *Clostridium difficile* infection?
1. Use alcohol-based hand gel before and after care.
2. Wash your hands with chlorhexidine after giving care.
3. Use double-gloving whenever body fluids are involved.
4. Wash with soap and water; scrub for at least 20 seconds.

14. To decrease the incidence of catheter-associated urinary tract infections (CAUTI), which nursing action is the **best**?
1. Query insertion of indwelling urinary catheter if condom catheter is an option.
2. Use a sterile technique for catheter insertion and a clean technique for daily care.
3. Advocate for automatic stop-order of indwelling urinary catheters.
4. Politely decline to take a verbal order for urinary catheter insertion.

15. The health care team is using the ventilator-associated pneumonia (VAP) bundle to care for a patient. To fulfill VAP bundle recommendations, the nurse will give the AP special instructions about which task?
1. Assisting the patient with bathing.
2. Assisting the patient with oral hygiene.
3. Helping the patient with urinary elimination.
4. Cleaning the perineum after bowel movements.

16. Which measure would the nurse use to reduce the risk of transmission to self when caring for a patient who has COVID-19?
1. Monitor self for fever and other signs/symptoms.
2. Use an N95 mask, gown, gloves, and eye protection.
3. Maintain physical distancing of at least 6 feet.
4. Perform hand hygiene before touching the patient.

17. A senior nursing student, who is scheduled to attend the final clinical experience before graduation, has a roommate who is showing symptoms of COVID-19; the test results are pending. Which action would the student take **first**?
    1. Take own temperature, assess self for symptoms, and initiate self-quarantine.
    2. Stay home, care for the roommate, and get tested as soon as possible.
    3. Call nursing instructor, explain circumstances, and ask for guidance.
    4. Attend clinical, wear an N95 mask, and physical-distance as much as possible.

18. In caring for patients who have or are suspected of having COVID-19, which aerosol-generated procedure creates the **greatest** risk for aerosol transmission?
    1. Bronchoscopy.
    2. Manual suction.
    3. Sputum induction.
    4. Endotracheal (ET) intubation.

19. Enhanced Multiple Response _____

Scenario: The nurse is reviewing evidence-based information about infection control and hand hygiene. According to the World Health Organization (WHO), health care workers are encouraged to practice MY 5 moments for hand hygiene. These five moments represent occasions during patient care where hand hygiene is recommended.

Which five tasks are part of the WHO recommendations?
Instructions: Place an X in the space provided or highlight each item that is included in MY 5 moments for hand hygiene. Select five that apply.
1. ____Before entering the patient's room
2. ____Before touching a patient
3. ____Before clean/aseptic procedures
4. ____After body fluid exposure/risk
5. ____After donning gloves
6. ____After touching a patient
7. ____After touching patient surroundings
8. ____After doffing gloves
9. ____At the end of every shift

20. Cloze._____

Scenario: Based on what is currently known about the modes of transmission for COVID-19, the nurse is responsible for recognizing portals of entry and reservoirs. The nurse follows recommendations from the Centers of Disease Control and Prevention (CDC) to break the chain of infection.

Instructions: Complete the sentences below by choosing the best option for the missing information that corresponds with the same numbered list of options provided.
In person-to-person contact, airborne virus enters the body through ____1__, ____2____, or _____3_____. A _____4_____ is the **most** likely reservoir of COVID-19.

Options for 1 & 2 & 3	Options for 4
1. Nose	1. Surface or object, such as a door handle that is frequently touched
2. Eyes	2. Bat or cat sickened with COVID-19 infection
3. Mouth	3. Person who does not social-distance or wear a mask in public
4. Damaged skin	4. Public toilet that is not disinfected after every usage
5. Parenteral route	5. Chair or table in a public waiting room
6. Sexual contact	6. Health care worker or first responder
7. Drinking contaminated water	7. Person who had COVID-19 but has recovered

 Answer Key for this chapter begins on p. 72

Answers

1. **Ans: 1, 4, 6**   The AP is frequently assigned to make the patient's environment comfortable. Toileting and hygiene are also within the AP's scope of practice. Securing the device can also be delegated, but the nurse must give instructions about the type of knot and where to secure it. Explanations to the patient/family and assessment and documentation cannot be delegated. **Focus:** Delegation, Supervision; **QSEN:** TC; **Concept:** Safety; **Cognitive Level:** Applying, **IPEC:** T/T

2. **Ans: 1**   When a person with alcohol addiction stops drinking, delirium tremens can occur. Early withdrawal symptoms include shaking or tremors, sweating, anxiety, and nausea/vomiting. If not recognized and treated, death can occur because of respiratory complications or cardiovascular collapse. Korsakoff syndrome is a chronic loss of memory. It is sometimes preceded by Wernicke encephalopathy, which is a medical emergency that is reversible with the administration of intravenous thiamine. When tolerance to opioids develops, larger doses are required to achieve the desired effect. Liver failure can occur after long-term usage of alcohol. Signs/symptoms of liver failure are insidious and include abdominal pain and tenderness, dry mouth, increased thirst, fatigue, jaundice, loss of appetite, and nausea. **Focus:** Prioritization; **QSEN:** EBP; **Concept:** Addiction, Safety; **Cognitive Level:** Applying

3. **Ans: 3**   When patients have unwitnessed and unexpected changes in level of consciousness, checking responsiveness is the first action. The nurse may suspect cardiac or respiratory arrest; however, checking responsiveness is the first step in cardiopulmonary resuscitation. If verbal and physical stimuli do not arouse the patient or stimulate spontaneous breathing, the nurse would check pulse and initiate chest compressions and rescue breathing. If the patient arouses or if spontaneous breathing occurs, the nurse would apply oxygen. Oral airways are used for airway management for patients who are unconscious and breathing (e.g., postseizure). **Focus:** Prioritization; **QSEN:** EBP; **Concept:** Clinical Judgment; **Cognitive Level:** Applying

4. **Ans: 1**   Gloves are the most commonly used items that contain latex and gloves are required for many procedures. Many other patient care items may also contain latex (e.g., catheters and straps that secure drainage bags, bandages, intravenous catheters, nasogastric tubes, condoms, stethoscopes, and the tubing of some blood pressure cuffs). **Focus:** Prioritization, Supervision; **QSEN:** EBP; **Concept:** Safety, Immunity; **Cognitive Level:** Analyzing

5. **Ans: 3**   AP-C needs a reminder that turning off all lights increases the risk of falls. Walkways to the bathroom need muted lighting. Leaving doors open is an additional safety measure. The other APs are performing actions that help to reduce falls. **Focus:** Delegation, Supervision; **QSEN:** S; **Concept:** Safety; **Cognitive Level:** Applying

6. **Ans: 2**   Care must be organized and performed efficiently to minimize exposure time. The dosimeter badge should be worn, but the purpose is to measure radiation exposure over time. It does not provide any direct protection. Lead shielding does provide protection, but the AP should wear the shield rather than place it over the patient's body. While distancing and shielding are important for self-protection, the health care team should try to avoid behaviors or actions that make the patient feel shunned. **Focus:** Delegation, Supervision; **QSEN:** S; **Concept:** Safety; **Cognitive Level:** Analyzing

7. **Ans: 4**   Electrical appliances that are brought into the health care facility must be inspected by maintenance personnel. In the home setting, the nurse would be more likely to help the patient and family to check for fraying cords and to encourage following the manufacturer's instructions and to use three-pronged plugs for grounding. **Focus:** Prioritization; **QSEN:** S; **Concept:** Safety; **Cognitive Level:** Analyzing

8. **Ans: 1**   The mnemonic RACE guides the priorities for a fire emergency. RACE stands for Rescue those in immediate danger; Activate the alarm; Confine the fire; Extinguish the fire. The nurse would instruct the AP to direct ambulatory residents away from the fire source. If the fire spreads, directing ambulatory residents out of harm's way increases the number of people saved, compared to helping one or two bedridden residents. Extinguishing the fire is the last step and should only be attempted if it is small and localized (e.g., trash can). Exit doors should always be open and freely accessible. Barrier doors should be closed to slow the progression of the fire. **Focus:** Delegation, Prioritization; **QSEN:** S, EBP; **Concept:** Safety; **Cognitive Level:** Applying; **IPEC:** T/T

9. **Ans: 2**   Raising the bed to the correct working height is the first action and this may be sufficient to accomplish the task. The nurse may use the other options, as needed, to reduce injury to self. **Focus:** Prioritization; **QSEN:** S, EBP; **Concept:** Safety; **Cognitive Level:** Applying

10. **Ans: 1, 3, 4, 5, 6**   Basic information includes the name of product, the suspected amount, time of ingestion (inhalation, injection, or exposure), signs/symptoms, name of caller and name of the person who is poisoned,

call back number, and details about the exposure, such as how it happened. Poison control has a large database of substances, so it is not necessary to explain the purpose of the medication. **Focus:** Prioritization; **QSEN:** S, EBP; **Concept:** Safety; **Cognitive Level:** Applying. **Test Taking Tip:** Young children and older people have the highest risk for accidental poisoning. Review the patient education for poison prevention in your fundamentals textbook. Prevention measures are likely to be tested during NCLEX.

11. **Ans: 1, 2, 3, 4, 6** All of these actions place the nurse at risk for needle or sharp injury, but if needlesticks occur while drawing medication, there is no transfer of blood-borne infection to the nurse. Recapping can be achieved by laying the sheath on a flat surface and sliding the tip of the needle into the sheath without exposing the nurse's fingers. (This technique is only used if recapping is necessary for safety and the needle is not contaminated with blood or body fluids.) Sharps containers should be changed before they become overloaded. Habitually removing sharps after use reduces exposure to injury. If blood must be drawn from a confused or uncooperative patient, adequate help reduces risk of injury to the patient and staff. If containers are used in the home setting, they must be puncture-proof and stablized and the opening must allow disposal without touching the rim of the container. **Focus:** Prioritization; **QSEN:** S, EBP; **Concept:** Safety; **Cognitive Level:** Analyzing

12. **Ans: 1** The AP assists with daily hygiene and hygiene after toileting. Removing gloves and hand hygiene prevents cross-contamination from a dirty area, such as the rectum, to a cleaner area, such as the labia. Invasive procedures, assessing, monitoring equipment, and advocating for the patient cannot be delegated to the AP. (Some states may allow APs to insert urinary catheters, but the AP would need additional training to perform this task. The nurse must be familiar with the AP's scope of practice for their state and facility and be sure that the AP has mastered the skill.) **Focus:** Delegation, Supervision; **QSEN:** EBP; **Concept:** Infection; **Cognitive Level:** Applying; **IPEC:** R/R

13. **Ans: 4** Hand washing must be performed using soap, water, and friction for at least 20 seconds. Alcohol-based hand gel is not effective against *C. difficile* spores. Chlorhexidine is a topical antiseptic used to clean the skin before an invasive procedure. Chlorhexidine is also an ingredient in some mouthwashes and reduces risk for VAP. Double-gloving may be used during some surgical procedures but is not commonly used for bedside care. **Focus:** Delegation, Supervision; **QSEN:** EBP; **Concept:** Infection; **Cognitive Level:** Applying

14. **Ans: 1** If the patient is a candidate for a condom catheter, then the best measure to prevent CAUTI would be to avoid catheter insertion. Sterile and clean techniques do help to reduce CAUTI, but the catheter provides an ongoing avenue for organisms to enter the body. Automatic stop-orders are preferred because prolonged indwelling time increases risk for infection. Verbal versus written orders will not prevent CAUTI, but the nurse can take the opportunity to discuss the need for catheterization with the HCP and ask for a stop-order as needed. **Focus:** Prioritization; **QSEN:** EBP; **Concept:** Infection; **Cognitive Level:** Analyzing; **IPEC:** IC

15. **Ans: 2** Oral hygiene is an important component of the VAP bundle and the task can usually be delegated to the AP. The care includes brushing the teeth, gums, and tongue at least twice a day with a soft bristle brush; applying moisturizer to the lips every 2 to 4 hours; rinsing the oral cavity with a mouthwash containing chlorhexidine; and using oral swabs with hydrogen peroxide to remove plaque from the tongue. Bathing and hygiene after elimination are general measures to decrease infection but are less specific to the VAP bundle. **Focus:** Delegation, Supervision; **QSEN:** EBP; **Concept:** Infection; **Cognitive Level:** Analyzing; **IPEC:** IC

16. **Ans 2** All of these actions are considered important for infection control related to COVID-19. However, for the protection of self, members of the health care team must wear an N95 mask or equivalent or higher respirator mask, gown, gloves, and eye protection. Monitoring self and self-quarantine are measures that protect others from someone who is potentially infected. Maintaining 6 feet physical distancing is recommended to the general public. For the nurse, physical distancing is not always possible, but the nurse would organize care to limit time spent in close proximity to infected patients. Performing hand hygiene reduces risk of passing infection to others and protects self if hands get contaminated. **Focus:** Prioritization; **QSEN:** S; **Concept:** Infection; **Cognitive Level:** Analyzing

17. **Ans: 1** A senior student would recognize the need to first assess for signs and symptoms and to self-quarantine. The next step would be to notify the instructor, report circumstances, and ask for guidance. Caring for the roommate may be necessary. Getting tested is an important step because of the potential exposure. In this circumstance, attending clinical would be ill advised because of the potential for exposing others. **Focus:** Prioritization; **QSEN:** S; **Concept:** Infection; **Cognitive Level:** Analyzing. **Test Taking Tip:** An important part of supervising, assigning, and delegating is to anticipate and understand the capabilities and skill level of members of the health care team. In this case, a senior nursing student who is about to graduate has a higher level of assessment skills, initiative, and decision-making, whereas a first-year student would call the instructor first because of less skill and experience in making clinical decisions.

18. **Ans: 4** Of the four aerosol-producing procedures, ET intubation creates the greatest risk. This procedure is often done in emergency situations and complete donning of personal protective equipment (PPE), patient education, and sedation are not always possible. Insertion of the ET tube stimulates coughing, gagging, and salivation. The HCP must look directly into the oral pharynx to visualize the vocal cords while inserting the tube. Generally, a respiratory therapist and a nurse stand close to the patient's head to assist with the intubation. During a bronchoscopy, a thin tube is passed into the nose or mouth for the purpose of visualizing the lungs and airways. The patient is educated and sedated prior to the procedure, which is then performed under controlled conditions. For manual suction, a rigid plastic tube can be used to quickly remove mucous from the mouth. Coughing and gagging will not occur if oral suctioning is correctly performed. Manual suction, using a thin flexible tube, is performed to remove secretions from an established ET tube. Coughing may occur, but the insertion and suction (limited to 10 seconds) are quickly accomplished. For sputum induction, the patient is given a nebulized saline solution and then coached to deep breath and cough. The team member who is performing the sputum induction uses patient education, PPE, and maximal physical distancing to reduce the risk of transmission. **Focus:** Prioritization; **QSEN:** S; **Concept:** Infection; **Cognitive Level:** Analyzing

19. **Ans: 2, 3, 4, 6, 7** The WHO gives guidance to a large audience who practice in a wide range of settings. The WHO guidelines are generalized and are intended to be easy to learn and remember. Facility policies may exceed MY 5 moments for hand hygiene in the number of steps and specific details. Thus hand hygiene before entering the patient's room and after doffing gloves may be included in facility procedure manuals. Hand hygiene is not generally recommended after donning gloves. Hand hygiene at the end of the shift is an excellent habit, but this is typically regarded as a personal responsibility rather than part of the facility's policies. **Focus:** Prioritization; **QSEN:** S; **Concept:** Infection, EBP; **Cognitive Level:** Applying; **Cognitive Skill**; Recognize Cues

20. **Ans:** In person-to-person contact, airborne virus enters the body through the **nose, eyes, or mouth. A person who does not social-distance or wear a mask in public** is the most likely reservoir of COVID-19. Person-to-person contact indicates that at least two people are present for transmission to occur. Airborne organisms enter the body through inhalation through the nose or mouth. Eyes are also vulnerable when droplets are sprayed by coughing, sneezing, or loud talking. Virus can also enter the eyes by rubbing with contaminated hands. A reservoir (host) is a place where infectious organisms, such as COVID-19, grow, multiply, and wait for an opportunity to be transmitted to another host. COVID-19 is being spread by persons who test positive for the virus, as well as persons who are presymptomatic or asymptomatic. Thus people who do not practice social distancing or wear a mask in public are the most common source for spreading the virus. Bats and other mammals can be infected with COVID-19. The virus is viable for various lengths of time on objects, such as doorknobs, toilets, and furniture; thus hand hygiene is important. Health care workers, first responders, and people who have recovered from the virus may be stigmatized as potential carriers of COVID-19, but if they follow CDC recommendations (distancing, masks, hand hygiene, self-quarantine for symptoms, etc.), the risk potential is similar to the general population. **Focus:** Prioritization; **QSEN:** S; **Concept:** Infection; **Cognitive Level:** Analyzing; **Cognitive Skill:** Recognizes Cues. **Test Taking Tip:** General knowledge of chain of infection can be applied to answer this type of question. If you lack knowledge about a specific organism, you can still make an educated guess by focusing on the key terms (person-to-person contact, airborne, reservoir).

QSEN Key: PCC, Patient-Centered Care; **TC,** Teamwork & Collaboration; **EBP,** Evidence-Based Practice; **QI,** Quality Improvement; **S,** Safety; **I,** Informatics.
IPEC Key: Domain 1 Values/Ethics (**V/E**); Domain 2 Roles/Responsibilities (**R/R**); Domain 3 Interprofessional Communication (**IC**); Domain 4 Teams/Teamwork (**T/T**).

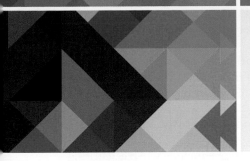

CHAPTER 11

Fluid, Electrolyte, and Acid–Base Balance

Questions

1. The nurse is providing care for a patient with symptoms of thirst, poor skin turgor, weight loss, weakness, dizziness, and dry mucous membranes. The patient's supine (lying) blood pressure is 112/70; standing blood pressure is 90/68. What is the nurse's **priority** concern?
   1. Fluid imbalance.
   2. Overhydration.
   3. Dehydration.
   4. Insensible fluid loss.

2. Which actions or interventions would the nurse safely delegate to the assistive personnel (AP) for an alert patient with dehydration? **Select all that apply.**
   1. Assessing the skin turgor while bathing the patient.
   2. Checking and recording the patient's temperature every 4 hours.
   3. Monitoring the patient's intravenous (IV) site for patency.
   4. Encouraging the patient to consume oral fluids every 2 hours.
   5. Administering the patient's hydroxyzine for nausea as needed.
   6. Providing mouth care after an episode of vomiting.

3. Which **priority** finding would the nurse instruct the AP to report immediately for a patient with dehydration?
   1. Temperature of 99.2°F (37.3°C).
   2. Difficulty swallowing breakfast cereal.
   3. Heart rate of 93 beats per minute.
   4. Dry skin on legs bilaterally.

4. The nurse is providing care for an 85-year-old patient with coronary artery disease who is receiving IV fluid normal saline (0.9%) for dehydration. Which assessment is **most** important?
   1. Urine output every 2 hours.
   2. Skin elasticity every shift.
   3. IV insertion site every 6 hours.
   4. Lung auscultation every 4 hours.

5. A patient with hypervolemia asks the nurse why her hematocrit is low. What is the nurse's **best** response?
   1. "Your hematocrit is low because of because extra fluid in your blood vessels dilutes the concentration of the red blood cells (RBCs)."
   2. "Usually when a person's hematocrit is low, it is related to bleeding somewhere in the body."
   3. "A low hematocrit can be caused by failure of your body to make enough RBCs."
   4. "Because of the extra fluid in your body, your RBCs may be breaking down more rapidly than usual."

6. Which actions or interventions will the nurse expect for a patient with overhydration? **Select all that apply.**
   1. Bed rest.
   2. IV fluids.
   3. Low-sodium diet.
   4. Diuretic therapy.
   5. Elastic stockings.
   6. Urinary catheter placement.

7. The nurse discovers that a patient's serum sodium level is 128 mEq/L. Which assessment findings will the nurse expect? **Select all that apply.**
   1. Headache.
   2. Dry mucous membranes.
   3. Nausea and vomiting.
   4. Low-grade temperature.
   5. Muscle cramps.
   6. Intense thirst.

8. Which action or intervention would the nurse safely delegate to an AP when providing care for a patient with a decreased serum calcium level (hypocalcemia)?
   1. Administering oral calcium 30 minutes before meals.
   2. Reminding patient to consume dietary sources such as cheese and broccoli.
   3. Assessing for Chvostek or Trousseau signs.
   4. Encourage increased fluid intake of 3–4 L/d.

9. The adult patient has a respiratory rate of 40 breaths per minute. Which acid–base imbalance is **most** likely to occur?
   1. Respiratory acidosis.
   2. Metabolic acidosis.
   3. Respiratory alkalosis.
   4. Metabolic alkalosis.

10. When the patient with chronic obstructive pulmonary disease (COPD) becomes a little short of breath while completing morning care, the AP asks the nurse if his oxygen flow can be increased above 3 L/min. What is the nurse's **best** response?
    1. "Before increasing a patient's oxygen flow rate, we should check the oxygen saturation by pulse oximetry."
    2. "That is a good idea because the patient is not receiving enough oxygen to carry to all cells and tissues."
    3. "I'll have to contact the health care provider (HCP) and ask for a prescription to increase the oxygen flow rate."
    4. "When a patient with COPD is on oxygen, it must be administered carefully because it can cause a respiratory arrest."

11. The nurse is providing care for a patient whose oral medications include hydrochlorothiazide (HCTZ) twice a day for hypertension and an antacid every 4 hours for reflux. Which acid–base abnormality will the nurse monitor for?
    1. Respiratory acidosis.
    2. Metabolic acidosis.
    3. Respiratory alkalosis.
    4. Metabolic alkalosis.

12. Which actions or interventions will the nurse safely delegate to the experienced AP when caring for a patient with a fluid imbalance of overhydration? **Select all that apply.**
    1. Checking and recording intake and output.
    2. Increasing the oxygen flow rate.
    3. Ambulating the patient to the bathroom.
    4. Assessing for bilateral breath sounds.
    5. Reminding the patient to drink extra fluids.
    6. Checking oxygen saturation by pulse oximetry.

13. For which action will the nurse intervene when an AP is checking and recording intake and output for a 78-year-old patient?
    1. AP reminds the patient to save all urine.
    2. AP calculates fluid intake from the meal tray.
    3. AP enters the room and immediately empties the patient's urinal.
    4. AP totals intake and output at the end of shift.

14. Which fluids must the nurse include when calculating a patient's daily output? **Select all that apply.**
    1. Diarrhea stools.
    2. Emesis.
    3. IV fluids.
    4. Wound drainage.
    5. Normal perspiration.
    6. Gastric drainage.

15. The nurse is providing care for a patient with renal failure. Which acid–base imbalance will the nurse monitor for?
    1. Respiratory acidosis.
    2. Metabolic acidosis.
    3. Respiratory alkalosis.
    4. Metabolic alkalosis.

16. Which instruction is **best** for the nurse to give the AP related to checking daily weights for a patient with dehydration?
    1. "Check the weight at the same time using the same scale, with the patient wearing the same clothing."
    2. "Check the weight using the same scale at any time in the morning before the patient has breakfast."
    3. "Check the weight at the same time every day with the patient wearing the same amount of clothing."
    4. "Check the weight using the same scale at the same time, before the patient voids every morning."

17. The patient with hypertension is prescribed a low-sodium diet. Which foods will the nurse teach the patient to avoid? **Select all that apply.**
    1. Hot dogs.
    2. Broccoli.
    3. Dried fruits.
    4. Lunch meats.
    5. Pickles.
    6. Fresh tomatoes.

18. The nurse is caring for a patient with fluid volume excess and assesses the finding in this picture. How will the nurse **best** document this finding?

1. Swelling of feet.
2. Swelling of ankles.
3. Pedal pitting edema.
4. Pedal edema with nonpalpable pedal pulses.

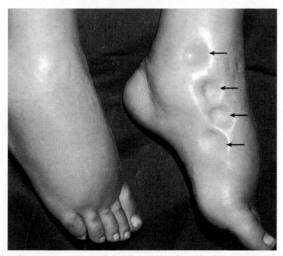

(Figure from Patton KT, Thibodeau GA. (2014) The Human Body in Health and Disease (6th ed.), Elsevier.)

19. Nextgen (Enhanced Hot Spot)

Scenario: A 75-year-old patient was admitted with a weight gain of 10 pounds, bilateral crackles in lower lobes of lungs, and visible neck veins when lying down. Vital signs are T 97.8°F (36.5°C), HR 56/min regular, RR 18/min, BP 178/90. The patient is lethargic but is able to respond to questions. The patient has bilateral 2+ edema to the ankles. History includes renal insufficiency and chronic obstructive pulmonary disease (COPD). Laboratory values include decreased serum sodium, normal serum potassium, and decreased hematocrit.

Instructions: Highlight or underline the findings that indicate the patient is at risk for overhydration.

20. Nextgen (Cloze).

Scenario: The nurse is caring for a patient with an electrolyte imbalance. The telemetry monitor technician reports the patient has cardiac dysrhythmias, so the nurse checks the patient's ___1___ laboratory value and finds that the patient has ___2___. The nurse expects the HCP to prescribe ___3___.

Instructions: Choose the *most likely* options for the information missing from the statement below by selecting from the lists of options provided.

Options for 1	Options for 2	Options for 3
A. Sodium	A. Hypokalemia	A. Furosemide
B. Calcium	B. Hypernatremia	B. Potassium supplement
C. Potassium	C. Hypocalcemia	C. Calcium supplement

Answer Key for this chapter begins on p. 78

Answers

PART 2   Common Health Scenarios

1. **Ans: 3**   All of these symptoms are found when a patient is dehydrated. The nurse would also want to check the patient's urine output, which is usually decreased as well as dark and concentrated. When the blood pressure drops when the patient moves from a supine to a standing position, the nurse would suspect postural hypotension, which occurs with dehydration. **Focus:** Prioritization; **QSEN:** PCC, S; **Concept:** Fluid and Electrolytes; **Cognitive Level:** Analyzing. **Test Taking Tip:** It is important to know classic signs and symptoms of dehydration and overhydration. Dehydration signs and symptoms show that the patient has a deficit of fluid volume.

2. **Ans: 2, 4, 6**   The scope of practice for an AP includes checking and recording vital signs, providing hygiene care (e.g., mouth care), and reminding or encouraging patients about what has already been taught by the nurse (e.g., consumption of oral fluids). Assessing, monitoring, and administering medications require additional skills of the professional nurse. **Focus:** Delegation, Supervision; **QSEN:** PCC, S; **Concept:** Care Coordination; **Cognitive Level:** Applying

3. **Ans: 2**   Difficulty with swallowing increases a patient's risk for aspiration and must be assessed immediately. While a low-grade temperature, a heart rate in the 90s, and dry skin need to be monitored, none are as urgent as difficulty swallowing. **Focus:** Delegation, Supervision; **QSEN:** PCC, TC, S; **Concept:** Clinical Judgment; **Cognitive Level:** Analyzing; **IPEC:** IC, R/R. **Test Taking Tip:** To respond to a question like this, it is essential to consider which finding indicates a risk of life or limb to the patient.

4. **Ans: 4**   Older adults with cardiac problems and dehydration must be rehydrated with care because they are at increased risk for fluid overload (overhydration) if IV fluids are infused too rapidly. The nurse assesses for signs and symptoms of this problem, which include abnormal breath sounds (e.g., crackles), that must be reported immediately to the HCP. The other findings are important but not as urgent as changes in lung sounds. **Focus:** Prioritization; **QSEN:** Clinical Judgment, S; **Concept:** Fluid and Electrolytes, Safety; **Cognitive Level:** Analyzing

5. **Ans: 1**   When a patient is overhydrated (hypervolemic) the hematocrit is low from hemodilution. Although bleeding, failure to make enough RBCs, and premature breakdown of RBCs can cause low hematocrit, these conditions are not usually related to overhydration. **Focus:** Prioritization; **QSEN:** PCC; **Concept:** Patient Education; **Cognitive Level:** Applying

6. **Ans: 1, 3, 4, 5**   Bed rest may be prescribed to facilitate the excretion of fluid because the kidneys function best when the body is supine. A low-sodium diet and diuretic drugs will help with the elimination of extra fluid. Elastic stockings or sequential compression devices help decrease edema. IV fluids would make overhydration worse, and urinary catheter placement increases a patient's risk for infection. **Focus:** Prioritization; **QSEN:** PCC, S; **Concept:** Fluid and Electrolytes, Safety; **Cognitive Level:** Applying

7. **Ans: 1, 3, 5**   A sodium level of 128 mEq/L is a low value indicating hyponatremia, a fairly common electrolyte abnormality with signs and symptoms that include headache, nausea and vomiting, and muscle cramps. Dry mucous membranes, low-grade temperature, and intense thirst are signs and symptoms of hypernatremia (elevated sodium level [greater than 145 mEq/L; normal range is 135–145 mEq/L]). **Focus:** Prioritization; **QSEN:** PCC, S; **Concept:** Fluid and Electrolytes, Clinical Judgment; **Cognitive Level:** Analyzing

8. **Ans: 2**   An AP can remind a patient about what has already been taught by the nurse. Administering medications and assessing patients requires additional skills and training appropriate to professional nurses. Option 4 is not correct. Increasing fluid intake is an intervention for a patient with increased calcium, not decreased calcium. **Focus:** Delegation; **QSEN:** PCC, S, TC; **Concept:** Fluid and Electrolytes, Safety; **Cognitive Level:** Applying; **IPEC:** IC, R/R

9. **Ans: 3**   When an adult's respiratory rate is 40 breaths per minute, the patient is hyperventilating (elevated respiratory rate). This leads to blowing off carbon dioxide (CO_2). The bicarbonate level remains the same and the pH decreases (acidosis). **Focus:** Prioritization; **QSEN:** PCC, S; **Concept:** Acid–Base Balance; **Cognitive Level:** Analyzing

10. **Ans: 4**   A patient with COPD has an altered respiratory drive mechanism and oxygen can act as a respiratory depressant, so it must be given cautiously (less than 2–3 L/min). Although uncommon, higher flow rates can cause a respiratory arrest. Checking the oxygen saturation is a good idea but does not answer the AP's question. Checking with the HCP is also a good idea but also does not answer the AP's question. **Focus:** Prioritization, Supervision; **QSEN:** PCC, S, TC; **Concept:** Acid–Base Balance, Leadership, Safety; **Cognitive Level:** Applying; **IPEC:** IC

11. **Ans: 4**   The most common cause of metabolic alkalosis is diuretic administration (e.g., HCTZ). In addition, this patient is receiving an antacid every 4 hours. Antacids can also cause metabolic alkalosis, especially when used excessively. **Focus:** Prioritization; **QSEN:** PCC, S; **Concept:** Acid–Base Balance, Clinical Judgment; **Cognitive Level:** Analyzing

12. **Ans: 1, 3, 6** The AP's scope of practice includes keeping track of intake and output and assisting patients with ambulating to the bathroom. The experienced AP would have been taught how to check oxygen saturation using pulse oximetry. Oxygen is considered to be a medication and should be increased by the nurse. Assessing breath sounds requires additional skills of a professional nurse. A patient with overhydration would likely be on a fluid restriction, not taking in extra fluids. **Focus:** Delegation, Supervision; **QSEN:** PCC, S, TC; **Concept:** Clinical Judgment, Safety; **Cognitive Level:** Analyzing; **IPEC:** IC

13. **Ans: 3** Before emptying a patient's urinal, the AP must put on clean gloves to decrease the risk of transferring microorganisms. The nurse would instruct the AP about using gloves when coming in contact with any patient fluids. The AP must also measure the urine before emptying the urinal. All of the other options are appropriate for measuring intake and output for a patient. **Focus:** Delegation, Supervision; **QSEN:** PCC, S; **Concept:** Leadership, Safety; **Cognitive Level:** Applying; **IPEC:** IC

14. **Ans: 1, 2, 4, 6** A patient's output would include urine, diarrhea stool, emesis, gastric drainage, wound drainage, and excessive perspiration. IV fluids are counted as intake. Normal perspiration is not considered output. **Focus:** Prioritization; **QSEN:** PCC; **Concept:** Fluid and Electrolytes; **Cognitive Level:** Applying

15. **Ans: 2** A deficit of bicarbonate ions or an increased production or retention of hydrogen ions leads to metabolic acidosis. The major causes include excessive loss of bicarbonate ions from diarrhea, renal failure, diabetic ketoacidosis (DKA), hyperkalemia, and sepsis. In kidney disease there is decreased excretion of acids and decreased production of bicarbonate, which causes metabolic acidosis. **Focus:** Prioritization; **QSEN:** PCC, S; **Concept:** Acid–Base Balance, Clinical Judgment; **Cognitive Level:** Analyzing

16. **Ans: 1** The AP would be instructed to check the patient's weight at the same time each morning using the same scale, with the patient wearing the same amount of clothing. The weight should be checked after the patient voids and before the patient eats breakfast. **Focus:** Delegation, Supervision; **QSEN:** PCC; **Concept:** Fluid and Electrolytes, Leadership; **Cognitive Level:** Applying; **IPEC:** IC

17. **Ans: 1, 3, 4, 5** Fresh fruits and vegetables are generally low in sodium. High-sodium products include regular canned meats, regular canned soups, hot dogs, lunch meats, dried fruits, pickles, olives, and salted snacks (e.g., popcorn, pretzels, chips). Prepared condiments such as ketchup and mustard are also high in sodium. The nurse would check with the registered dietician nutritionist (RDN) for the list of foods that the patient can choose from and that should be avoided. **Focus:** Prioritization; **QSEN:** PCC, S; **Concept:** Fluid and Electrolytes, Patient Education; **Cognitive Level:** Applying; **IPEC:** IC

18. **Ans: 3** Edema is excessive accumulation of fluid in the interstitial tissue that is a sign of fluid overload. The arrows point to indentations in the swelling of the left foot, which is pitting edema. Patients accumulate fluid in dependent areas. The nurse presses his or her thumb into the skin over a bony prominence and holds for 5 seconds. If a depression forms and remains after the pressure is released, the patient has pitting edema. **Focus:** Prioritization; **QSEN:** PCC; **Concept:** Clinical Judgment; **Cognitive Level:** Applying

19. **Ans:**

> **Scenario:** A 75-year-old patient was admitted with a weight gain of 10 pounds, bilateral crackles in lower lobes of lungs, and visible neck veins when lying down. Vital signs are T 97.8°F (36.5°C), HR 56/min regular, RR 18/min, BP 178/90. The patient is lethargic but is able to respond to questions. The patient has bilateral 2+ edema to the ankles. History includes renal insufficiency and chronic obstructive pulmonary disease (COPD). Laboratory values include decreased serum sodium, normal serum potassium, and decreased hematocrit.

> **Instructions: Highlight or underline the findings that indicate the patient is at risk for overhydration.**

Rationale: Older adults are at increased risk for fluid imbalances. Signs and symptoms of overhydration include weight gain, crackles in the lungs, visible neck veins when supine (jugular venous distention), bradycardia, hypertension, lethargy, and peripheral edema. Renal insufficiency is also a risk factor. Laboratory values include decreased serum sodium and hematocrit. **Focus:** Prioritization; **QSEN:** PCC, S; **Concept:** Fluid and Electrolytes, Clinical Judgment; **Cognitive Level:** Analyzing; **Cognitive Skills:** Generate Solutions

20. Ans: The nurse is caring for a patient with an electrolyte imbalance. The telemetry monitor technician reports the patient has cardiac dysrhythmias, so the nurse checks the patient's ___1-C___ laboratory value and finds that the patient has ___2-A___. The nurse expects the HCP to prescribe ___3-B___.

Options for 1	Options for 2	Options for 3
A. Sodium	A. Hypokalemia	A. Furosemide
B. Calcium	B. Hypernatremia	B. Potassium supplement
C. Potassium	C. Hypocalcemia	C. Calcium supplement

Rationale: The presence of cardiac dysrhythmias on a telemetry tracing can indicate a low potassium level (hypokalemia). The HCP would most likely prescribe a potassium supplement to increase the potassium level. **Focus:** Prioritization; **QSEN:** PCC, S; **Concept:** Fluid and Electrolytes, Clinical Judgment; **Cognitive Level:** Analyzing; **Cognitive Skills:** Generate Solutions

QSEN Key: **PCC,** Patient-Centered Care; **TC,** Teamwork & Collaboration; **EBP,** Evidence-Based Practice; **QI,** Quality Improvement; **S,** Safety; **I,** Informatics.

IPEC Key: Domain 1 Values/Ethics (**V/E**); Domain 2 Roles/Responsibilities (**R/R**); Domain 3 Interprofessional Communication (**IC**); Domain 4 Teams/Teamwork (**T/T**).

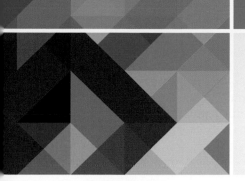

CHAPTER 12
LPN/LVN in the Rehabilitation Setting

Questions

1. Which nursing concepts are the **priorities** in the philosophy of rehabilitation nursing?
   1. Sensory perception and safety.
   2. Functional ability and self-management.
   3. Mood and affect and mobility.
   4. Family dynamics and stress and coping.

2. A recent stroke caused the patient to have left-sided paralysis and facial drooping. Which instruction would be **best** to give to the assistive personnel (AP) to promote the long-term goal of independence?
   1. Be supportive and do whatever the patient asks you to do.
   2. Wait and see what the patient will do for himself; then offer to help.
   3. Do passive range-of-motion exercises on the patient's left side.
   4. Keep the patient in bed and offer the bed pan frequently.

3. For a patient in a cardiac rehabilitation program, which lunch tray would be the **best**?
   1. Ham and cheese on whole wheat bread.
   2. Grilled salmon with steamed vegetables.
   3. Egg salad sandwich and watermelon.
   4. Low-fat cheese nachos and a diet soda.

4. A speech therapist is **most** likely to be included as a member of the rehabilitation team for which patient?
   1. Patient has arthritis and uses adaptive devices, such as foam build-ups for self-feeding.
   2. Patient had a supraglottic laryngectomy with difficulty adjusting to the tracheostomy.
   3. Patient is having "phantom sensations" after amputation of the dominant hand.
   4. Patient had a myocardial infarction and is experiencing depression and anxiety.

5. The health care team is preparing a patient for transfer from the hospital to a rehabilitation center. Which task is **best** performed by the LPN/LVN?
   1. Performing a pain assessment and neurovascular checks on the extremities.
   2. Helping the patient to pack belongings and dress in seasonal appropriate clothing.
   3. Completing a detailed patient summary sheet for the receiving facility.
   4. Giving a verbal phone report to the admitting nurse at the rehabilitation center.

6. In which rehabilitation setting is the nurse **most** likely to administer methadone to help the patients accomplish the goals of therapy?
   1. Cardiac rehabilitation.
   2. Stroke rehabilitation.
   3. Pulmonary rehabilitation.
   4. Drug addiction rehabilitation.

7. A patient in a pulmonary rehabilitation program experienced mild shortness of breath while performing prescribed ambulation in the hallways. The AP who was helping the patient reports the postexercise vital signs: BP 170/120 mm Hg, P 110/min, R 38/min, T 101.8°F (38.8°C). What should the nurse do **first**?
   1. Alert the supervising registered nurse (RN) and call the health care provider (HCP).
   2. Instruct the AP to assist the patient into bed and repeat the vital signs.
   3. Recheck vital signs, do a pulse oximeter reading, and assess respiratory status.
   4. Check flow sheet for trends in vital signs and assess for signs of infection.

8. The patient is prescribed disulfiram as part of the treatment in an alcohol rehabilitation program. Which patient comment is the **most** serious and needs to be reported to the RN for additional follow-up and medication teaching?
   1. "The medication is not doing anything, and the support group is a waste of time."
   2. "I got really drunk last night and my wife slipped the medicine into my glass."
   3. "I cannot remember when I am supposed to go for my liver function test."
   4. "I had a beer this morning and I did get nauseated, but that's my own fault."

9. For a patient who is in a cardiac rehabilitation program, which laboratory values are the **most** important when monitoring adherence to the dietary recommendations?
   1. Prealbumin and albumin.
   2. Potassium and calcium.
   3. Triglycerides and cholesterol.
   4. Hemoglobin and hematocrit.

10. The older patient has a history of chronic illness that necessitated a below the knee amputation. He acts helpless and depressed. Which action would the nurse use **first** to meet a short-term goal that helps the patient to progress toward independence?
    1. Helping the patient to inspect and clean the stump and prosthesis.
    2. Talking to the patient about setting a goal to walk independently.
    3. Allowing the patient to independently do some components of hygiene.
    4. Encouraging the patient to exercise and strengthen unaffected limbs.

11. A patient in a renal rehabilitation program is selecting a protein item for lunch. Which item is the **best** choice?
    1. Baked honey-glazed ham.
    2. Barbequed sausage.
    3. Thinly sliced lunchmeat.
    4. Grilled chicken breast.

12. The patient who was admitted to a rehabilitation unit for right-sided weakness after a stroke says, "I'm never going to be able to take care of myself." To promote independence, which instruction would the nurse give to the AP about helping with bathing?
    1. Show the patient how to use the left hand to clean the right side of the body.
    2. Bathe the right side of the body and observe the patient's ability to clean the left side.
    3. Give the patient a clean moist washcloth and encourage her to wash her face.

    4. Take the patient to the bathroom, provide privacy, and return to check on the patient.

13. A patient who experienced a major burn is transferred to a rehabilitation unit. Which treatments does the rehabilitation nurse anticipate?
    1. Fluid resuscitation, circulatory support, and prevention of shock.
    2. Pressure garments, physical therapy, and regular exercise.
    3. Respiratory support with humified oxygen, coughing, and turning.
    4. Wound treatment, escharotomy, debridement, and grafting.

14. A patient who has paraplegia secondary to a spinal cord injury is admitted to the rehabilitation unit. To prevent the complication of venous thrombosis, which instruction will the nurse give to the AP?
    1. Assist the patient with applying compression stockings before getting out of bed.
    2. Gently massage the legs during bathing and when assisting the patient to bed.
    3. Make sure that the patient takes the dose of oral anticoagulant as prescribed.
    4. Encourage the patient to use a reclining position whenever sitting in a wheelchair.

15. A patient with quadriplegia has been in the rehabilitation unit for 1 month. His progress has been slower than anticipated and he is depressed. He tells the nurse, "I wish I had died in the accident; I just can't go on like this." Which response is the **most** therapeutic?"
    1. "I'm sorry, but I can't keep this confidential. I have to tell your doctor what you said."
    2. "Let's try the deep breathing exercises; yesterday you did a great job with that task."
    3. "You seem upset. Tell me more about what you mean by, 'I can't go on like this.'"
    4. "I'm glad that you didn't die. You can overcome this disability if you keep trying."

16. A transgender woman who is admitted for cognitive rehabilitation secondary to a traumatic brain injury needs assistance with personal hygiene and bathing. Which instruction is **best** to give to the AP?
    1. Treat the patient with kindness and avoid references to gender identity.
    2. Patient self-identifies as a female and should be treated as such.
    3. Regardless of how you feel or what you see, maintain a neutral expression.
    4. Give the same care that you would to any other patient; act naturally.

17. Matrix. _____

Scenario: The 68-year-old male patient was hospitalized for an acute exacerbation of chronic obstructive pulmonary disease (COPD) and then transferred to the rehabilitation unit for pulmonary rehabilitation. He lives alone and hopes to return to his own home as soon as possible. The report from the hospital indicates that he is alert and independently ambulatory but desaturates with minor exertion. He is reluctant to start using portable oxygen and thinks that his inhaler and other medications are enough. He has been smoking since adolescence and expresses doubts about being able to quit but is willing to try. He has had three hospitalizations for pneumonia within the past 4 years and has frequent episodes of upper respiratory tract infections that require oral antibiotics.

Instructions: For each potential health care provider order, place an X in the box to indicate whether it is essential, nonessential, or contraindicated.

Potential Order	Essential	Nonessential	Contraindicated
Plan a regular walking routine			
Teach correct use of metered dose inhaler			
Monitor vital signs to check cardiopulmonary effects during and after exercise			
Teach energy conservation			
Remind patient to get an annual chest x-ray			
Wash hands often; teach avoidance of respiratory infections			
Include routine steroid medications in daily pill reminder box			
Offer smoking cessation information			
Offer information about support group and/or counseling			

     Answer Key for this chapter begins on p. 84

Answers

1. **Ans: 2** The goal of rehabilitation is to help the patient achieve the highest possible level of function and to achieve/maintain as much independence as possible. Additional nursing concepts are used, as needed, to create individualized care plans. **Focus:** Prioritization; **QSEN:** PCC; **Concept:** Functional Ability, Self-Management; **Cognitive Level:** Applying

2. **Ans: 3** Interventions such as passive range-of-motion exercises are immediately started to facilitate the long-term goal of recovering as much function and independence as possible. The nurse must give the AP specific instructions about what to do for the patient and how to respond if the patient asks the AP to do something that is not part of the care plan. Patients are generally assisted with getting out of bed as soon as possible unless the health care provider gives specific orders to maintain bed rest. **Focus:** Prioritization, Supervision; **QSEN:** PCC; **Concept:** Functional Ability, Self-Management; **Cognitive Level:** Analyzing

3. **Ans: 2** All of these lunch options contain some foods that would be recommended for a heart-healthy diet. However, fish, poultry, low-fat dairy, and high-fiber foods would be first choices. Red meat; eggs; high-fat dairy products; and convenience, prepackaged, processed, and fast foods should generally be avoided. **Focus:** Prioritization; **QSEN:** EBP; **Concept:** Nutrition; **Cognitive Level:** Applying

4. **Ans: 2** Following a laryngectomy and tracheotomy the patient loses verbal communication and has a risk for aspiration. A speech therapist can teach exercises that facilitate swallowing and help to restore some form of speech. Occupational therapists assist patients with arthritis, who need adaptive devices. Patients with phantom limb pain may get relief with transcutaneous electrical nerve stimulation; physical therapists can assist with this therapy. For depression and anxiety related to myocardial infarction, patients may be referred to support groups or prescribed antidepressants or anxiolytic medication by the health care provider. **Focus:** Prioritization; **QSEN:** PCC; **Concept:** Communication; **Cognitive Level:** Applying; **IPEC:** R/R

5. **Ans: 1** Transferring a patient from one facility to another is a time-consuming responsibility that can be shared by several members of the health care team. The skills of the LPN/LVN are best utilized in performing the focused assessments. This data can be added to the final transfer summary. The AP can help the patient pack and dress. Completing the summary sheet and giving the phone report should be done by the RN, because the supervising RN would be responsible for problems that occur if information is missing, incorrect, or poorly communicated. **Focus:** Assignment, Delegation; **QSEN:** TC; **Concept:** Collaboration; **Cognitive Level:** Analyzing; **IPEC:** T/T

6. **Ans: 4** Methadone is a medication that is prescribed for opioid use disorder. This long-acting opioid allows patients with opioid addiction to perform normal daily activities. **Focus:** Prioritization; **QSEN:** PCC; **Concept:** Addiction; **Cognitive Level:** Applying

7. **Ans: 3** First, the nurse would assess the patient by repeating the vital signs, taking a pulse oximeter reading, and assessing the respiratory status to include breath sounds, respiratory effort, use of accessory muscles, body position, color of skin and mucous membranes, capillary refill, and accompanying signs and symptoms, such as diaphoresis or chest pressure. Based on the assessment findings, the nurse may also use the other options. **Focus:** Prioritization; **QSEN:** EBP; **Concept:** Gas Exchange; **Cognitive Level:** Applying

8. **Ans: 2** The combination of large amounts of alcohol and disulfiram is potentially fatal. All of these comments indicate that the patient and the family need additional medication teaching and follow-up on the understanding and commitment to the treatment plan. **Focus:** Prioritization; **QSEN:** S; **Concept:** Safety, Addiction; **Cognitive Level:** Analyzing

9. **Ans: 3** Dietary recommendations for cardiovascular disease include a reduction of fats, cholesterol, and sodium. Three types of cholesterol are monitored: high-density lipoprotein (HDL), low-density lipoprotein (LDL), and very-low-density lipoprotein (VLDL). HDL is the "good" cholesterol, which cleans fatty deposits from blood vessels. LDL, the "bad" cholesterol, contributes to fatty accumulation. VDRL carries triglycerides, which are associated with coronary artery disease. Prealbumin and albumin reflect nutritional protein status. Potassium and calcium are involved in many body functions, including heart muscle contraction. Hemoglobin and hematocrit are monitored for anemia or blood loss. **Focus:** Prioritization; **QSEN:** PCC; **Concept** Nutrition; **Cognitive Level:** Analyzing. **Test Taking Tip:** Clinical application of pathophysiology can be difficult; however, understanding the pathophysiology of coronary artery disease allows an educated guess about this type of question.

10. **Ans: 3** Short-term goals should be relatively easy to accomplish. Independently performing small, familiar hygienic tasks such as brushing teeth or shaving builds confidence toward functioning in daily activities. Dealing with the stump and prosthesis may be difficult and discouraging, particularly if the patient is depressed or having trouble coping with loss of a body part. Setting a goal to independently walk is preceded by many other small steps. Exercising unaffected limbs is a preparatory step; some patients may be anxious to start these exercises; other patients may need additional time to recognize how general exercise fits into the long-term goal of independently ambulating with a prosthesis. **Focus:** Prioritization; **QSEN:** PCC; **Concept:** Functional Ability, Self-Management; **Cognitive Level:** Analyzing

11. **Ans: 4** Patients with renal failure will often be advised to restrict protein intake and select high-quality proteins such as fish, meats, and eggs. Processed meats such as ham, sausage, or lunch meat should generally be avoided, because sodium content is high and sodium intake is also restricted according to the progression of renal failure. **Focus:** Prioritization; **QSEN:** EBP; **Concept:** Nutrition; **Cognitive Level:** Applying

12. **Ans: 3** Since the patient is expressing doubt, the nurse would instruct the AP to start with a simple and easily accomplished task. When the patient shows readiness, the nurse or the occupational therapist would show the patient how to use the left hand. The nurse should observe the patient's ability to accomplish bathing. At this stage, leaving the patient alone in the bathroom is incorrect; this is a long-term goal. Abilities for self-care will gradually increase as the patient learns to cope and builds self-confidence. **Focus:** Assignment, Supervision; **QSEN:** PCC; **Concept:** Self-Management, Functional Ability; **Cognitive Level:** Analyzing; **IPEC:** IC

13. **Ans: 2** The long-term goals for burn rehabilitation are reentry into social, work, and family roles. Pressure garments are used to reduce disfiguring scars. Physical therapy and exercise are used to gain and maintain mobility. The other treatments are more likely to happen in the acute care hospital. Fluid resuscitation and oxygenation treatments are used in the emergent phase. Wound treatment starts immediately to prevent fluid loss and infection and to minimize pain. Escharotomy (incision) is performed if the burn eschar is encircling the chest or extremity and preventing respiration or perfusion. Debridement is the removal of dead tissue; this promotes new tissue growth. Grafting (own skin, other person's skin, animal skin, or artificial skin) is performed to cover the burned

area. **Focus:** Prioritization; **QSEN:** N/A; **Concept:** Functional Ability; **Cognitive Level:** Applying. **Test Taking Tip:** During your studies, pay attention to acute versus chronic stages of patients' conditions. This will help you identify the priorities of care as acuity changes over time.

14. **Ans: 1** Helping the patient to apply compression stockings before getting out of bed is a measure that helps to prevent venous thrombosis. Massaging the legs is contraindicated because there is a possibility of dislodging a clot. APs are usually not responsible for administering or ensuring that patients take their medication. (Certified medication assistants do administer routine medications in some settings. Be familiar with the state board of nursing recommendations and facility policies, which will vary.) The reclining position can be used if patients are having trouble with orthostatic hypotension. **Focus:** Prioritization, Supervision; **QSEN:** S; **Concept:** Perfusion; **Cognitive Level:** Applying

15. **Ans: 3** Acknowledging the underlying feeling is therapeutic and "tell me more about" encourages the patient to expand on feelings and is also a means to assess for suicidal ideation and plan. The nurse would explain the need to share the comment with other members of the health care team, but this is not the first thing that the nurse would say. Focusing on previous success is also therapeutic, but in this situation, it would be considered a nontherapeutic comment that abruptly changes the subject. "I'm glad" shifts the focus to the nurse and "overcome disability by trying" could be interpreted as false reassurance. **Focus:** Prioritization; **QSEN:** PCC; **Concept:** Communication; **Cognitive Level:** Applying

16. **Ans: 2** It is the nurse's responsibility to identify the person's preferences and concerns. These preferences are then clearly conveyed to the AP. Patients should always be treated with kindness; references to gender identity (e.g., that is a pretty dress) should not be avoided because they are an important part of self-image. Rather than telling the AP to maintain a neutral expression, encourage him or her to verbalize feelings to the nursing staff and prepare the AP for what might be observed (transgender persons may have had partial or complete surgical reconstruction of genitalia and hormonal therapy can also affect the appearance of the genitalia). "Give the same care and act naturally" functions as a platitude. This instruction suggests that all patients are the same and that all APs have the same emotional response to patients. **Focus:** Prioritization, Supervision; **QSEN:** PCC; **Concept:** Culture, Communication; **Cognitive Level:** Analyzing; **IPEC:** IC

17. Ans:

Potential Order	Essential	Nonessential	Contraindicated
Plan a regular walking routine	X		
Teach correct use of metered dose inhaler	X		
Monitor vital signs to check cardiopulmonary effects during and after exercise	X		
Teach energy conservation	X		
Remind patient to get an annual chest x-ray		X	
Wash hands often; teach avoidance of respiratory infections	X		
Include routine steroid medications in daily pill reminder box			X
Offer smoking cessation information	X		
Offer information about support group and/or counseling	X		

Patients in pulmonary rehabilitation programs are encouraged to: walk for exercise, correctly use metered dose inhalers, monitor pulse and breathing rates during and after exercise, conserve energy to prevent fatigue, use hand hygiene and other measures to prevent respiratory infections (e.g., keeping immunizations updated and avoiding crowds), participate in smoking cessation programs, and use counseling or support groups.

Annual chest x-rays are not necessary; however, x-rays would be taken if a new condition, such as pneumonia, is suspected. Steroids are usually prescribed only for acute exacerbations. Steroids have multiple side effects, so other medications are preferred for chronic COPD. **Focus:** Prioritization **QSEN:** PCC; **Concept:** Gas Exchange; **Cognitive Level:** Analyzing; **Cognitive Skill:** Generate Solutions.

QSEN Key: PCC, Patient-Centered Care; **TC,** Teamwork & Collaboration; **EBP,** Evidence-Based Practice; **QI,** Quality Improvement; **S,** Safety; **I,** Informatics.

IPEC Key: Domain 1 Values/Ethics (**V/E**); Domain 2 Roles/Responsibilities (**R/R**); Domain 3 Interprofessional Communication (**IC**); Domain 4 Teams/Teamwork (**T/T**).

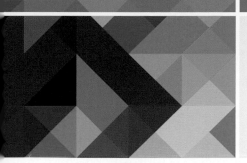

CHAPTER 13

LPN/LVN in the Long-Term Care Setting

Questions

1. A resident in a long-term care center seems to be falling once or twice a month. Which action would the nursing staff take **first**?
   1. Ask the health care provider (HCP) to prescribe restraints until a long-term plan is in place.
   2. Talk to the family about the need for a hired sitter to stay at the bedside.
   3. Ensure that an assistive personnel (AP) is assigned to check on the resident once an hour around-the-clock.
   4. Check records and discuss behaviors or descriptions of events associated with falls.

2. An older woman was recently transferred from an orthopedic rehabilitation unit to the long-term care center. The daughter says, "My mom has had mild dementia for years. I keep telling the doctors that she has never hallucinated or acted lethargic, but they will not listen to me." Which question is the nurse **most** likely to ask to differentiate dementia from delirium?
   1. "Does she make up answers or give vague responses?"
   2. "When did you first notice the changes in her behavior?"
   3. "Does she recognize you and know where she is at?"
   4. "If you tell her to do a simple action, can she do it?"

3. A newly graduated LPN/LVN just completed orientation in a long-term care facility. Which residents would be assigned to this new nurse? **Select all that apply.**
   1. Resident who was recently admitted and is often belligerent and confused.
   2. Resident who needs assistance while recovering from hip surgery.
   3. Resident who had a stroke several years ago with residual right-sided paralysis.
   4. Resident with chronic pain and decreased mobility secondary to arthritis.
   5. Resident with several chronic health problems and a change of mental status.
   6. Resident with dementia who is in the manic phase of bipolar disorder.

4. An older resident in a long-term care center, who has been immobile for several weeks, suddenly displays confusion, anxiety, and respiratory distress with dyspnea. What would the nurse do **first**?
   1. Check the vital signs.
   2. Raise the head of the bed.
   3. Call the HCP.
   4. Reorient and reassure the resident.

5. What is the nurse's responsibility, in a long-term care facility, where certified medication assistants (CMAs) administer the routine and scheduled medications?
   1. Perform the six rights of medication administration for the CMA.
   2. Assess for pouching or difficulty with swallowing after CMA gives medication.
   3. Assume liability if the CMA administers medication to the wrong resident.
   4. Monitor for therapeutic response and side effects after CMA gives medication.

6. The AP tells the nurse that a resident keeps calling for assistance to the bathroom after he has already soiled himself and his pants are usually partially undone. What does the nurse suspect **first**?
   1. Stress incontinence.
   2. Functional incontinence.
   3. Overflow incontinence.
   4. Neurologic incontinence.

7. The nurse notices that the AP is spending an excessive amount of time with one resident and neglecting other residents. The nurse suspects that the AP may have professional boundary issues. What would the nurse do **first**?
   1. Reassign the AP to a different group of residents in another part of the facility.
   2. Gently remind the AP that the other residents also need care and attention.
   3. Report the AP's behavior, with specific times and incidents, to the nurse manager.
   4. Ask the AP about what is happening during the time spent with the resident.

8. Which AP needs a reminder about the prevention of pressure injuries?
   1. AP-A checks on bedridden residents every 1 to 2 hours for toileting and hygiene.
   2. AP-B encourages protein foods, as ordered, when assisting residents with eating.
   3. AP-C puts incontinence pants on every resident to prepare them for bed.
   4. AP-D reminds residents who are sitting in the dayroom to frequently change position.

9. Two male residents who live in the long-term care center ask the nurse if they could move into the same room. They openly express their desire to be treated as a couple. Which response is **best**?
   1. "Sharing a room is not allowed, but closed-door visits would be respected."
   2. "I am not sure that unmarried couples can room together, but I'll find out."
   3. "You can ask the HCP to write an order for the shared room."
   4. "If your family has been informed, you can move when a double room is available."

10. Which long-term care resident would be **best** to assign to an inexperienced AP who has recently graduated from a training program?
    1. Resident who has chronic joint pain in the morning related to arthritis.
    2. Resident who gets anxious and aggressive during stressful events.
    3. Resident with mild dementia who fell yesterday in the bathroom.
    4. Resident who needs total assistance with activities of daily living (ADLs).

11. Which recommendations related to COVID-19 do the Centers for Disease Control and Prevention (CDC) give for nursing homes and long-term care facilities? **Select all that apply.**
    1. At least one individual with training in infection control should be assigned to provide on-site management of the infection prevention control (IPC) program.
    2. Nurses and AP should wear cloth face coverings at all times and cluster care to minimize personal exposure.
    3. Residents should not be allowed to mingle in common areas or leave their rooms unless there is a medical emergency.
    4. Residents, healthcare personnel, and visitors should be educated on COVID-19, precautions being taken, and actions they should use to protect themselves.
    5. Weekly reports should be sent to the National Healthcare Safety Network (NHSN) Long-Term Care Facility (LTCF) COVID-19 Module and include information about COVID-19 cases, staffing, and supplies.
    6. Visitors are allowed to visit briefly, if they are asymptomatic, agree to wear cloth face coverings, and the resident is defined as needing compassionate care (end-of-life).

12. The nurse is working with a new AP who recently graduated from a training program. It is her first day to work independently and she seems unsure of what to do. Which resident will the nurse instruct the AP to assist **first**?
    1. Resident immediately needs to go to the bathroom to urinate.
    2. Resident is crying and urgently calling for a glass of water.
    3. Resident is angry because it is time for her scheduled shower.
    4. Resident is confused and trying to exit the building.

13. The nurse is talking to a resident who wants to understand why the COVID-19 pandemic has caused restrictions to be placed on visits with her grandchildren. Which response is the **most** accurate?
    1. "Children are more likely to be asymptomatic or have mild symptoms, so they could expose you to the virus."
    2. "Younger children cannot be expected to wear masks, practice social distancing, or conform to correct hand hygiene."
    3. "Children of all ages often have false negatives with COVID-19 testing, and this increases exposure risk to older people."
    4. "Children have extremely high risk for serious complications from the virus that lead to chronic health problems."

14. The supervising registered nurse (RN) says, "The HCP phoned in a one-time order for a placebo. Tell the resident that she is getting morphine and do not document the placebo dose, just call the HCP in 1 hour to report the response." Which action would the nurse take **first**?
    1. Ask for clarification of the instructions and then administer the placebo.
    2. Refuse to administer the dose because the supervising RN took the phone order.
    3. Seek an explanation for the use of a placebo and omitting the documentation.
    4. Go up the chain of command and report exactly what the supervising RN said.

15. Which instruction will the nurse give to the AP related to the care of an older resident who has Crohn's disease?
    1. Offer the resident extra fluids between meals.
    2. Help the resident to fill out the bland diet menu form.
    3. Encourage the resident to ambulate five to six times each day.
    4. Prevent the resident from smoking tobacco.

16. Which residents in a long-term care center have risk for falls? **Select all that apply.**
    1. A frail 81-year-old woman with poor food and fluid intake.
    2. A 65-year-old man who was recently started a new antihypertensive drug.
    3. An older adult resident who has end-stage Alzheimer's disease.
    4. A confused resident who intermittently forgets to use the call bell.
    5. An older resident who recently slipped and fell because the floor was wet.
    6. A 73-year-old man who takes daily walks in the enclosed garden space.

17. The long-term care team includes an LPN/LVN who is the team leader, a CMA, two experienced AP, and an AP in orientation. Which task is **best** to assign to the AP in orientation?
    1. Collecting a midstream urine specimen from a female resident.
    2. Assisting a thin, fragile resident to take a shower.
    3. Taking and reporting vital signs on a resident.
    4. Observing while a resident swallows pills and water.

 18. Matrix.

Scenario: The resident had a fall and sustained an obvious bump on the head. She was transferred to the emergency department and was seen, evaluated, and transported back to the long-term care center with standard head injury instructions. The HCP was notified about the injury and received the medical report from the emergency department. The HCP gives the nurse additional orders and the nurse initiates nursing interventions that are related to the standard head injury instructions.

Instructions: For each potential HCP order or nursing intervention listed below, check to specify whether the order/intervention is anticipated, nonessential, or contraindicated.

Potential HCP Orders and Nursing Interventions	Anticipated	Nonessential	Contraindicated
Raise head of the bed 20 to 30 degrees.			
Keep neck in flexed midline position.			
Vital signs and neuro checks every hour for 4 hours, then every 4 hours for the next 24 hours.			
Encourage coughing and deep breathing.			
Wake the resident every 2 hours and assess orientation.			
Report nausea, mild headache, or dizziness to HCP.			
Maintain bed rest and do passive range of motion.			

PART 2   Common Health Scenarios

                    Answer Key for this chapter begins on p. 91

19. Enhanced Multiple Response. _____

Scenario: The HCP recently increased the furosemide to 40 mg/day and added telmisartan 40 mg/day to improve control of the resident's blood pressure. The nurse recognizes that these medications changes could cause the resident to experience orthostatic hypotension. The care plan is modified, and the supervising RN performs patient teaching related to the medications and the fall prevention measures. The nurse is assigned to supervise and delegate fall prevention interventions to the AP. Which interventions related to orthostatic hypotension can be delegated to the AP? **Select all that apply.**

Instructions: Place an X in the space provided or highlight each nursing intervention that would be delegated to the AP. Select all that apply.

1. _____Instruct the resident to rise slowly from a lying or sitting position.
2. _____Have the resident sit for at least 1 minute before standing.
3. _____Remind the resident to flex and extend and rotate feet before standing.
4. _____Assist the resident with donning soft slippers or warm socks before standing.
5. _____Support the resident in a standing position for 1 minute.
6. _____Remind the resident to turn head and visually sweep while walking.
7. _____If dizziness occurs while walking, stay with the resident and call for help.
8. _____Assess dizziness and ask about factors that trigger light-headedness.
9. _____Assist the resident with ambulating immediately after eating snacks or meals.

20. Enhanced Multiple Response. _____

Scenario: The nurse is on a safety committee of a long-term care center. A primary goal of the committee is to ensure that COVID-19 prevention measures are in place to protect the residents, staff, and visitors. The nurse was given the task of gathering information about factors that are known to contribute to the spread of COVID-19 in long-term care centers. In the early phase of the pandemic (spring of 2020), which factors **most** likely contributed to the devastating spread of COVID-19 throughout long-term care and nursing home facilities in the United States?

Instructions: Place an X in the space provided or highlight each factor that contributed to the spread of COVID-19 in long-term care centers in the United States during the early phase of the pandemic. Select all that apply.

1. _____Lack of access to personal protective equipment (PPE) such as masks and gowns.
2. _____Frequent physical contact between residents and staff.
3. _____Understaffing.
4. _____Employees who worked in more than one nursing center.
5. _____Visitors failed to wear masks and social distance.
6. _____Residents shared rooms.
7. _____Opposition to taking influenza or other vaccinations.
8. _____Vulnerability of the residents.
9. _____Transfers of residents from hospitals and other settings.
10. _____Deficiencies in infection control and prevention that predated COVID-19.

Answer Key for this chapter begins on p. 91

Answers

1. **Ans: 4** The staff would first try to identify patterns associated with the falls. For example, there are known safety issues around shift change. Also, residents may fall in the bathroom or fall while attempting to get to the bathroom. Sundowner syndrome occurs in the late afternoon or evening and results in increased confusion. Once these types of patterns are identified, targeted interventions can be employed. Restraints are inappropriate and may contribute to injury. A bedside sitter or frequent around-the-clock observation would be ideal for the resident, but expense and multiple staff duties are obstacles. **Focus:** Prioritization; **QSEN:** S; EBP; **Concept:** Safety; **Cognitive Level:** Analyzing

2. **Ans: 2** Delirium and dementia affect cognitive function and many of the signs and symptoms will occur in both disorders. The most significant difference is the onset of symptoms. Delirium is associated with rapid onset, whereas dementia develops slowly. Making up answers or vague responses are more associated with dementia. Incoherent or garbled speech occurs more with delirium. Disorientation and inability to follow simple commands can occur in both disorders. **Focus:** Prioritization; **QSEN:** S; **Concept:** Cognition, Psychosis; **Cognitive Level:** Analyzing. **Test Taking Tip:** Delirium is treatable once the cause is identified. Older adults with dementia are often viewed as having chronic and untreatable symptoms, so the nurse is responsible for advocating for the person when subtle changes in behavior are detected.

3. **Ans: 2, 3, 4** A new nurse should be assigned to care for stable residents that have relatively straightforward health concerns that require common nursing interventions. For example, hip surgery, stroke, and arthritis create problems with mobility and self-care. Persons who are postsurgical and those with arthritis require pain management. Recently admitted residents, especially those who are having problems with adjustment, would be assigned to experienced staff. A change of mental status is an acute situation and an RN should care for this person while the cause is investigated. Comorbidities, such as dementia and other mental health disorders, require experienced assessment; an RN should care for the resident while the manic behavior is evaluated and treated. **Focus:** Assignment; **QSEN:** TC; **Concept:** Care Coordination; **Cognitive Level:** Analyzing; **Cognitive Level:** Analyze Cues; **IPEC:** R/R

4. **Ans: 2** Raising the head of the bed is a quick intervention that helps the resident to breathe. After using emergency interventions to relieve respiratory distress, such as applying oxygen, suctioning, repositioning, or clearing the airway, the nurse would use the other options. **Focus:** Prioritization; **QSEN:** S; **Concept:** Gas Exchange; **Cognitive Level:** Applying. **Test Taking Tip:** While knowledge of potential medical diagnosis (e.g., pulmonary emboli, bronchospasm, foreign body airway obstruction) is useful, this question can be answered by using the ABCs (airway, breathing, circulation) to identify the problem and the priority action.

5. **Ans: 4** The nurse has pharmacologic knowledge and is responsible for monitoring response and medication side effects. The CMA must perform the six rights prior to administering the medication and is responsible for observing and reporting problems that occur during the medication process, such as pouching or difficulty swallowing. The CMA is also responsible for personal actions that are within the scope of CMA practice. The nurse would be liable if the CMA reports information and the nurse fails to take appropriate action. **Focus:** Assignment; **QSEN:** TC; **Concept:** Health Care Law; **Cognitive Level:** Analyzing; **IPEC:** R/R

6. **Ans: 2** The resident is recognizing the urge to void, calling for help, and trying to manipulate his clothing, so the nurse suspects that he has functional incontinence related to the inability to act quickly enough to get to the toilet. The resident could also be experiencing urge incontinence, which is a sudden urge and an uncontrollable loss of urine. Stress incontinence is loss of urine during coughing, sneezing, or exercise. Overflow incontinence in older males can occur because of an enlarged prostate. In overflow incontinence the urge to void may or may not accompany dribbling or leakage. Neurologic incontinence is associated with neurologic disorders, such as spinal cord injury. **Focus:** Prioritization; **QSEN:** EBP; **Concept:** Elimination; **Cognitive Level:** Applying

7. **Ans: 4** First, the nurse would assess the situation. Professional boundaries can blur when care requires a lot of time, and the AP might believe that spending extra time is therapeutic. Issues to investigate include: "Is the resident fulfilling a personal need for the AP?" and "Can the resident's needs be met if less time is spent?" If the answer to either of these questions is yes, then it is likely that a boundary problem exists. The nurse and the nurse manager can assist the AP with making a plan that allows the AP to complete care and fosters healthy professional relationships with all assigned residents. **Focus:** Prioritization, Supervision; **QSEN:** PCC; **Concept:** Professional Identity; **Cognitive Level:** Analyzing; **IPEC:** V/E, IC

8. **Ans: 3** Putting incontinence pants on every resident is an example of using an intervention for staff convenience. Incontinence pants increase friction and moisture against the skin and increase the risk for skin breakdown. The pants are an option for uncontrollably leakage and dribbling or passing small amounts of urine during sleep. However, the pants should not be used for residents who are able to get up to go to the bathroom and for those who are not incontinent. **Focus:** Prioritization, Supervision; **QSEN:** S; **Concept:** Tissue Integrity; **Cognitive Level:** Applying; **IPEC:** IC. **Test Taking Tip:** Older patients with immobility problems are at risk for skin breakdown. Care of older patients and measures to prevent pressure injuries are topics that are likely to be tested during NCLEX.

9. **Ans: 2** The nurse's best response is to acknowledge their desire to be a couple and a promise to seek an answer. Institutional policies related to sexuality vary greatly by facility. Marital status, sexual preference, and gender identity may or may not be part of the administrative decision-making. Older adults are frequently stigmatized as having cognitive limitations that affect their choices. In addition, family, friends, and staff may have real or imagined concerns about consensual desire versus the potential for sexual abuse. **Focus:** Prioritization; **QSEN:** PCC; **Concept:** Sexuality, Health Disparities; **Cognitive Level:** Analyzing; **IPEC:** V/E

10. **Ans: 1** A resident with arthritis and chronic pain will have experience in self-management and can direct the inexperienced AP to assist in ways that minimize effort and pain. An experienced AP will be more familiar with stressful triggering events for the anxious resident and total assistance with ADLs requires organization and proficiency. Recent falls increase fall risk and the resident may be fearful. In addition, an experienced AP is more likely to recognize occult injuries from yesterday's fall that should be immediately reported. **Focus:** Assignment; **QSEN:** PCC, S; **Concept:** Care Coordination; **Cognitive Level:** Analyzing

11. **Ans: 1, 4, 5** The CDC recommends having at least one trained individual for on-site management of the IPC program. Education about precautions and prevention should be provided for residents, staff, and visitors. Weekly reports to the NHSN are recommended. Clustering care is a good strategy, but cloth masks do not provide adequate protection for health care staff. Comingling in common areas is not encouraged but leaving the room is still a personal decision; however, there are large variations in facilities' policies. CDC recommendations related to visitors include the use of cloth masks and screening for fever and symptoms of COVID-19. Visitation is not limited to residents defined as needing compassionate care. However, in the case of compassionate care, the facility

is more likely to allow leniency for the length of time spent and the number and frequency of visitors. **Focus:** Prioritization; **QSEN:** S; **Concept:** Infection, Health Policy; **Cognitive Level:** Analyzing. **Test Taking Tip:** The CDC is a source of updated information on COVID-19: https://www.cdc.gov/coronavirus/2019-ncov/hcp/long-term-care.html#core-practices.

12. **Ans: 4** The nurse reminds the AP that the first concern is safety. So the confused resident should be directed away from the door. Next, the AP should assist the resident who needs to go to the bathroom. The nurse would point out that timely assistance prevents having to help the resident clean up and change clothes. If the AP feels able to cope with the angry resident, the nurse can give praise and allow her to proceed. If the AP feels threatened by the resident's anger, the nurse can talk to the resident. The nurse would assess the resident who is crying and calling for water to determine if there is an emotional or physical problem. **Focus:** Delegation, Prioritization; **QSEN:** S; **Concept:** Care Coordination; **Cognitive Level:** Analyzing

13. **Ans: 1** Most children have mild or no symptoms if they contract COVID-19, but there is a risk of spreading the virus to others. Initially, many nursing homes did not allow any visitors because of the high mortality rate among residents. Children under 2 years old are exempt from wearing masks because of the risk for suffocation; however, parents are encouraged to role-model social distancing and assist with hand hygiene as needed. False negatives for COVID-19 can occur if there is a low viral load at the time of testing. Children are less likely to have a severe course of illness; however, there is evidence of multisystem inflammatory syndrome in children. It is considered rare and usually resolves with medical care. **Focus:** Prioritization; **QSEN:** S; **Concept:** Care Coordination; **Cognitive Level:** Analyzing. **Test Taking Tip:** The CDC offers additional and updated information about children and COVID-19: https://www.cdc.gov/coronavirus/2019-ncov/groups/families-children.html?CDC_AA_refVal=https%3A%2F%2Fwww.cdc.gov%2Fcoronavirus%2F2019-ncov%2Fdaily-life-coping%2Fchildren%2Fsymptoms.html.

14. **Ans: 3** First, the nurse would ask for an explanation. Giving placebos is generally considered an unethical practice, but there are a few circumstances where a placebo may be used (e.g., double-blind research study or for diagnosis). The resident (or patient) should be informed about the possibility of receiving a placebo. Asking for the clarification of instructions and requesting to see the order in writing would be reasonable. Going up the chain of command is an option if the nurse feels there is an ethical or legal violation of the resident's rights. **Focus:** Prioritization; **QSEN:** PCC; **Concept:** Ethics; **Cognitive Level:** Analyzing; **IPEC:** V/E, IC

15. **Ans: 1** Fluids are encouraged for diarrhea or constipation. In general, older adults are at risk for dehydration because of limited fluid reserves, decreased subjective thirst, and functional limitations (e.g., unable to reach or obtain fluids). Institutionalized persons have an even greater risk for dehydration. Crohn's disease is usually diagnosed in early adulthood. The expected symptoms include abdominal pain, diarrhea, weight loss, anemia, and fatigue. Older adults are more likely to experience weight loss, bleeding, fever, and paradoxical constipation. A regular diet and avoidance of personal "trigger" foods are usually recommended. Ambulating stimulates peristalsis and is encouraged for constipation; however, the nurse would assess for fatigue and modify the instructions to the AP accordingly. Smoking can worsen symptoms but preventing smoking would be a violation of the resident's rights. **Focus:** Delegation, Supervision; **QSEN:** PCC; **Concept:** Fluid and Electrolytes, Elimination; **Cognitive Level:** Analyzing; **IPEC:** IC

16. **Ans: 1, 2, 4, 5** Frailty, poor nutrition and fluid intake, antihypertensives (especially newly prescribed), confusion, inconsistent use of the call bell, and a history of falls are risk factors. While anyone can slip and fall on a wet floor, the staff would be advised that a recent fall event places the long-term care resident in a higher risk category. The resident with end-stage Alzheimer's disease is less likely to fall because of loss of volition and strength. Daily walks increase strength and balance and would help to prevent falls. **Focus:** Prioritization; **QSEN:** PCC; **Concept:** Safety; **Cognitive Level:** Analyzing; **Cognitive Skill:** Analyze Cues

17. **Ans: 3** One of the first skills that APs are taught is taking vital signs. In addition, if the new AP is instructed to report all vital signs, this eliminates the need for the new AP to discriminate normal from abnormal. Collecting a midstream urine sample from a female requires some problem solving if the person has cognitive or fine motor problems. When assisting with daily showering or bathing, the APs are responsible for observing for and reporting problems with the skin and any changes in the baseline ability to independently accomplish ADLs. A new AP should receive supervision before being assigned to do the task alone. Observing residents for swallowing medications or fluids would be assigned to the CMA. **Focus:** Assignment, Delegation; **QSEN:** TC; **Concept:** Care Coordination; **Cognitive Level:** Applying; **IPEC:** R/R

18. **Ans:**

Potential Orders	Anticipated	Nonessential	Contraindicated
Raise head of the bed 20 to 30 degrees.	X		
Keep neck in flexed midline position.			X
Vital signs and neuro checks every hour for 4 hours, then every 4 hours for the next 24 hours.	X		
Encourage coughing and deep breathing.			X
Wake the resident every 2 hours and assess orientation.			X
Report nausea, mild headache, or dizziness to HCP.		X	
Maintain bed rest and do passive range-of-motion.		X	

Raising the head of the bed and keeping the neck in a neutral (not slightly flexed) position facilitates venous drainage. Vital signs and neuro checks should be done at least once an hour for 4 hours and then every 4 hours for the next 24 hours. If the resident decompensates or if intracranial pressure (ICP) is increasing, vital signs and neuro checks should be done more frequently (e.g., every 15 minutes). Coughing is not encouraged because this can increase ICP. Waking the resident every 2 hours is not necessary and disrupting sleep patterns may increase confusion and obscure assessment of cognitive changes. Nausea, mild headache, or dizziness are expected symptoms that should be documented. The HCP would be notified for projectile vomiting, worsening headaches, or dizziness that causes falls or loss of balance. Bed rest and passive range-of-motion are not necessary for residents who can move independently. **Focus:** Prioritization; **QSEN:** S; **Concept:** Intracranial Regulation; **Cognitive Level:** Analyzing; **Cognitive Skill:** Analyze Cues

19. **Ans: 1, 2, 3, 5, 7** Rising slowly, 1-minute pauses between position changes, stimulating feet and ankle joints before standing, and staying with the resident are fall prevention measures that would be delegated to the AP. Shoes with supportive soles are safer than soft slippers or socks. Turning the head with a sweeping motion could increase dizziness. (Turning the head back and forth to visually sweep the area is an intervention that is used for patients who have lost large portions of the visual field.) Ambulation is deferred at least 30 to 60 minutes after eating because digestion diverts blood flow to the gastrointestinal system. If dizziness occurs, the nurse would assess the resident and ask about trigger factors. **Focus:** Delegation; **QSEN:** S; **Concept:** Perfusion; **Cognitive Level:** Analyzing; **Cognitive Skill:** Take Action

20. **Ans: 1, 2, 3, 4, 6, 8, 9, 10** Long-term care centers and nursing homes provide services for a vulnerable group of people. The care requires close and prolonged contact. These facilities are frequently understaffed, and staffing is supplemented by agency (per diem, or temporary) personnel who work at multiple locations. Residents frequently share rooms and transfers from hospitals, homes, or rehabilitation centers are common. Preexisting lack of PPE and deficiencies in infection control and prevention contributed to the spread. Masks and social distancing were initiated after the rapid spread was recognized. Unfortunately, by that time, many older adults in nursing homes had died and visitors were prohibited. Opposition to vaccinations did not contribute to the early spread of COVID-19, but there is a concern that resistance to COVID-19 vaccination will contribute to further spread of the virus through the general population. **Focus:** Prioritization; **QSEN:** S; **Concept:** Infection, Health Policy; **Cognitive Level:** Analyzing; **Test Taking Tip:** The CDC is a source for updated information on COVID-19: https://www.cdc.gov/coronavirus/2019-ncov/hcp/long-term-care.html#core-practices.

QSEN Key: PCC, Patient-Centered Care; **TC,** Teamwork & Collaboration; **EBP,** Evidence-Based Practice; **QI,** Quality Improvement; **S,** Safety; **I,** Informatics.

IPEC Key: Domain 1 Values/Ethics (**V/E**); Domain 2 Roles/Responsibilities (**R/R**); Domain 3 Interprofessional Communication (**IC**); Domain 4 Teams/Teamwork (**T/T**)

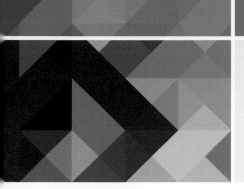

CHAPTER 14
LPN/LVN in the Urgent Care Setting

Questions

1. The nurse explains that acuity and level of care differentiate the urgent care clinic from the emergency department (ED). Which ailments should the nurse inform the student need to be triaged to the ED? **Select all that apply**
   1. Chest pain.
   2. Allergic reaction.
   3. Immunizations.
   4. Sexually transmitted disease (STD).
   5. Severe abdominal pain.
   6. Sudden paralysis or numbness in face or extremities.
   7. Colds/flu.

2. The nurse in the urgent care unit is assisting the health care provider (HCP) with school physicals. Which vaccines are state mandated and legally required in 50 states for school-aged children in kindergarten through 12th grade? **Select all that apply.**
   1. Tetanus, diphtheria, whooping cough (Tdap).
   2. Polio (IPV).
   3. Human papilloma virus (HPV).
   4. Chickenpox (Varicella).
   5. Meningococcal disease (MenACWY).
   6. Hepatitis B.

3. The nurse is caring for a patient who presents with a bee sting on her right upper forearm. The area is red, swollen, and itching. The patient has no known allergies but there is a family history of anaphylactic reactions. Which medication should the nurse make sure is available to administer immediately?
   1. Diphenhydramine 50 mg/mL.
   2. Epinephrine 1:1000 1 mg/mL.
   3. Hydrocortisone sodium succinate 250 mg/2 mL.
   4. Famotidine 20 mg/50 mL.

4. A patient presents to the urgent care clinic with complaints of nausea, chest pain, and dizziness. He states that he was playing golf when the symptoms occurred about 15 minutes ago. Vital signs are T 37°C (98.6°F), pulse 98 irregular, R 22, BP 100/60, O_2 Sat 94%. He is alert, oriented, has no allergies, and has a history of coronary artery disease (CAD). What is the **first** action of the nurse?
   1. Call 911.
   2. Apply oxygen at 2 L per nasal cannula.
   3. Perform a 12-lead EKG.
   4. Insert a saline lock.

5. The nurse assigned to urgent care is caring for a 29-year-old male who sustained superficial partial-thickness burns to the palm of his right hand from an exploding firecracker. Vital signs are stable and he reports 7/10 pain in his right hand. Which action should the nurse take **first**?
   1. Medicate the patient for pain.
   2. Remove the patient's ring and bracelet.
   3. Irrigate the hand under cool water for 10 minutes.
   4. Place a sterile dressing over the burn.

6. A 24-year-old male has been diagnosed with a ruptured eardrum by the HCP. Which statement made by the patient would cause the nurse to repeat the discharge instructions given by the HCP?
   1. "I will seek followup care with my family physician."
   2. "I will wear earplugs when playing my drums."
   3. "I will not blow my nose until my eardrum has healed."
   4. "I can shower or bathe as usual."

7. The HCP asked the nurse to perform a visual acuity test on a patient with a corneal abrasion. Which is the correct procedure for the nurse to use when using the Snellen eye chart?
   1. At a distance of 40 feet from the chart, both eyes are tested together.
   2. At a distance of 20 feet from the chart, both eyes are tested together.
   3. At a distance of 20 feet from the chart, the right eye is tested, then the left eye is tested.
   4. At a distance of 20 feet from the chart, each eye is tested separately, then both eyes are tested together.

8. The HCP has prescribed cyclobenzaprine hydrochloride for a patient with back spasms. Which medical condition should the nurse remind the HCP about before filling the prescription?
   1. Asthma.
   2. CAD.
   3. Diabetes mellitus.
   4. Narrow-angle glaucoma.

9. A 55-year-old male patient is being treated for gastroenteritis. He reports nausea, vomiting, abdominal cramping, and diarrhea for 24 hours. The HCP has prescribed sublingual ondansetron to relieve the nausea and vomiting. Which instructions will the nurse reinforce before discharging the patient? **Select all that apply.**
   1. Do not eat or drink anything until the vomiting has stopped for several hours.
   2. Brush your teeth after vomiting.
   3. Sip small amounts of soda or fruit juices for 12 to 24 hours.
   4. Suck ice chips or electrolyte popsicles for 12 to 24 hours.
   5. Once vomiting stops, add bananas, rice, applesauce, tea, and toast.
   6. If the diarrhea continues once vomiting stops, you can take an over-the-counter antidiarrheal.

10. The nurse is assigned to telephone triage at an urgent care center. A patient calls the triage line and states that he thinks he may have COVID-19. The nurse determines that the patient is 30 years old, has a fever of 37.7°C (100°F), cough, headache, and fatigue. He has no underlying medical conditions and states he is not short of breath. Which recommendation is best for the nurse to offer?
    1. Direct the patient to the lab for a COVID-19 antibody test.
    2. Direct the patient to the ED.
    3. Offer the patient a telehealth appointment with the urgent care HCP.
    4. Tell the patient to wear a mask at all times, wash his hands frequently, and practice social distancing.

11. An LPN/LVN from the ED has floated to the urgent care center to assist the registered nurse and assistive personnel (AP) for the day. Which nursing duties can be safely and efficiently assigned to the float nurse? **Select all that apply.**
    1. Update patient information.
    2. Collect patient data.
    3. Administer oral medications.
    4. Telephone patients to follow up on their condition.
    5. Clean and sterilize equipment.
    6. Schedule appointments.

12. Matrix. _____

A 60-year-old patient walked into the urgent care and stated she twisted her left ankle when she was stepping off a curb on her way to an Alcoholics Anonymous meeting. She has a history of osteoporosis and type 2 diabetes. The ankle is not deformed and is red and swollen with a small abrasion on the left lateral side with good pulses and adequate circulation and sensation. The patient states her pain level is a 7/10 and she is lightheaded. Vital signs are T 37°C (98.7°F), pulse 110, R 20, BP 150/88, O_2 Sat 95% on room air.

For each potential HCP prescription, place an X in the box to indicate whether it is anticipated, nonessential, or contraindicated

Nursing Action	Anticipated	Nonessential	Contraindicated
X-ray left ankle			
Oxygen at 2 L per minute via nasal cannula			
Hydrocodone 5 mg by mouth			
Finger stick blood glucose			
Vitamin D level			
Tetanus toxoid vaccine IM			
Warm water soak and heat pack left ankle			
Compression wrap left ankle			
Crutches			

13. Extended Multiple Response

Case Study: An adult male patient presents to the urgent care with several dog bites on his left hand. The puncture wounds are draining serosanguinous fluid. He states the dog was not his and came out of nowhere to attack him as he walked to the mailbox. Vital signs are stable and he has no known allergies.

Question: Which actions can the nurse delegate to the medical assistant or AP? (Circle the answers.)

1. Clean the wound and irrigate.
2. Administer a tetanus toxoid vaccine.
3. Record vital signs.
4. Notify animal control.
5. Administer ibuprofen 400 mg by mouth.
6. Provide a written discharge instruction sheet.
7. Obtain insurance and billing information.
8. Telephone the HCP antibiotic prescription to the pharmacy.
9. Arrange for an appointment with the patient's primary care provider for wound followup.

14. Nextgen Drag and Drop

Scenario: In the afternoon several clients come to the clinic for walk-in care. The AP has placed several urgent care patients in four separate rooms.

Instructions:
Prioritize the following patients in the order in which they should be seen by the HCP in order to ensure safe and efficient patient care.

Patients to be seen

A. A 38-year-old female with moderate intermittent right shoulder and mid-epigastric pain vomiting yellow bile. She is afebrile.
B. A 26-year-old female with a sudden onset of fatigue, aches, and cough. Temperature is 37.7°C (100°F).
C. A 13-year-old boy with lethargy with right lower quadrant pain, nausea, vomiting, lack of appetite, and a fever of 37.7°C (100°F).
D. A 67-year-old woman who reports burning in her throat and gnawing stomach discomfort that is worse between meals. She is afebrile.

Place the letter of the patient from the column on the left in the correct order to be seen below.

1. _____
2. _____
3. _____
4. _____

PART 2   Common Health Scenarios

Answer Key for this chapter begins on p. 98

Answers

Common Health Scenarios

PART 2

1. **Ans: 1, 5, 6** Chest pain needs to be evaluated and treated immediately in a hospital with a cardiac catheterization lab and/or emergency medications to rapidly restore blood flow to the heart. Severe abdominal pain needs to be evaluated and treated in a hospital with surgical services. Sudden paralysis or numbness in the face or extremities needs to be evaluated and treated in a hospital so medications can be given in a timely manner to restore brain blood flow. All other conditions mentioned can be treated in an urgent care center. **Focus:** Prioritization; **QSEN:** T/C, PCC; **Concept:** Communication; **Cognitive Level:** Analyzing; **IPEC:** IC

2. **Ans: 1, 2, 4** According to the CDC, in 2014 all 50 states and the District of Columbia approved mandatory vaccination programs for diphtheria, tetanus, pertussis, polio, measles, and rubella. Some states require additional vaccinations for children. HPV, MenACWY, and hepatitis B are not mandatory in all 50 states but are recommended by the CDC. Nurses should make parents aware of all vaccines that are available and be prepared to answer questions about them. Information on all vaccinations can easily be found on the CDC website. **Focus:** Prioritization; **QSEN:** PCC, S; EBP; **Concept:** Safety, Patient Education; **Cognitive Level:** Analyzing

3. **Ans: 2** Allergies and anaphylactic reactions can run in families. All the medications listed are likely to be given to a patient with an anaphylactic reaction but the first medication that must be given is epinephrine 1:1000 IM. Epinephrine prevents upper airway constriction by bronchodilation and prevents hypotension and shock through vasoconstriction. **Focus:** Prioritization; **QSEN:** PCC, S, EBP; **Concept:** EBP; **Cognitive Level:** Analyzing. **Test Taking Tip:** Remember there are two dilutions of epinephrine: epinephrine 1:1000/ mL and epinephrine 1:10,000/10 mL. Epinephrine 1:10,000 dilution is given intravenously for cardiac arrest.

4. **Ans: 1** The nurse should call 911 for transport as it is likely the patient is having a myocardial infarction. The urgent care is not equipped to fully take care of this type of illness, so transport to a hospital with a coronary catheterization lab is vital. Oxygen can be applied after calling 911. If there is time to insert a saline lock and perform a 12-lead EKG without delaying transport, it can be completed in the clinic; otherwise, it should be completed in the ambulance on the way to the hospital. **Focus:** Prioritization; **QSEN:** PCC, S; **Concept:** Perfusion; **Cognitive Level:** Analyzing

5. **Ans: 2** Capillary permeability after a burn causes plasma to leak out from capillaries to interstitial spaces. Capillary permeability and leaking plasma are greatest in the first 8 hours of a burn and continue for 48 hours. If rings and bracelets are not removed immediately, obstruction to blood flow can cause permanent damage to the hand. **Focus:** Prioritization; **QSEN:** PCC, EBP; **Concept:** Perfusion, Safety; **Cognitive Level:** Analyzing

6. **Ans: 4** The ear should be kept dry with petroleum jelly applied to a cotton ball while bathing or showering to avoid infection. A ruptured eardrum should heal on its own in several weeks but if hearing worsens, a physician should be consulted. The ear should be protected from acoustic injury like loud noises or explosions. Increased pressure from nose blowing, flying in airplanes, or diving should be avoided so reinjuring the ear does not occur. **Focus:** Prioritization; **QSEN:** PCC; **Concept:** Safety; **Cognitive Level:** Analyzing

7. **Ans: 4** The patient either sits or stands 20 feet from the chart and the right eye is tested with the left eye covered, then the left eye is tested with the right eye covered, then both eyes are tested together. **Focus:** Prioritization; **QSEN:** PCC; **Concept:** Sensory Perception; **Cognitive Level:** Analyzing

8. **Ans: 4** Cyclobenzaprine hydrochloride has an anticholinergic effect, which can worsen increased intraocular pressure in patients with narrow closure glaucoma and urinary retention. **Focus:** Prioritization; **QSEN:** PCC, S; **Concept:** Safety; **Cognitive Level:** Analyzing

9. **Ans: 1, 4, 5** Eating and drinking too soon after vomiting can reintroduce vomiting. Ice chips and electrolyte popsicles will help prevent dehydration. Brushing your teeth after vomiting can ruin the enamel on your teeth because vomit contains stomach acids that are corrosive. Soda and fruit juice contain a high sugar content that can worsen dehydration. Fruit juice has acid that may worsen nausea and vomiting when added to stomach acid. Generally, it is best not to stop diarrhea unless the cause is known. If diarrhea continues after 3 or 4 days, a stool sample should be taken to find the causative agent. **Focus:** Prioritization; **QSEN:** PCC; **Concept:** Fluid and Electrolytes; **Cognitive Level:** Analyzing

10. **Ans: 3** According to the CDC, COVID-19 symptoms are suspected in this patient but his symptoms are not emergent, so he should be offered a telehealth appointment with the HCP. In order to diagnose COVID-19, a nasopharyngeal swab

polymerase chain reaction (PCR) test is done. Antibody testing is best done a week or 2 weeks after the resolution of COVID-19 symptoms to find out if an immune response to the virus has occurred. The patient should be quarantined and not simply social-distance himself until a definitive COVID-19 nasopharyngeal swab PCR test is completed. **Focus:** Prioritization; **QSEN:** PCC; **Concept:** Gas Exchange; **Cognitive Level:** Analyzing

11. **Ans: 2, 3, 4** Updating patient information, cleaning and sterilizing equipment, and scheduling appointments are duties best left to the AP or medical assistants for consistency and efficiency. A float nurse could perform these duties but would be unfamiliar with the unit procedures and protocols and this would be an inefficient use of nursing time. **Focus:** Assignment; **QSEN:** PCC; **Concept:** Care Coordination; **Cognitive Level:** Analyzing

12. **Ans:**

Nursing Action	Anticipated	Nonessential	Contraindicated
X-ray left ankle	X		
Oxygen at 2 L per minute via nasal cannula		X	
Hydrocodone 5 mg by mouth			X
Finger stick blood glucose	X		
Vitamin D level		X	
Tetanus toxoid vaccine IM	X		
Heat pack to the left ankle			X
Compression wrap left ankle	X		
Crutches		X	

This patient has osteoporosis, so it is reasonable to anticipate the HCP may order an x-ray of her left ankle to rule out a fracture; however, soft tissue injuries do not show up on an x-ray. Hydrocodone is contraindicated in recovering alcoholics unless absolutely necessary. Pain from strains and sprains can be relieved with acetaminophen or ibuprofen, as well as elevation and ice application for 15 to 20 minutes every 2 hours, along with the application of a compression bandage. Heat will aggravate the pain and cause more swelling to the initial injury and should not be used.

It would be prudent to check a blood glucose as the patient has diabetes and complains of being lightheaded. She may have stumbled from hypoglycemia. Crutches are nonessential at this time as weight-bearing has been shown to help heal ankle sprains and strains more quickly. A tetanus toxoid should be given and the abrasion should be cleaned and dressed as necessary. **Focus:** Prioritization; **QSEN:** PCC; **Concept:** Inflammation; **Cognitive Level:** Analyzing

13. **Ans: 3, 4, 7, 9** In general, APs or medical assistants working in the urgent care clinic can record vital signs and complete administrative tasks such as intake information, assisting in the HCP or nurse with examinations, ordering supplies, updating records, and assisting with followup appointments. **Focus:** Delegation; **QSEN:** PCC, T/C; **Concept:** Safety; **Cognitive Level:** Analyzing; **IPEC:** R/R

14. **Ans: C, A, B, D** C: The 13-year-old exhibits symptoms of appendicitis and should be seen first and sent to either the ED or an on-call surgeon immediately. A: The 38-year-old female exhibits signs of gallbladder disease and should be evaluated next so a decision on whether or not it requires emergency treatment can be made by the HCP. B: The 26-year-old female may have the flu and should be given a mask to wear to protect anyone coming in contact with her before she is seen by the HCP. D: The 67-year-old woman exhibits symptoms of gastrointestinal reflux and indigestion, which is not urgent. She can be given a prescription and a followup appointment with her family HCP for a complete medical examination. **Focus:** Prioritization; **QSEN:** PCC; **Concept:** Care Coordination; **Cognitive Level:** Analyzing

QSEN Key: PCC, Patient-Centered Care; **TC,** Teamwork & Collaboration; **EBP,** Evidence-Based Practice; **QI,** Quality Improvement; **S,** Safety; **I,** Informatics.

IPEC Key: Domain 1 Values/Ethics (**V/E**); Domain 2 Roles/Responsibilities (**R/R**); Domain 3 Interprofessional Communication (**IC**); Domain 4 Teams/Teamwork (**T/T**).

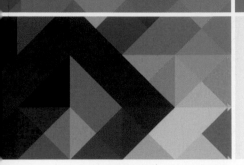

Questions

1. The nurse is caring for a 38-year-old patient who was recently admitted to the medical-surgical unit from the emergency department (ED). The patient sustained multiple abrasions and contusions from a motor vehicle rollover crash. Which observation by the nurse would warrant a call to the health care provider (HCP)?
   1. The patient refuses to eat.
   2. The patient's urine is dark reddish brown.
   3. The patient is lethargic and confused.
   4. The patient pulled out his central line catheter.

2. An older patient has small blisters on his mid-back that extend to his stomach. The lesions are itching and he states his pain level is 6/10. The HCP has diagnosed the patient with shingles. Which nursing actions should be taken to relieve pain in a patient with shingles? **Select all that apply.**
   1. Do not allow patient contact with pregnant women.
   2. Request opioid analgesics from the HCP.
   3. Administer famciclovir 500 mg every 8 hours by mouth.
   4. Apply cold compresses with Burrow solution.
   5. Place the patient on airborne and contact precautions.
   6. Give the patient a crossword puzzle book.

3. The nurse is working on a busy medical-surgical unit. There have been several admissions and the nurse still has several tasks that should be completed quickly. Which tasks can the nurse safely delegate to experienced assistive personnel (AP) on the unit? **Select all that apply.**
   1. Bathe and change the linen on a patient who recently vomited.
   2. Observe for redness or swelling of an intravenous line (IV) and report to the nurse.
   3. Document vital signs.
   4. Turn and position a patient with a stage 3 pressure injury.
   5. Test the urine of a patient with suspected urinary tract infection (UTI) using a reagent strip.
   6. Ambulate a frail elderly gentleman in the hallway.

4. All patients on the telemetry floor are currently stable. Which cardiac rhythm would require the nurse to call the rapid response team (RRT)?

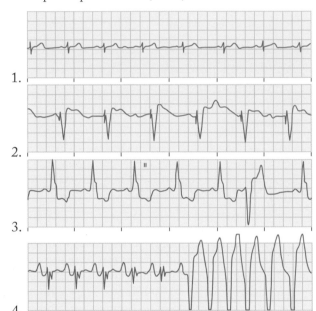

Figures from Aehlert B. (2018). *ECGs Made Easy.* 6th ed., Elsevier.

5. Which instructions will the nurse give to the AP for a cancer patient undergoing brachytherapy? **Select all that apply.**
   1. Place a sign on the door that prohibits pregnant women and children from entering the room.
   2. Stay at least 3 feet away from the patient unless performing personal care.
   3. Leave all food trays and linen in the room in the designated containers.
   4. Observe and report signs of sadness and loneliness.
   5. Flush patient wastes and body fluids down the toilet.
   6. Wear a dosimeter for protection when giving close personal care.

6. A patient with a spinal fracture at level T6 from a skiing accident reports a pounding headache. What action will the nurse take **first**?
   1. Medicate the patient with ibuprofen for headache.
   2. Take the patient's blood pressure.
   3. Check the bladder residual with ultrasound.
   4. Instruct the AP to darken the room.

7. A diabetic patient with venous and arterial insufficiency injured her ankle on the bedside stand while getting out of bed. The nurse notes a small partial thickness skin tear the size of a dime above the right ankle. Which nursing interventions are appropriate to implement? **Select all that apply.**
   1. Apply a moist dressing and elastic bandage to the wound.
   2. Apply a hydrocolloid dressing every 3 to 7 days or as needed.
   3. Notify the HCP.
   4. Apply moisturizing lotion around the area.
   5. Elevate the leg above the heart.
   6. Observe the patient for fever, chills, redness, and swelling.

8. A patient who is taking levetiracetam for epilepsy is scheduled for a total hip replacement in the morning. Which nursing interventions are important for the nurse to establish? **Select all that apply.**
   1. Set up a suction canister and tubing with a Yankauer catheter.
   2. Pad the side rails and headboard of the patient's bed.
   3. Remove potential safety hazards from the room.
   4. Set up oxygen with flow meter and green "Christmas tree" adapter.
   5. Have a nonrebreather mask readily available.
   6. Tape a padded tongue blade on the wall above the bed.

9. The nurse is caring for a 56-year-old female who returned from surgery after an above-the-knee amputation (AKA) sustained in a motorcycle accident. Which nursing action is the priority?
   1. Placing the patient in a prone position for 30 minutes every 4 hours.
   2. Elevating the stump for 48 hours.
   3. Examining the stump dressing for fresh bleeding.
   4. Administering prescribed antibiotics.

10. The nurse has been assigned two new admissions that require her immediate attention. Which nursing duties can be safely delegated to the AP in the unit? **Select all that apply.**
    1. Observe the buttocks of an incontinent patient for redness or skin tears.
    2. Provide a package of witch hazel cooling pads to a patient with hemorrhoids.
    3. Observe the outer surface of an abdominal dressing.
    4. Assist a patient with a new hip replacement to the bathroom.
    5. Perform a venipuncture for blood glucose.
    6. Discontinue an IV on a patient who is on coumadin.

11. A patient with renal failure is receiving peritoneal dialysis. The nurse would supervise a newly graduated AP in the performance of which task?
    1. Observe the patient for abdominal bloating, pain, and tenderness.
    2. Meticulously record intake and output record.
    3. Obtain vital signs every 4 hours.
    4. Obtain patient weight before and after dialysis.

12. The nurse is assigning patients for two APs on her team. Which patient should **not** be assigned to the pregnant AP?
    1. An 87-year-old female with influenza.
    2. A 27-year-old male patient with systemic lupus erythematosus (SLE).
    3. A 58-year-old male patient with cancer receiving palliative care.
    4. A 76-year-old female with a hip fracture.

13. A 36-year-old female patient had a right total mastectomy with removal of 20 axillary nodes two days ago. Which procedure could increase the risk for developing lymphedema?
    1. Taking blood pressure in the left arm.
    2. Applying an ice pack to the right arm.
    3. Elevation of the right arm above the level of the heart for 45 minutes twice a day.
    4. Application of compression stockings to lower extremities.

14. A 24-year-old male patient with a tumor on his adrenal medulla (pheochromocytoma) has been admitted to the unit for an adrenalectomy that is scheduled for the next morning. Vital signs are T 37°F (98.7°C), pulse 125 regular, R 20, BP 180/90, O$_2$ Sat 96% on 2 L of oxygen. He reports headache and is sweating. Which class of medication might the nurse expect the HCP to order for lowering both the heart rate and blood pressure?
    1. A beta-blocker combined with an alpha-blocker.
    2. A calcium channel blocker.
    3. Angiotensin receptor blockers.
    4. Angiotensin-converting enzyme (ACE) inhibitors.

Answer Key for this chapter begins on p. 104

PART 2 Common Health Scenarios

Common Health Scenarios   PART 2

15. An 88-year-old patient with heart failure is receiving a unit of packed red blood cells (PRBCs). Vital signs are T 98.7°F (37°C), pulse 74 regular, R 18, BP 110/60, O₂ Sat 96% on 2 L of oxygen. Which nursing action is **most** important to carry out while infusing the blood on this patient?
1. Record vital signs every 15 minutes during the first hour of transfusion.
2. Assess respiratory effort and lung sounds every 30 minutes.
3. Adjust infusion time for blood to be delivered within 4 hours.
4. Monitor hourly urine output.

16. A 34-year-old patient with leukemia is receiving chemotherapy and the nurse notes that the patient's platelet count is 20,000. What is the **priority** action of the nurse?
1. Advise the registered nurse (RN) team leader so that the patient can be placed in reverse isolation to prevent infection.
2. Notify the HCP immediately.
3. Place the patient on bleeding precautions.
4. Assure the patient is wearing compression stockings to prevent a blood clot.

17. A patient is receiving total parental nutrition (TPN) through a central venous line. Which nursing action is **most** important during the infusion?
1. Monitor liver function studies.
2. Monitor serum glucose levels.
3. Maintain strict aseptic technique when changing the central line.
4. Closely monitor vital signs.

18. Drag and Drop _____

Scenario: The AP reports that a diabetic patient is sweating profusely. Vital signs are T 37°C (98.7°F), pulse 84 regular, R 18, BP 120/80, O₂ Sat 98% on room air, blood sugar is 75 mg/dL. The nurse notes that the patient received glyburide, labetalol, and digoxin at 8:00 a.m. and ate 25% of her breakfast tray at 8:30 a.m. What is the order of nursing actions that the nurse will take?

Instructions:
Place the letter for the correct sequence of nursing actions to be taken for this patient.

Nursing Actions

A. Have the patient eat some cheese and crackers.

B. Repeat blood sugar and vital signs.

C. Notify the HCP.

D. Have the patient drink ½ cup of apple juice.

Order of Nursing Actions

19. Matrix. _____

A 34-year-old female patient is being admitted with reports of sudden 8/10 sharp mid-back pain and pink-tinged urine. She has a history of a gastric ulcer that is healed, gastroesophageal reflux disease (GERD), which is controlled with famotidine and calcium carbonate, and hypertension controlled with hydrochlorothiazide (HCTZ) 25 mg. She has an allergy to povidone-iodine and adhesive tape, which became apparent when she had a right knee replacement last year. She has lost 100 lb since being on a high-protein diet for a year. Vital signs are T 100°F (37.7°C), pulse 84 regular, R 18, BP 150/90, O2 Sat 96% on room air. For each potential HCP order, place an X in the box to indicate whether it is anticipated, nonessential, or contraindicated.

Potential Order	Anticipated	Nonessential	Contraindicated
Hydrocodone 10 mg by mouth every 4 hours for severe pain			
Ibuprofen 400 mg by mouth twice a day for pain			
Urinalysis with culture and sensitivity			
CT scan with contrast			
Kidney, ureter, bladder (KUB) x-ray			
Increase fluids to 2 L a day			
Strain all urine			
Furosemide 40 mg every day by mouth			

Answer Key for this chapter begins on p. 104

20. Extended Multiple Response

Case Study: The LPN/LVN is paired with the RN in a COVID-19 unit and is responsible for delivering skilled treatments, passing medications, and supervising personal patient care provided by AP who are on the team.

Question: Which nursing actions or interventions are the responsibility of the LPN/LVN?

Select all that apply by circling or highlighting your answers.

1. Encouraging nutritional intake.
2. Collaborating with social services to provide the patient and family with counseling and arrange for visitation.
3. Assessing laboratory values.
4. Administering prescribed medications and monitoring for effect.
5. Following hospital protocol for changing IV tubing and sites.
6. Monitoring vital signs as ordered for changes in baseline.
7. Assisting with intubation and mechanical ventilation as directed.
8. Scheduling patient care activities to allow uninterrupted periods of rest.
9. Performing chest physiotherapy as ordered by the HCP.

Answer Key for this chapter begins on p. 104

Answers

1. **Ans: 3** The HCP should be notified immediately of lethargy and confusion as these signs can signal a head injury. Signs of a traumatic brain injury can sometimes take days to weeks to appear. Refusing to eat could be a side effect of stress and anxiety. The nurse can offer the patient soft, palatable foods in small portions throughout the day. Urine that is reddish brown is normal for this patient, who suffered multiple contusions and is the result of myoglobin from the muscle injury that can cause rhabdomyolysis, which can lead to kidney failure. Strict intake and output should be initiated. The nurse should obtain an order to have the midline catheter replaced and fortified, so it cannot be easily removed again. **Focus:** Prioritization; **QSEN:** EBP; **Concept:** Cognition; **Cognitive Level:** Analyzing

2. **Ans: 3,4, 6** Methods to relieve pain include administering famciclovir, which can shorten the duration of pain, applying cold compresses of Burrow solution or calamine lotion, and using diversional activities. Guided imagery, puzzles, and other distraction techniques can also assist with pain relief. Pregnant women and persons who have not had varicella or been immunized should not have contact with the patient, but this will not help relieve the pain for the patient, nor will correctly placing the patient on airborne and contact precautions. Opioids should only be requested if the above solutions do not relieve pain as opioids can lead to addiction, constipation, and falls in the older adult. **Focus:** Prioritization; **QSEN:** EBP; **Concept:** Pain; **Cognitive Level:** Analyzing

3. **Ans: 1, 2, 3, 4, 5** An LPN/LVN can only delegate duties to an AP that are within both of their job descriptions. The AP can bathe, change linen, document vital signs, perform routine care, turn and position a patient, and test urine using a reagent strip. The experienced AP in the unit may also observe for redness and swelling and report back to the nurse. Ambulating a frail, morbidly obese patient or an otherwise unstable patient is best accomplished by the nurse as the LPN/LVN is accountable for the care that is delegated. **Focus:** Delegation; **QSEN:** PCC, S; **Concept:** Safety; **Cognitive Level:** Analyzing

4. **Ans: 4** This rhythm is a sinus rhythm that progresses to a wide complex tachycardia or ventricular tachycardia, which is a medical emergency. The nurse should stay with the patient, activate the RRT immediately, and call for a crash cart. Option 1 is a normal sinus rhythm, option 2 is a ventricular paced rhythm, and option 3 is a normal sinus rhythm with a widened QRS and a premature ventricular complex (PVC). **Focus:** Prioritization; **QSEN:** EBP, S; **Concept:** Perfusion; **Cognitive Level:** Analyzing

5. **Ans: 1, 2, 3, 4, 5** Brachytherapy involves radiation implants that are placed inside the patient near the tumor site. The patient's body will give off radiation. Pregnant women and children under 18 should not enter the room. Time limits and distance from the patient are designated by hospital policy but are always limited, so entrance into the room is prohibited unless it is necessary. Everything in the room must stay there and is placed in designated containers and removed by specialty personnel. The patient must remain alone the majority of the time and can become depressed. Wastes and fluids from bedpans can be discarded in the toilet in the room. Wearing a lead apron provides protection but a dosimeter does not. **Focus:** Assignment/Supervision; **QSEN:** S; **Concept:** Cellular Regulation, Safety; **Cognitive Level:** Analyzing

6. **Ans: 2** Autonomic dysreflexia is a life-threatening emergency that can occur in spinal cord injuries at T6 and above. The patient will not have feeling below the level of their injury, but the nerves still send signals back to the brain when there are noxious stimuli below the area of injury. Usually, the first symptom of autonomic dysreflexia is a headache. The blood pressure can go dangerously high due to a reflex sympathetic discharge, which leads to vasoconstriction and can cause stroke or heart attack. An overdistended bladder, irritation to the bowel, constipation, or pressure against the skin are the most common causes of autonomic dysreflexia. If the blood pressure needs to be lowered immediately, the patient must be placed in a sitting position or the head of the bed elevated to 45 degrees. Removing the source of the irritation will prevent occurrence. **Focus:** Prioritization; **QSEN:** EBP, PCC, S; **Concept:** Safety, Perfusion; **Cognitive Level:** Analyzing

7. **Ans: 2, 3, 4, 6** The patient has arterial and venous insufficiency. A compression bandage and elevation above the heart will worsen arterial blood supply to the area. Hydrocolloid dressings provide moisture and a barrier to the wound and are changed every 3 to 7 days or sooner if necessary. Infection can develop quickly, so the HCP should be notified. The patient should be closely observed for signs of infection. **Focus:** Prioritization; **QSEN:** PCC, EBP; **Concept:** Perfusion, Infection; **Cognitive Level:** Analyzing

8. **Ans: 1, 2, 3, 4, 5** Safety is the priority for the patient with a history of seizure activity. The patient's mouth should never be pried open and nothing should be placed in the patient's mouth during the seizure because once the jaw clamps down, teeth may be broken, and the airway could become obstructed. All other interventions listed are appropriate. **Focus:** Prioritization; **QSEN:** S; **Concept:** Safety; **Cognitive Level:** Analyzing

Common Health Scenarios PART 2

PART 2 Common Health Scenarios

9. **Ans: 3** The priority problem after an amputation is bleeding. Fresh bleeding should be reported to the HCP immediately. Elevating the stump helps prevent edema, which affects the fitting of a prosthesis and healing. Placing the patient in a prone position helps prevent hip contractures. Antibiotics are usually given prophylactically to prevent infection

10. **Ans: 1, 2, 3** The AP is able to observe the skin condition and the condition of an abdominal dressing and report the finding to the nurse. The nurse can then retriage her duties as needed. If the skin condition needs immediate care or the abdominal dressing needs to be changed or reapplied, the nurse can assign the care to another nurse as needed. Witch hazel cooling pads are considered a nursing order and giving them to the patient who is uncomfortable is good care. The patient with a hip replacement should be assisted by the nurse because it will likely be a painful and fearful experience for the patient. The scope of practice for an AP does not include venipuncture. Discontinuing an IV on a patient with coumadin is performed by the nurse because of increased bleeding time. **Focus:** Delegation; **QSEN:** S, T/C; **Concept:** Safety, Care Coordination; **Cognitive Level:** Analyzing; **IPEC:** R/R, T/T

11. **Ans: 1** Although AP are allowed to observe patients for changes in condition, a newly graduated AP's observation skills may not be keen enough to result in an accurate observation of peritonitis. The nurse should observe and assess the patient with the new AP to educate and foster teamwork. Recording intake and output, taking vital signs, and obtaining weight are skills that a new AP should be able to independently perform with minimal guidance. **Focus:** Assignment/Delegation; **QSEN:** PCC, T/C; **Concept:** Care Coordination; **Cognitive Level:** Analyzing; **IPEC:** T/T, R/R

12. **Ans: 1** Pregnant women are more susceptible to infection and at higher risk of developing severe illness if exposed to corona viruses or influenza. Pregnant women who get the flu are more likely to have preterm labor and premature birth than women who don't get the flu. Although personal protective equipment (PPE) is worn to mitigate the risks, it is prudent not to expose a pregnant coworker to respiratory illnesses if at all possible. The rest of the patients are considered safe for a pregnant woman to care for with usual standard precautions. **Focus:** Assignment; **QSEN:** S, T/C; **Concept:** Care Coordination, Safety; **Cognitive Level:** Analyzing; **IPEC:** T/T, V/E

13. **Ans: 2** Lymph nodes act as a drain and if the drain is removed, fluid will back up and cause lymphedema. An ice pack to the right arm can vasoconstrict blood vessels and further block the flow of fluids. Blood pressure cuffs, ice packs, tight bands, or jewelry should not be applied on the same arm as nodal removal. **Focus:** Prioritization; **QSEN:** S; **Concept:** Fluid and Electrolytes, Safety; **Cognitive Level:** Analyzing

14. **Ans: 1** A pheochromocytoma is a tumor on the adrenal gland. The adrenal medulla secretes the hormones epinephrine and norepinephrine. One effect of epinephrine stimulates beta-1 receptors and increases heart rate. Norepinephrine stimulates the alpha receptors and vasoconstricts blood vessels, raising the blood pressure. Labetalol is an example of a nonselective beta-adrenergic blocker and a selective alpha-adrenergic blocker and is frequently used in patients with pheochromocytoma. **Focus:** Prioritization; **QSEN:** S; **Concept:** Perfusion, Safety; **Cognitive Level:** Analyzing

15. **Ans: 2** The older patient with heart failure is at risk for congestive heart failure from fluid overload. Assessment of respiratory effort and lung sounds every 30 minutes is the most important nursing action for this patient who is receiving a unit of blood so that fluid overload can be recognized before interfering with oxygenation. Adjusting the infusion time to run slower will help prevent fluid overload. Temperature rise greater than or equal to 1° C (or 2°F), tachycardia, and hypotension are indications of a transfusion reaction. Urine output should be at least 0.5 mL/kg/h to assure renal perfusion. LPNs cannot start blood transfusions but can monitor blood transfusions. **Focus:** Prioritization; **QSEN:** PCC, EBP; **Concept:** Gas Exchange, Perfusion; **Cognitive Level:** Analyzing. **Test Taking Tip:** Physiological needs are those necessary for survival and are the first step in Maslow's hierarchy of needs. Whenever deciding on physiological priorities, follow the ABCs of airway before breathing before circulation.

16. **Ans: 2** The HCP should be notified immediately of the dangerously low platelet count, which leaves the patient vulnerable to spontaneous hemorrhage. The next step is to place the patient on bleeding precautions. **Focus:** Prioritization; **QSEN:** S; **Concept:** Perfusion; **Cognitive Level:** Applying

17. **Ans: 2** Although all the nursing actions are important to care for the patient receiving TPN, the priority is to monitor serum glucose levels. Glucose levels are usually checked every 6 hours with an order for sliding scale insulin administration to prevent hyperglycemia. Hyperglycemia can result in increased incidence of infection. **Focus:** Prioritization; **QSEN:** EBP; **Concept:** Cellular Regulation, Fluids and Electrolytes; **Cognitive Level:** Analyzing

18. **Ans: D, A, B, C** The patient is hypoglycemic. Beta-blockers prevent the sympathetic nervous system from allowing the liver to make glucose. The usual symptoms of shakiness, anxiety, and hunger are being masked. Diaphoresis is unmasked and is usually the only sign of hypoglycemia in patients taking beta-blockers. The priority action is to raise the blood sugar by providing ½ cup of juice or soda that is not diet and have the patient eat some cheese and crackers for a longer-acting source of glucose. The next step is to reevaluate the blood sugar and recheck vital signs. The nurse should then notify the HCP **Focus:** Prioritization; **QSEN:** PCC, S; **Concept:** Cellular Regulation; **Cognitive Level:** Analyzing

19. Ans:

Potential Order	Anticipated	Nonessential	Contraindicated
Hydrocodone 5 mg by mouth every 4 hours for severe pain	X		
Ibuprofen 400 mg by mouth twice a day for pain			X
Urinalysis with culture and sensitivity (C&S)	X		
CT scan with contrast			X
Kidney, ureter, bladder (KUB) x-ray	X		
Increase fluids to at least 2 L a day	X		
Strain all urine	X		
Furosemide 40 mg everyday		X	

Severe, acute, mid-back pain with pink-tinged urine, a high-protein diet, calcium carbonate intake, and a history of being overweight provide some clues that the patient may have a kidney stone. Ibuprofen is contraindicated due to the history of a gastric ulcer, and the patient is allergic to iodine, so a CT scan with contrast is also contraindicated. A KUB will reveal the size and location of stone. Increasing fluids will help flush out the stones and all urine should be strained for stones. Furosemide is nonessential for this patient as she is on HCTZ, which is a diuretic that also reduces calcium in the urine. A urinalysis with C&S can reveal mineral levels as well as rule out infection. **Focus:** Prioritization; **QSEN:** EBP; **Concept:** Elimination; **Cognitive Level:** Analyzing

20. Ans: 1, 4, 6, 8, 9 The RN is responsible for assessment and specialty skills; an assessment of the spiritual and emotional status of both the patient and the family must be completed before collaborating with social services, so this must be done by the RN. The LPN can monitor the labs for abnormalities but the RN must assess the abnormalities so that further action can be taken. The LPN can monitor IV sites but changing tubing and sites is a skill that should be done by the RN. The RN should assist with intubation and mechanical ventilation. **Focus:** Assignment; **QSEN:** S; **Concept:** Care Coordination; **Cognitive Level:** Analyzing; **IPEC:** R/R

QSEN Key: PCC, Patient-Centered Care; **TC,** Teamwork & Collaboration; **EBP,** Evidence-Based Practice; **QI,** Quality Improvement; **S,** Safety; **I,** Informatics.

IPEC Key: Domain 1 Values/Ethics (**V/E**); Domain 2 Roles/Responsibilities (**R/R**); Domain 3 Interprofessional Communication (**IC**); Domain 4 Teams/Teamwork (**T/T**).

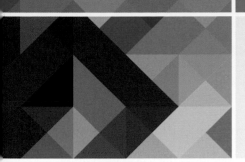

CHAPTER 16
LPN/LVN in the Postpartum Setting

Questions

1. The patient is 1 day postpartum and experiencing sore nipples while breastfeeding. Which action would **best** demonstrate evidence-based practice?
   1. Inform the mother that a certain amount of soreness is normal.
   2. Observe the mother–baby couplet for nursing position and latch and correct as indicated.
   3. Advise the use of a breast pump until the soreness is resolved.
   4. Advise alternating breastfeeding and pumping to avoid excess sucking at the nipple.

2. A 26-year-old gravida 1 para 1 patient delivered via cesarean section 24 hours ago and is having trouble breastfeeding. Which of the following tasks for this patient could be delegated to the assistive personnel (AP)? **Select all that apply.**
   1. Provide the mother with an ordered abdominal binder.
   2. Assist the mother with breastfeeding.
   3. Take the mother's vital signs.
   4. Check the amount of lochia present.
   5. Assist the mother with ambulation.
   6. Check the incision site.

3. The nurse is assessing a gravida 2 para 2 patient who is 16 hours postpartum and notes a large amount of vaginal bleeding. Which nursing action would be the **priority**?
   1. Check the vital signs.
   2. Notify the health care provider (HCP).
   3. Firmly massage the uterine fundus.
   4. Put the baby to breast.

4. The new nurse on the locked postpartum unit observes an experienced nurse open the door for a middle-aged woman without a visitor badge and then leave the unit for lunch. The new nurse sees the woman wandering in the hall. In what order would the following actions be performed?
   1. Find the nurse who allowed the woman in and question her to see if she knows the woman and why she let her in.
   2. Ask the supervisor to clarify the access policies for the postpartum unit.
   3. Go up to the woman and ask if you can help her. Confirm which patient she is visiting and request that she get a visitor's pass.
   4. Ask the unit desk secretary to closely monitor the infant security system.

5. A patient being admitted to the postpartum unit after delivery has a diagnosis of latent tuberculosis (TB). She had a chest x-ray during pregnancy showing no active TB in the lungs and has no current symptoms. Which types of isolation precautions are needed for this patient?
   1. Isolate the mother, initiate droplet precautions.
   2. Separate the mother and baby and do not allow breastfeeding at this time.
   3. Place a face mask on the mother when she is outside of her room.
   4. No isolation precautions are needed at this time.

6. The patient underwent a primary cesarean section 24 hours ago. Which assessment finding would be of the **most** concern?
   1. Small amount of lochia rubra
   2. Temperature of 99°F (37.2°C)
   3. Edema with slight pain and redness of left calf
   4. Pain rated as 3/10 at the incision site

7. A patient who delivered 3 hours ago is being admitted to the postpartum unit. She has a diagnosis of varicella. Which statement by the student nurse to the patient would require intervention by the nurse?
   1. "You may keep your baby in your room with you."
   2. "You should pump your milk and discard it."
   3. "Your family members should be vaccinated against varicella."
   4. "You must wear a face mask when outside your room."

8. Which finding on the newborn's umbilical cord on the 3rd day of life should be reported to the HCP?
   1. The plastic cord clamp is not present.
   2. The base of the umbilical cord is moist.
   3. The end of the umbilical cord is brown and dry.
   4. There is edema at the base of the umbilical cord.

9. The mother of the patient is at the bedside and instructs the new mother to place her baby face down in the bassinet and to cover her with a warm blanket. How would the nurse respond?
   1. "That is exactly how I was first taught to place a baby in her crib, but let me share with you some newer information regarding the safest position for sleep."
   2. "The baby looks very comfortable like that."
   3. "If you place the baby in that position, there is a higher risk the baby will die."
   4. "If you place the baby face down in the crib, be sure to turn her head to one side or the other."

10. The patient is 6 hours postpartum after an uncomplicated vaginal birth and complains of lower abdominal discomfort. On examination of the abdomen, the nurse notes that the uterine fundus is 2 centimeters above the umbilicus and deviated to the right side. Which intervention would be done **first**?
    1. Notify the HCP.
    2. Administer ibuprofen as ordered for pain.
    3. Assist the patient to the washroom if she is able to walk and encourage her to void.
    4. Perform straight catheterization of the urinary bladder.

11. Due to the COVID-19 pandemic, the hospital has limited visitors in the postpartum area and is allowing only the support person who was present during labor and delivery to be on the unit. The patient is 1 day postpartum and is angry because she wants her mother to be present to help her as she says her husband who is at the bedside is not good with babies. How would the nurse respond?
    1. Tell the patient the rule is nonnegotiable. Explain that the pandemic is serious, and the rule's purpose is to reduce the risk of the virus in the hospital.
    2. Explore what needs the patient and her husband have at this time. Utilize technology to include her mother in the discussion if desired.
    3. Ask the supervisor if the patient's mother can come in as the husband is unwilling to help.
    4. Take the baby to the nursery so the patient can rest and not need to care for the infant at this time

12. The nurse on the postpartum unit has received report and has several challenging patients to care for. Which tasks could be delegated to the experienced AP? **Select all that apply**
    1. Review new lab results for the preeclamptic patient.

2. Check vital signs of the patient who experienced a postpartum hemorrhage.
3. Remove the indwelling bladder catheter of the patient who had an emergency cesarean section and hysterectomy 1 day ago.
4. Assess the knowledge of the patient whose baby has a cleft lip.
5. Teach the patient with bipolar disorder basic baby care.
6. Call the Women, Infants and Children (WIC) office to obtain the paperwork needed for a homeless mother.

13. The postpartum patient with preeclampsia has orders for magnesium sulfate 2 g/h IV. Which symptom would be expected with this medication?
    1. Hot flashes.
    2. Headaches.
    3. Leg pain.
    4. Shortness of breath.

14. The newborn was born at 40 weeks gestation and weighed 7 lb 4 oz (3289 g) at delivery. At 2 days of life, the HCP has discharged the baby home with a weight of 6 lb 10 oz (3005 g). The breastfeeding mother is upset that the baby has lost weight and asks if she should supplement the baby with formula. How would the nurse respond?
    1. Yes, supplement the baby with formula after each breastfeeding to prevent further weight loss.
    2. No, it is not necessary to supplement the baby at this time. Continue to breastfeed the baby every 2 to 3 hours and monitor her urine and stool output.
    3. No, a breastfed baby should not be supplemented with formula. Continue to breastfeed and follow up at your pediatrician's office in 2 weeks.
    4. Yes, supplement the baby with 1 ounce of formula prior to each breastfeeding to be sure she is getting enough.

15. The 34-year-old woman is a gravida 1 para 1 who delivered her first baby by cesarean section due to the failure of the baby to descend during the second stage of labor. The patient is 4 hours postpartum and has been on her phone constantly talking with her friends about her birth experience. She does not show interest in caring for her baby at this time. Which nursing intervention would be appropriate at this time?
    1. Contact the social worker to assess the mother for no evidence of bonding.
    2. Advise the mother that it is time to begin learning how to care for her baby.
    3. Advise the mother that her baby needs her attention at this time.
    4. Allow the mother time to talk with her friends and discuss her experiences.

16. The nurse has noted how exhausted and overwhelmed many of the new mothers on the postpartum unit are and how this impacts their abilities to take on the care of their newborns. Which changes would the nurse propose at the next unit meeting? **Select all that apply.**
    1. Discontinue night vital signs to allow rest.
    2. Institute quiet hours on the postpartum unit to minimize environmental noise.
    3. Create signage that can be placed on patient doors to eliminate nonessential personnel from coming in to the room.
    4. Teach parents how to limit visitors.
    5. Work with AP to cluster care and minimize disruption of rest.
    6. Encourage mothers to place infants in the nursery at night to allow rest.

17. The new father has refused to allow the nurse to give the newborn an ordered injection of vitamin K. What is the **best** response?
    1. "What is the reason you do not want your baby to have vitamin K?"
    2. "Vitamin K is needed by all newborns to prevent bleeding."
    3. "If you do not want me to give the shot, I will not give it."
    4. "Vitamin K is the first of many shots your baby will need to get."

18. The patient is a 17-year-old who is 6 hours postpartum. The AP reports to the nurse that her blood pressure is 160/110 and she is complaining of a headache. Which action would the nurse perform at this time?
    1. Administer acetaminophen 1000 mg as ordered and recheck blood pressure after 20 minutes. If still elevated, report to HCP.
    2. Darken room, encourage rest, and recheck blood pressure in 20 minutes. If still elevated, report to HCP.
    3. Advise the AP to provide the patient with a cool cloth to the forehead and determine if the patient is stressed about something.
    4. Report findings immediately to the HCP.

19. Enhanced Multiple Response.

    > **Scenario:** The nurse has received orders to initiate phototherapy on a 36-hour-old breastfeeding newborn with an elevated bilirubin level. The nurse asks the student nurse working with her to explain how she will administer the treatment.

    Which actions would be expected from the student nurse?

Select all that apply. Highlight or circle the correct answers.
1. Cover the infant's eyes with a mask.
2. Monitor the infant's temperature closely.
3. Keep the infant nothing by mouth (NPO) during treatment.
4. Apply ointment to the infant's skin prior to light exposure.
5. Offer the infant only sterile water feedings during the treatment.
6. Instruct the mother to pump her breasts because the infant will not be breastfeeding during the treatment.
7. Clothe infant in shirt and diaper only.
8. Remove eye coverings when the parent is feeding the infant.

20. Matrix.
    The postpartum breastfeeding patient has the following lab results.

Hemoglobin	Blood Type	Rh Factor	Varicella	Rubella
11.5	A	Negative	Immune	Nonimmune

Answer Key for this chapter begins on p. 111

Common Health Scenarios PART 2

The patient will be discharged home today. For each potential HCP prescription, place an X in the box to indicate whether it is anticipated, nonessential, or contraindicated.

	Anticipated	Nonessential	Contraindicated
Rubella vaccine IM			
Varicella vaccine subcutaneous			
Rho(D) immune globulin IM			
Ferrous sulfate 325 mg daily PO			

Answer Key for this chapter begins on p. 111

Answers

1. **Ans: 2**   Improper latch and position are the most common cause of nipple soreness and can be corrected with assessment and assistance to the mother. This practice supports the Perinatal Core Measure of increasing the percentage of newborns who are fed breast milk exclusively. Advising the mother that soreness can be normal does not provide assistance to the mother with her problem. Utilizing a breast pump may be appropriate at some times during lactation, but the first priority is to assess and correct the issue that may be causing the soreness. **Focus:** Prioritization; **QSEN:** EBP; **Concept:** Evidence; **Cognitive Level:** Applying

2. **Ans: 1, 3, 5**   The AP could provide an abdominal binder, measure the vital signs of the patient, and assist her in ambulating. The nurse would be responsible for evaluating the normality of vital signs. The AP should be given parameter limits for vital signs and told to report values outside the limits to the nurse. Assisting a new mother in breastfeeding is a very important nursing function because the nurse needs to give consistent evidence-based advice to enhance success at breastfeeding. A common complaint of postpartum patients is inconsistent help with and advice on breastfeeding. The nurse should also be the one to check the amount of lochia as that must be carefully evaluated to assess for signs of postpartum hemorrhage. The surgical incision also needs to be evaluated by the nurse for any signs of infection or dehiscence. The nurse's assistance with breastfeeding supports the perinatal core measures of increasing the percentage of newborns that are fed breast milk exclusively. The nurse's careful assessment of lochia also supports the perinatal core measurement of reducing the likelihood of harm due to maternal hemorrhage. **Focus:** Delegation; **QSEN:** TC, EBP, PCC; **Concept:** Collaboration; **Cognitive Level:** Applying; **IPEC:** R/R. **Test Taking Tip:** For a delegation question, consider the five rights of delegation: Right circumstance? Right task? Right person? Right direction/communication? Right supervision?.

3. **Ans: 3**   Uterine fundal massage would be the priority nursing action because it helps the uterus to contract firmly and reduces bleeding. The first two answer choices are appropriate nursing actions but do nothing to stop the immediate bleeding. They would be appropriate next steps after fundal massage. Putting the baby to the breast does release oxytocin, which causes uterine contraction and can help slow bleeding, but the response will be slower than fundal massage. **Focus:** Prioritization; **QSEN:** S, EBP; **Concept:** Clinical Judgement; **Cognitive Level:** Applying

4. **Ans: 1, 2, 3, 4**   The nurse should simply ask the unauthorized visitor to identify herself and her purpose on the unit. If any hostility or combativeness is encountered, security should be immediately called. Alerting the desk secretary to maintain close attentiveness to the infant security system would enhance patient safety and allow a security code to be quickly called if an infant were missing. After patient safety is assured, it is then the professional responsibility of the nurse to look at the system issues that caused the breach. The other nurse should be asked why the unauthorized visitor was allowed into the unit. A new nurse should not feel unable to respectfully question the actions of a more experienced nurse when appropriate for patient safety. A review of policies with the staff by the unit leadership would then further remind all staff of the need for constant vigilance and adherence to security systems in place to avoid risk to the patients in their care. **Focus:** Prioritization; **QSEN:** S, TC, QI; **Concept:** Safety, Collaboration; **Cognitive Level:** Evaluating; **IPEC:** T/T. **Test Taking Tip:** In a prioritization question, place the action that most directly assures patient safety first.

5. **Ans: 4**   The key information in the question is that the diagnosis is latent TB and a chest x-ray examination showed no evidence of active TB processes in the lungs. The patient is therefore not considered infectious to other patients, staff, or her newborn. Her breast milk is not infectious. The nurse should always consult the Infection Control department or supervising nurse for policies regarding isolation if unsure. **Focus:** Prioritization, Assignment; **QSEN:** S, EBP; **Concept:** Infection, Health Promotion; **Cognitive Level:** Evaluating; **IPEC:** IC, T/T

6. **Ans: 3**   Slight redness and pain in the left calf could be suggestive of thrombophlebitis and requires further investigation. The other findings are within normal limits for this point in the postpartum and postoperative course. **Focus:** Prioritization; **QSEN:** S; **Concept:** Safety; **Cognitive Level:** Analyzing

7. **Ans: 2**   The nurse would need to correct the statement that the mother would need to dump her milk. This is not necessary because the varicella infection is not found in the breast milk. The information should be promptly corrected so that the mother has no misconceptions or guilt. The other advice given by the student nurse is correct. The newborn should have received varicella-zoster immune globulin and may room with the mother in isolation from other patients. The mother should prevent the infant's skin from contact with varicella lesions, and the pediatrician should

be notified of maternal varicella. A mother with varicella should have standard, airborne, and contact precautions. Consultation with the Infection Control department or supervising nurse should also be done to check policies. **Focus:** Supervision, **QSEN:** S, EB; **Concept:** Safety, Evidence; **Cognitive Level:** Analyzing; **IPEC:** IC, T/T

8. **Ans: 4**   Edema at the base of the umbilical cord could indicate infection and should be reported to the HCP. The plastic umbilical cord clamp is normally removed about 24 hours after birth. The base of the cord may remain moist for a few days while the end of the cord becomes drier and brownish black in the early newborn period. **Focus:** Prioritization; **QSEN:** S; **Concept:** Infection, Health Promotion; **IPEC:** R/R; **Cognitive Level:** Analyzing

9. **Ans: 1**   The newborn should always be placed on her back to sleep with no pillows, blankets, or other items in the crib. The use of this sleep position has reduced the incidence of Sudden Infant Death Syndrome (SIDS). The nurse in this option does not insult the mother and affirms that the instruction given by the mother was at one time acceptable. The nurse then shares updated information with the mother of the patient and the patient and appeals to their shared goal of infant safety. Telling the mother that the baby looks comfortable or giving instruction on positioning the newborn's head while in the prone position implies approval of the position, which is contrary to infant safety. Bluntly telling the mother that the baby is more likely to die in this position is not effective teaching. It also undermines the role of the mother of the patient as a resource for the younger mother. **Focus:** Prioritization; **QSEN:** EBP, S; **Concept:** Patient Education, Communication; **Cognitive Level:** Analyzing

10. **Ans: 3**   The physical exam findings suggest that the urinary bladder is full and displacing the uterine fundus upward and to the right and causing discomfort to the woman. This can also increase vaginal bleeding because the uterus is prevented from contracting effectively, which decreases vaginal bleeding. The first action would be to assist the patient with emptying her bladder. Most patients can do so without the use of a catheter, which increases the risk of infection. If the patient is unable to void, which sometimes happens in the early postpartum period due to the use of anesthesia or urethral trauma at delivery, then a catheter would be used to empty the bladder. After assisting the patient with voiding, the nurse would reassess the abdomen to assure that the uterus is involuting normally and reassess the patient's pain level. Ibuprofen would be administered as ordered if pain persists. The HCP would be notified if the above measures did not resolve the problem. **Focus:** Prioritization; **QSEN:** EBP, S; **Concept:** Elimination, Pain, Clinical Judgement; **Cognitive Level:** Evaluation

11. **Ans: 2**   When a patient is angry, the nurse will explore what the source of the anger is and try to address it. The patient and her husband may be exhausted and sleep deprived. They may be unhappy with the way the birth occurred. They may be feeling inadequate in how to care for their newborn. They may be experiencing increased anxiety due to the pandemic and feel alone in facing the care of the newborn. The use of technology can allow the nurse to bring the family together virtually to help dispel some of these feelings. It would not be appropriate at this time to lecture the patient on the seriousness of the pandemic nor to try to circumvent infection control rules in place. Bringing the baby to the nursery would not help the parents gain confidence in the care of their infant. A break from the baby, though, may be helpful if the parents are exhausted and the baby is fussy. **Focus:** Prioritization; **QSEN:** PCC, S; **Concept:** Stress and Coping, Fatigue, Communication; **Cognitive Level:** Analyzing

12. **Ans: 2, 3, 6**   The AP can do assigned tasks such as vital signs, removal of a catheter, and calling to get paperwork faxed. The nurse would supervise the overall care of each patient and must be the one to review data such as lab reports and vital signs. The nurse would need to have a solid knowledge of what values are normal and to consult appropriately for abnormal findings. The nurse would also evaluate knowledge deficits in a patient and determine teaching effectiveness. **Focus:** Delegation; **QSEN:** TC; **Concept:** Leadership, Professional Identity; **IPEC:** R/R, IC; **Cognitive Level:** Evaluating

13. **Ans: 1**   Hot flashes are a common side effect with magnesium sulfate. Headaches could indicate worsening preeclampsia. Leg pain or shortness of breath would be symptoms needing prompt evaluation as they could indicate thrombosis. **Focus:** Prioritization; **QSEN:** S; **Concept:** Safety; **Cognitive Level:** Applying

14. **Ans: 2**   It is normal for a healthy, full-term breastfed newborn to lose 7–10% of their birth weight. It is usually regained by 2 weeks of age. The mother should be reassured that this is normal as well as given parameters for urine and stool output in the next few days. She should be taught signs of dehydration and given specific instructions regarding follow-up with a pediatric HCP. It would not be correct to advise the mother to start supplementing with formula either before or after breastfeeding at this time as this may interfere with the successful establishment of breastfeeding. It would be incorrect to tell the mother that a breastfed baby is never supplemented because there may be problems with breastfeeding where formula supplementation is needed. Many newborns are seen for follow-up by the HCP within 2–3 days of discharge, especially if weight loss has been an issue. **Focus:** Prioritization; **QSEN:** PCC, EBP, S; **Concept:** Nutrition, Patient Education; **Cognitive Level:** Evaluating

15. **Ans: 4** The mother is demonstrating behavior typical of the taking in the phase of new motherhood, where the woman may need to discuss the events she experienced in her birth, which may have been surprising or traumatic for her. She will typically progress then to the taking hold phase in which she is interested and able to take on care of the newborn. It would not be appropriate to call a social worker for this normal developmental phase. It also would not be appropriate to rush the mother through this phase and make her feel inadequate for not immediately being ready to focus on the newborn. The nurse would need to be sure the newborn's needs are met but would have an understanding of the mother's needs as well. The nurse would continue her care and observation of the mother–baby couplet to be sure the mother eventually feels ready and able to take on the care of the newborn. **Focus:** Prioritization; **QSEN:** PCC; **Concept:** Development, Family Dynamics; **Cognitive Level:** Analyzing

16. **Ans: 2, 3, 4, 5** Minimizing environmental noise, creating signage to designate when a patient is resting, empowering parents to restrict visitors when needing rest and working with the team to cluster care can all help to allow the postpartum family to get the rest they need. Adequate rest and sleep are restorative and help the family's emotional state. Nighttime vital signs cannot be eliminated for all patients because the immediate postpartum period is a time requiring great vigilance for complications in both the mother and the newborn. Moving the newborn to the nursery is not a recommended intervention, especially for the breastfeeding infant, as the infant needs to feed frequently. The mother can be helped to really rest between feedings. Part of the role of the nurse is to notice problems on the unit and work collaboratively to improve the systems in place. **Focus:** Prioritization, Delegation; **QSEN:** PCC, TC, EBP, QI; **Concept:** Sleep, Fatigue; **IPEC:** IC, T/T; **Cognitive Level:** Creating

17. **Ans: 1** The nurse would first explore what the reasons are for the father's refusal. Assessing his knowledge, beliefs, and fears about the injection would help direct to the nurse on next steps in education. He may ultimately still refuse the shot, but the nurse has a responsibility to explore the reason for refusal, listen to the father respectfully, and provide accurate education about the purpose of the injection. It would not be appropriate to simply state what the shot does. Accepting his refusal without exploring the situation does not demonstrate professionalism. **Focus:** Prioritization; **QSEN:** PCC, S; **Concept:** Patient Education; **Cognitive Level:** Analyzing

18. **Ans: 4** The findings that the AP has reported to the nurse are suggestive of preeclampsia with severe features and require immediate reporting to the HCP. The other responses delay the report of the abnormal findings. A delay in the recognition and appropriate treatment of postpartum pre- eclampsia can be associated with maternal seizure, stroke, or death. It would not be appropriate to delegate further evaluation to the AP at this time. **Focus:** Delegation, Prioritization; **QSEN:** TC, S; **Concept:** Communication, Safety; **IPEC:** R/R, IC, T/T; **Cognitive Level:** Evaluating

19. **Ans: 1, 2, 8** During phototherapy, the infant's eyes must be protected and the temperature carefully monitored to avoid both hypothermia and hyperthermia. Breastfeeding should be continued to avoid dehydration and to encourage passage of meconium, which helps to excrete bilirubin. The eye coverings should be removed when the parent is holding the infant to feed. This allows normal visual stimulation for the infant and normal face-to-face interaction with the parent. Ointments or lotions should not be applied to the skin during phototherapy as they may cause burns. The infant should be unclothed as much as possible during phototherapy to allow the benefit of the light directly to the skin. Encouraging continued breastfeeding and teaching the family the benefits of breastfeeding in this scenario helps support the Perinatal Core Measure of increasing the percentage of infants who are fed breast milk only. **Focus:** Supervision; **QSEN:** S; **Concept:** Leadership; **Cognitive Level:** Evaluating; **IPEC:** R/R

20. **Ans:**

	Anticipated	Nonessential	Contraindicated
Rubella vaccine IM	X		
Varicella vaccine subcutaneous			X
Rho (D) immune globulin injection 300 mcg IM	X		
Ferrous sulfate 325 mg daily PO		X	

The lab results indicate that the patient's blood type is Rh negative, and therefore if the baby's blood type is positive, the mother would need Rho(D) immune globulin. The purpose of Rho(D) immune globulin is to prevent the mother from developing antibodies in her blood, which could adversely affect a future pregnancy. She would also need a rubella vaccine because her results indicate she is not immune to rubella. This vaccine can safely be given to a breastfeeding patient prior to discharge. A varicella vaccine would be contraindicated because the patient's lab results indicate that she is immune to varicella. A ferrous sulfate supplement at this time would be nonessential because the patient's hemoglobin level is normal for the postpartum period. An iron supplement at this time could increase constipation, which is already a problem for many postpartum patients. **Focus:** Prioritization; **QSEN:** PCC, EBP, S; **Concept:** Health Promotion, Immunity; **Cognitive level:** Analyzing

QSEN Key: PCC, Patient-Centered Care; **TC,** Teamwork & Collaboration; **EBP,** Evidence-Based Practice; **QI,** Quality Improvement; **S,** Safety; **I,** Informatics.

IPEC Key: Domain 1 Values/Ethics (**V/E**); Domain 2 Roles/Responsibilities (**R/R**); Domain 3 Interprofessional Communication (**IC**); Domain 4 Teams/Teamwork (**T/T**).

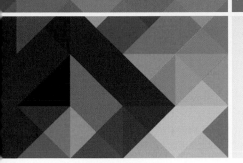

CHAPTER 17

LPN/LVN in the Pediatric Clinic Setting

PRIORITIZATION. DELEGATION, AND ASSIGNMENT

The LPN/LVN is working in a large pediatric clinic. The clinic provides pediatric care, which includes well visits and acute/sick visits.

Questions

1. A 7-year-old arrives at the health center complaining of tooth pain. The nurse observes the child to have frank caries. Which action is a **priority**?
   1. Take the child's temperature.
   2. Apply fluoride varnish.
   3. Administer ibuprofen.
   4. Inspect the oral cavity.

2. A 10-year-old arrives at the health center complaining of right eye pain. The right sclera is injected (red) and the child is complaining of pain and photophobia. The mother reports that the child was playing outside in the woods and poked his right eye with a tree branch. Which action is a **priority**?
   1. Administer ibuprofen.
   2. Flush the eye with saline.
   3. Set up a tray with fluorescein for the health care provider (HCP).
   4. Apply a cool compress for 10 minutes.

3. A 6-year-old girl arrives at the health center after sustaining a dog bite on the left lower leg. The child reports she was riding her bike when the neighbor's dog chased her and bit her on the left lower leg. The child immediately fell off the bike but quickly got back on and rode home. The father immediately brought the child to the pediatric clinic. The nurse observes multiple puncture wounds in the shape of a bite and multiple abrasions with road debris on the left lower leg. Which action is a **priority**?
   1. Contact the animal control officer.
   2. Administer human rabies immune globulin (HRIG).
   3. Apply a topical antibiotic ointment.
   4. Scrub the wound vigorously with soap and water.

4. A 2-year-old girl is brought to the pediatric clinic by her mother. The child had the first digit on her right hand "accidentally slammed in the car door." The nurse observes a subungual hematoma on the first digit of the right hand. The child is sitting on her mother's lap crying and holding her finger. Which action is a **priority**?
   1. Contact the child protection authorities.
   2. Set up cautery for the HCP.
   3. Apply a cold pack for 20 minutes.
   4. Determine the child's tetanus vaccine status.

5. An 18-month-old boy is brought to the pediatric clinic by his father. The child is crying and holding his left arm extended, internally rotated and adducted. The father relates that he does not know what happened. He was crossing the street with the child and holding his left hand. He helped the child jump up onto the curb and the child began crying shortly thereafter and refusing to move the left arm. Which action is a **priority**?
   1. Inform the HCP of the situation as this will likely require reduction.
   2. Ask the father when the last time the child ate, as anesthesia may be necessary.
   3. Apply an appropriately sized sling until the HCP is able to see the child.
   4. Apply ice to the arm and administer ibuprofen.

6. A 12-year-old boy arrives at the pediatric clinic with hives on the face and trunk. RR is 24 breaths/minute. Lung sounds are clear. There is no swelling of the face or lips. What action should the nurse take?
   1. Administer oxygen via face mask.
   2. Administer diphenylamine hydrochloride.
   3. Prepare the child for transport to the emergency room.
   4. Prepare to administer epinephrine.

7. A 6-week-old boy arrives at the pediatric clinic for a scheduled two-week follow-up after a surgical pyloromyotomy. The parents report that the child has experience vomiting once or twice a day for the past 3 days. The child is formula fed. The child has gained weight. On assessment, the child has 1 second capillary refill, an oral mucosa that is pink and moist, and tears with crying. What action should the nurse take?
   1. Reassure the parents the child is fine and vomiting will resolve over time.
   2. Suggest the parents keep the child upright 30 minutes after feeding.
   3. Inform the HCP as further assessment is required.
   4. Suggest the parents consider a formula change.

8. There are several children in the pediatric clinic who have procedures ordered by the HCP. Which action related to a child's care should the LPN/LVN delegate to the assistive personnel (AP)?
   1. Allergy shots for a 7-year-old child who is receiving them for the first time.
   2. Ear lavage for a 2-year-old with impacted cerumen in the right ear.
   3. Racemic epinephrine nebulizer treatment for an 18-month-old with croup.
   4. Administration of polyethylene glycol via gastrostomy for child with cerebral palsy.

9. The nurse is providing vision screen using the HOTV chart for a 3-year-old child. Which of the following would warrant a referral for further evaluation to an ophthalmologist?
   1. 20/30 vision in the right eye and 20/20 vision in the left eye.
   2. 20/20 vision in the right eye and 20/40 vision in the left eye.
   3. 20/30 vision in the right eye and 20/30 vision in the left eye.
   4. 20/40 vision in the right eye and 20/30 vision in the left eye.

10. The nurse is preparing a 9-month-old infant for a well-child visit with the HCP. When performing a developmental screening, the nurse records the highest level of developmental milestones the child has achieved. Which of the following assessments should be brought to the attention of the HCP?
   1. Babbles and coos; rolls from stomach to back; grasps objects.
   2. Says "ma-ma" and "da-da"; bangs objects together; sits without support.
   3. Understands "no"; feeds self; pulls to stand.
   4. Copies sounds; drops objects.

11. The HCP is evaluating an infant with developmental hip dysplasia. The nurse is preparing to provide parent education regarding the treatment of this condition. Which of the following teaching points should the nurse anticipate?
   1. Instruction for application of triple diapering.
   2. Instruction for passive range of motion.
   3. Instruction for pain relief measures.
   4. Instruct for application of a Pavlik harness.

12. The HCP is evaluating a 2-year-old who experienced a febrile seizure. The nurse is preparing to provide parent education regarding the treatment of this condition. Which of the following teaching points should the nurse anticipate?
   1. Instruction on safety measures if the child experiences another seizure.
   2. Instruction on the administration of phenobarbital.
   3. Instruction on alternating ibuprofen with acetaminophen whenever the child appears ill.
   4. Instruction on activity restrictions required for children with seizures.

13. A 7-year-old with head lice arrives at the pediatric health clinic with his mother. The child resides with his mother, father, and three other siblings. The nurse is preparing to provide education on head lice. What should be included in the teaching plan?
   1. The entire family will need to be treated with a pediculicide.
   2. The child cannot return to school until all of the nits are gone.
   3. Combs and brushes should be washed with a pediculicide.
   4. Apply olive oil or petrolatum to the hair to suffocate the lice.

14. A 16-year-old girl arrives at the pediatric clinic with her mother after sustaining a head injury during a soccer game. The girl headed the ball and is now complaining of a headache. What is a **priority** assessment question the nurse should ask?
   1. Can you describe what happened?
   2. Did anyone else witness the event?
   3. Did you vomit after the injury?
   4. How would you rate your pain on a scale from 1 to 10?

Answer Key for this chapter begins on p. 118

15. A child with iron deficiency anemia is receiving supplemental iron therapy. The father calls the nurse at the pediatric clinic concerned because the child's stools have become dark. What advice should the nurse provide?
   1. Continue supplemental iron therapy as ordered.
   2. Check the child's stool for the presence of occult blood.
   3. Discontinue supplemental iron therapy as this is a serious complication.
   4. Administer the iron supplementation every other day.

16. A 6-month-old infant who is not yet walking arrived at the health center with bruises on the lower extremities. How does the nurse interpret these findings?
   1. This is a normal finding for a 6-month-old infant.
   2. Further evaluation is needed to determine if there has been abuse.
   3. The infant may have a bleeding disorder.
   4. The bruises may be an indication of family stress.

17. Drag and Drop._____
Instructions: Indicate which staff member in the left column is appropriate for each intervention. In the right-hand column, write in the best staff member for each intervention. Note that all responses will be used and may be used more than once.

Staff Members	Interventions
RN	_____A 17-year-old with a migraine accompanied by nausea and vomiting who just received intravenous prochlorperazine requires repeat vital signs and mouth care.
LPN/LVN	_____A 2-year-old child with myelomeningocele (spina bifida) whose parents need reinforcement on clean intermittent catherization (CIC).
AP	_____A 14-year-old adolescent in sickle cell crisis who requires intravenous hydration and morphine patient-controlled analgesic (PCA).
	_____A 10-year-old child with acute lymphoblastic leukemia requires a blood transfusion.
	_____A 12-year-old child with type 1 diabetes mellitus requires observation using an insulin pump.
	_____A 2-month-old infant with cystic fibrosis whose parents require teaching regarding disease management.
	_____A 3-year-old child with grade IV vesicoureteral reflux and a urinary tract infection requires an intramuscular injection of ceftriaxone.
	_____A 6-year-old child with moderate asthma is experiencing an exacerbation and requires monitoring and an albuterol nebulizer treatment.
	_____An 18-month-old with croup is experiencing stridor and needs nebulized racemic epinephrine.
	_____A 13-year-old with moderate factor VIII deficiency requires intravenous recombinant human coagulation factor VIII replacement therapy.

18. A 4-year-old with severe atopic dermatitis arrives at the health center with several ill-distinct erythematous crusted plaques on the lower extremities. The parent reports the child is experiencing interrupted sleep as a result of itching. Which of the following teaching points should the nurse anticipate? **Select all that apply.**
   1. Wet wraps.
   2. Bleach baths.
   3. Vaccine recommendations.
   4. Emollient therapy.
   5. Daily administration of melatonin.
   6. Topical steroid application.
   7. Administration of an oral antibiotic.

19. A 6-year-old child who is experiencing an asthma exacerbation arrives at the health center. Which task can the LPN/LVN delegate to AP?
   1. Administering an albuterol nebulizer treatment.
   2. Obtaining vital signs.
   3. Administering oral prednisone.
   4. Administering oxygen via nasal cannula.

 Answer Key for this chapter begins on p. 118

Answers

PART 2 Common Health Scenarios

1. **Ans: 1** The priority assessment in this situation is to determine if there is an infection, specifically an abscess. Fever is an indicator of infection which may warrant urgent treatment. Ibuprofen may be administered after taking the temperature as well as inspecting the oral cavity and applying fluoride varnish. **Focus:** Prioritization; **QSEN:** PCC, EBP; **Concept:** Infection; **Cognitive Level:** Applying

2. **Ans: 3** The history of the incident and complaints of photophobia and pain are consistent with a corneal abrasion. The HCP will need fluorescein dye and a Wood's lamp in order to ascertain if a corneal abrasion is present. The nurse would not flush the eye until an assessment is performed by the HCP and the HCP orders this treatment. Ibuprofen for pain may be helpful but an evaluation by the HCP is a priority. A cool compress is unlikely to relieve the pain because the damage is not in the area of the orbit. **Focus:** Prioritization; **QSEN:** EBP, S; **Concept:** Infection, Tissue Integrity, Inflammation; **Cognitive Level:** Applying

3. **Ans: 4** According to the American Academy of Pediatrics Committee on Infectious Diseases, the first action is to thoroughly clean the wound to remove debris and bacteria. Until a thorough assessment is completed by the HCP, the need to call the animal control officer or administer HRIG cannot be determined. A topical antibiotic ointment should not be applied until the wound is cleaned and the HCP has completed the evaluation. **Focus:** Prioritization; **QSEN:** EBP, S; **Concept:** Infection; Tissue Integrity; **Cognitive Level:** Applying

4. **Ans: 2** A subungual hematoma is a common childhood injury. The nurse would want to obtain more information about the incident but pain relief is the priority. Trephination of subungual hematomas (i.e., making a hole in the nail) using cautery drains the blood and relieves the pain. This must be performed by a HCP. Tetanus is not of concern as this is a clean closed wound/injury. **Focus:** Prioritization; **QSEN:** EBP, S; **Concept:** Infection, Pain; **Cognitive Level:** Applying

5. **Ans: 1** This injury is consistent with nursemaid's elbow, a common childhood injury that often occurs when an adult holds the child's hand and suddenly pulls on the arm to avoid a dangerous situation or to help the child onto a step or curb. Reduction of nursemaid's elbow is an outpatient procedure that does not require anesthesia. Neither a sling nor ice is indicated. With reduction the pain is relieved immediately and ibuprofen is not warranted. **Focus:** Prioritization; **QSEN:** EBP, S; **Concept:** Pain; **Cognitive Level:** Applying

6. **Ans: 2** The child is not exhibiting any signs of anaphylaxis, which would require transport to the emergency room, oxygen, and administration of epinephrine. Diphenylamine hydrochloride is an over-the-counter antihistamine that can provide symptomatic relief. **Focus:** Prioritization; **QSEN:** EBP, S; **Concept:** Safety; **Cognitive Level:** Applying

7. **Ans: 3** A pyloromyotomy is a surgical procedure used to correct hypertrophic pyloric stenosis. This surgical procedure involves an incision to cut the thickened pylorus muscle, which causes the mechanical obstruction associated with hypertrophic pyloric stenosis. The child is now 2 weeks postsurgery. It is not expected that the child would continue to have vomiting. Vomiting can be related to the surgery or another underlying condition such as gastroesophageal reflux. However, this assessment needs to be completed by the HCP. **Focus:** Prioritization; **QSEN:** EBP, S; **Concept:** Clinical Judgement; **Cognitive Level:** Applying

8. **Ans: 2** Postassessments and monitoring during the procedure are required for first-time allergy shots, administration of racemic epinephrine, and gastrostomy administration of polyethylene glycol. This is beyond the scope of practice for an AP. An AP can perform an ear lavage independently as postassessment is not required by the AP. **Focus:** Delegation; **QSEN:** S; **Concept:** Safety, Care Coordination; **Cognitive Level:** Applying; **IPEC:** R/R

9. **Ans: 2** Three-year-old children do not have 20/20 vision. Recommendations for referral include 20/50 or worse in either eye or a two-line difference between eyes. **Focus:** Prioritization; **QSEN:** EBP; **Concept:** Sensory Perception, Development; **Cognitive Level:** Analyzing

10. **Ans: 1** Answers 2, 3, and 4 are all expected milestones for a 9-month-old. Babbling and cooing is achieved at 2 to 6 months; rolling from stomach to back is achieved at 4 months; and banging objects together is achieved at 6 months. These findings indicate a developmental delay and warrant further evaluation by the HCP. **Focus:** Prioritization; **QSEN:** EBP; **Concept:** Development; **Cognitive Level:** Applying. **Test Taking Tip:** NCLEX is likely to test your knowledge of growth and development because early recognition and intervention of developmental delays is associated with better patient outcomes.

11. **Ans: 4** The treatment for developmental hip dysplasia is a Pavlik harness. Triple diapering does not ensure consistent or sufficient hip abduction needed to provide a therapeutic effect. Passive range-of-motion is not indicated for developmental hip dysplasia. Developmental hip dysplasia has not been associated with pain; hence ibuprofen is not required for this condition. **Focus:** Prioritization **QSEN:** EBP; **Concept:** Patient Education **Cognitive Level:** Applying

12. **Ans: 1** Educating parents about what to expect with a febrile seizure and how to keep the child safe is a priority. Febrile seizures generally occur in children 6 months to 5 years old. Phenobarbital is not recommended for the prevention of febrile seizures. The efficacy of alternating ibuprofen with acetaminophen for fever in general has not been established. Advising parents to administer these medications whenever the child appears ill can result in excessive use when not warranted and may have adverse effects. Activity restrictions are not required for febrile seizures. **Focus:** Prioritization; **QSEN:** EBP; **Concept:** Safety; **Cognitive Level:** Applying

13. **Ans: 3** Cleaning brushes and combs with pediculicides reduces transmission and reinfestation. All household members and other close contacts should be checked for head lice but only those persons with evidence of an active infestation should be treated. The American Academy of Pediatrics (AAP) and the National Association of School Nurses (NASN) advocate that "no-nit" policies should be discontinued because nits are empty shells, not viable lice. Olive oil and petrolatum are not effective pediculicides. **Focus:** Prioritization; **QSEN:** EBP; **Concept:** Infection; **Cognitive Level:** Applying. **Test Taking Tip:** Professional organizations, such as AAP and NASN, are good sources for EBP and frequently have updated guidelines and recommendations for practice.

14. **Ans: 1** Asking the patient to describe the incident allows the nurse to determine if the patient lost consciousness and orientation level. The other questions may add to the assessment but establishing if a loss of consciousness occurred and orientation is a priority. **Focus:** Prioritization; **QSEN:** EBP; **Concept:** Intracranial Regulation; **Cognitive Level:** Applying. **Test Taking Tip:** When an injury or accident occurs, asking about the mechanism of injury helps the health care team to anticipate and monitor for occult damage.

15. **Ans: 1** Supplemental iron can result in dark stools. This does not indicate blood in the stool and the iron supplementation should be continued. **Focus:** Prioritization; **QSEN:** EBP; **Concept:** Nutrition; **Cognitive Level:** Applying

16. **Ans: 2** The bruises are inconsistent with the developmental level of a 6-month-old who is not yet walking. These findings raise the question of abuse. Additional assessment is required as it is possible that there may be an alternate explanation for the bruising such as an undiagnosed bleeding disorder. **Focus:** Prioritization; **QSEN:** S, PCC; **Concept:** Development; **Cognitive Level:** Applying

17. **Ans:**

Staff Members	Interventions
RN	__AP_____ A 17-year-old with a migraine accompanied by nausea and vomiting who just received intravenous prochlorperazine requires repeat vital signs and mouth care.
LPN/LVN	__LPN/LVN___ A 2 year old child with myelomeningocele (spina bifida) whose parents need reinforcement on clean intermittent catherization (CIC).
AP	___RN_____ A 14-year-old adolescent in sickle cell crisis who requires intravenous hydration and morphine patient-controlled analgesic (PCA).
	___RN_____ A 10-year-old child with acute lymphoblastic leukemia requires a blood transfusion.
	__LPN/LVN___ A 12-year-old child with type 1 diabetes mellitus requires observation using an insulin pump.
	___RN_____ A 2-month-old infant with cystic fibrosis whose parents require teaching regarding disease management.
	__LPN/LVN___ A 3-year-old child with grade IV vesicoureteral reflux and a urinary tract infection requires an intramuscular injection of ceftriaxone.
	__LPN/LVN___ A 6-year-old child with moderate asthma is experiencing an exacerbation and requires monitoring and an albuterol nebulizer treatment.
	___RN_____ An 18-month-old with croup is experiencing stridor and needs nebulized racemic epinephrine.
	___RN_____ A 13-year-old with moderate factor VIII deficiency requires intravenous recombinant human coagulation factor VIII replacement therapy.

An LPN/LVN is licensed to deliver oral and intramuscular injections and is allowed to reinforce patient education that the RN previously delivered. The LPN/LVN is also allowed to observe how well a patient performs a skill. The RN must deliver intravenous fluids and medications and deliver patient teaching about disease management. The RN should deliver the racemic epinephrine to a child with croup as this represents a medical emergency and the child needs serial assessments and response to treatment. The AP can take vital signs and provide mouth care. **Focus:** Assignment, Prioritization; **QSEN:** S, PCC; **Concept:** Safety, Care Coordination; **Cognitive Level:** Analyzing; **Cognitive Skill:** Take Action

18. **Ans: 1, 2, 4, 6, 7** Atopic dermatitis is a chronic inflammatory disease in which there is a defect in filaggrin protein. This defect results in a more permeable stratum corneum (the outer layer of the skin), which results in water loss to the skin and easier entry of pathogens. Wet wraps combined with emollient therapy are occlusive and return moisture to the skin. Topical steroids are the mainstay of treatment for inflammation associated with atopic dermatitis. The crusting is indicative of a staphylococcus infection, which requires an oral antibiotic to treat the current infections and bleach baths to eradicate colonization of staphylococcus on the skin. There are no vaccines to prevent staphylococcus infections of the skin. Melatonin is a hormone that may improve sleep but does not relieve itching associated with atopic dermatitis. An antihistamine is recommended for itching. **Focus:** Prioritization; **QSEN:** S, PCC, EBP; **Concept:** Safety, Patient Teaching, Tissue Integrity; **Cognitive Level:** Analyzing

19. **Ans: 2** Administering medications requires assessment of effectiveness and potential adverse reactions. Albuterol, prednisone, and oxygen are medications. This is not within the scope of practice for AP. Obtaining vital signs can be delegated to AP under the supervision of an LPN/LVN. **Focus:** Delegation; **QSEN:** S; **Concept:** Safety; **Cognitive Level:** Applying

QSEN Key: PCC, Patient-Centered Care; **TC,** Teamwork & Collaboration; **EBP,** Evidence-Based Practice; **QI,** Quality Improvement; **S,** Safety; **I,** Informatics.

IPEC Key: Domain 1 Values/Ethics (**V/E**); Domain 2 Roles/Responsibilities (**R/R**); Domain 3 Interprofessional Communication (**IC**); Domain 4 Teams/Teamwork (**T/T**).

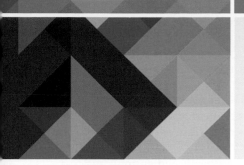

Pharmacology

Questions

1. The nurse administers a patient's morning oral dose of lisinopril. Which finding indicates to the nurse that the drug is having its intended action?
   1. Patient's heart rate is 72 beats per minute.
   2. Patient's blood pressure is 124/80.
   3. Patient's lungs are clear to auscultation.
   4. Patient's urine output increases.

2. Which instruction is **most** important when the nurse gives a patient the first dose of an antihypertensive drug?
   1. "Your blood pressure will be checked twice a shift today."
   2. "Drink extra fluids during the day today."
   3. "Be sure to call for assistance when you first get out of bed."
   4. "Save all urine for measurement of output today."

3. What is the **most** important instruction for the nurse to provide for the assistive personnel (AP) when providing care for a male patient who is receiving an intravenous dose of furosemide?
   1. "Make sure that his urinal is available and remind him to save all urine because we will be measuring his urine output."
   2. "Keep the patient on bed rest until we know whether the drug is working like it should."
   3. "Check the patient's blood pressure and heart rate every 2 hours and report any changes that you find."
   4. "Encourage the patient to drink a glass of water every 2 hours and be sure that his water pitcher is kept full."

4. A patient with atrial fibrillation is prescribed atenolol 50 mg orally once a day. The AP reports these vital signs to the nurse: T 99.8°F (37.7°C), HR 48/min, RR 20/min, BP 102/78. Which **priority** actions will the nurse take before administering this medication? **Select all that apply.**
   1. Administering acetaminophen 650 mg for elevated temperature.
   2. Instructing the AP to recheck the patient's vital signs in 30 minutes.
   3. Checking an apical pulse on the patient to confirm the heart rate.
   4. Holding the dose of atenolol.
   5. Notifying the health care provider (HCP).
   6. Asking the patient to sit down and rechecking the blood pressure.

5. According to research, which are the two most common mistakes patients make when using a metered-dose inhaler?
   1. Using an inhaler without inhaling first and not waiting long enough between puffs.
   2. Not using a spacer and exhaling before medication absorbs into lung tissue.
   3. Using the inhaler with the cap in place and improper use of the mouthpiece.
   4. Using an inhaler without exhaling first and failing to shake the inhaler before use.

6. The RN supervisor is responsible for the care of eight patients in a medical care unit. Which tasks would be **best** for the RN to assign to the LPN/LVN? **Select all that apply.**
   1. Administer sliding scale (SS) insulin to a patient with type 1 diabetes.
   2. Perform a urinary catheter insertion on a patient with acute renal failure.
   3. Assist a patient with morning mouth care and bath.
   4. Give a patient an acetaminophen suppository.
   5. Check vital signs on a patient who was admitted with dizziness.
   6. Feed a patient who had a stroke 4 days ago.

7. The nurse is to give a patient heparin 4000 units subcutaneously. The 1 mL vial contains heparin 5000 units. How many mL will the nurse administer?
   1. 0.2 mL.
   2. 0.4 mL.
   3. 0.6 mL.
   4. 0.8 mL.

Copyright © 2023 by Elsevier, Inc. All rights reserved.

8. Which patient care action would the nurse safely delegate to an AP when administering beclomethasone by multidose inhaler (MDI) to a patient with asthma?
   1. Teach the patient how to clean the inhaler.
   2. Assist the patient with rinsing the mouth with water or mouth wash after inhaler use.
   3. Assess the patient's mouth for white patches on the tongue.
   4. Listen to the lungs for abnormal breath sounds before and after MDI use.

9. The nurse is administering promethazine 12.5 mg orally to a patient experiencing nausea and vomiting. For which common side effect will the nurse be sure to monitor?
   1. Increased heart rate.
   2. Hyperactive bowel sounds.
   3. Drowsiness.
   4. Constipation.

10. A patient is prescribed atorvastatin 40 mg orally each day for hypercholesterolemia. Which statement by the patient requires that the nurse notify the HCP immediately?
    1. "I'm feeling a little stomach upset today."
    2. "I woke up with a headache this morning."
    3. "I'm very thirsty and hungry today."
    4. "I'm having pain in my calf muscle now."

11. Which actions or interventions will the nurse give as instructions to the AP when providing care for a patient who takes a drug that affects blood clotting? **Select all that apply.**
    1. Report any signs of bleeding in the patient's urine or stool.
    2. Provide the patient with a stiff toothbrush for cleaning teeth.
    3. Shave the patient using an electric razor.
    4. Recheck the patient's vital signs and oxygen saturation.
    5. Remove any extra or unused equipment from the patient's room.
    6. Teach the patient the importance of avoiding high-impact exercise.

12. Which statement by a patient prescribed enoxaparin indicates the need for additional teaching?
    1. "I will be sure to get regular follow-up laboratory clotting studies."
    2. "I will inform my HCP if I notice blood in my urine."
    3. "I will remove all throw rugs from my home."
    4. "I will avoid taking aspirin or aspiring-containing products."

13. A patient is prescribed loperamide 2 mg orally as needed. Which finding indicates that the drug has been effective?
    1. The patient reports a bowel movement with a small hard stool.
    2. The patient reports relief from nausea and vomiting.
    3. The patient reports no further diarrheal stools.
    4. The patient reports relief from gastric reflux.

14. The nurse is administering oral memantine 5 mg to a 72-year-old patient with Alzheimer's disease. His wife asks about the purpose of the drug. What is the nurse's **best** response?
    1. "Taken twice a day, memantine will cure your husband's illness over time."
    2. "Memantine may temporarily slow the progression of dementia symptoms."
    3. "This drug will help to control some of your husband's symptoms."
    4. "Memantine was developed for Parkinson disease but may also help your husband."

15. A patient is prescribed amitriptyline for the treatment of depression. Which question will the nurse ask related to the action of this drug?
    1. "How long have you experienced symptoms of depression?"
    2. "Do you often feel anxious in certain situations?"
    3. "Do you smoke cigarettes and if so, how much do you smoke?"
    4. "Do you currently take over-the-counter ginseng?"

16. Which patient will the nurse assess **first** before giving his or her prescribed medication?
    1. 56-year-old prescribed furosemide whose 24-hour urine output was 1220 mL.
    2. 67-year-old prescribed amlodipine whose blood pressure is 142/80.
    3. 74-year-old prescribed docusate who reports constipation.
    4. 82-year-old prescribed digoxin whose heart rate is 52/min and irregular.

17. A patient diagnosed with overactive bladder is prescribed oxybutynin XL. Which action will the nurse safely delegate to the AP?
    1. Teaching the patient not to crush, chew, break, or open the capsule.
    2. Weighing the patient and reporting a weight gain of more than 2 pounds per day.
    3. Instructing the patient to report urinary urgency or frequency to the HCP.
    4. Assessing the patient for dry eyes, dry mouth, headache, dizziness, or constipation.

18. The nurse is providing care for a patient with hypothyroidism who is prescribed levothyroxine 75 mcg daily. For which side effects will the nurse monitor? **Select all that apply.**

1. Difficulty sleeping.
2. Lack of energy.
3. Fine tremors of the hands.
4. Decreased heart rate.
5. Increased blood pressure.
6. Feeling cold all the time.

19. Nextgen (Cloze) _____

Scenario: The nurse is providing care for a patient with erectile dysfunction. The patient will be discharged with a prescription for a _____1_____ drug for the treatment of this disorder. The nurse will instruct the patient about _____2_____. A contraindication for use of this drug would be _____3_____. The nurse will tell the patient to contact the HCP for ___4___ and ___5___.

Instructions: Complete the sentences below by choosing the best option for the missing information that corresponds with the numbered list of options provided below.

PART 2

Common Health Scenarios

Options for 1	Options for 2	Options for 3	Options for 4 & 5
Beta-blocker antihypertensive	Need for sexual stimulation for drug to work	Over-the-counter use of ginkgo biloba	Erection that lasts more than 4 hours
Loop diuretic	Need to take the drug 4 hours before sexual activity	Concurrent use of a nitrate drug	Occurrence of headache
Phosphodiesterase-5 inhibitor	Need to monitor blood pressure and heartrate before and after sex	Diagnosis of hypothyroidism	Prolonged and painful erection
Testosterone replacer	Need for surgery to insert a penile implant	Family history of coronary artery disease	Gastrointestinal upset

20. Nextgen (Hot Spot) _____

Scenario: The patient diagnosed with a bacterial pneumonia is prescribed amoxicillin 250 mg orally every 6 hours. On assessment, it is discovered that the patient is experiencing nausea and vomiting and chills. The AP reports that the patient's vital signs are T 101.4°F (38.5°C), HR 88/min, RR 28/min, BP 132/84. A rash is seen on the patient's face and chest and the patient does not know his current location.

Instructions: Highlight or underline the findings in the scenario that indicate the patient is experiencing a side effect or adverse effect of a penicillin drug.

    Answer Key for this chapter begins on p. 124

Answers

1. **Ans: 2** Lisinopril is an angiotensin-converting-enzyme (ACE) inhibitor. These drugs are antihypertensives with the action of relaxing arterial vessels and lowering blood pressure. **Focus:** Prioritization; **QSEN:** EBP, PCC, S; **Concept:** Clinical Judgment, Perfusion; **Cognitive Level:** Analyzing; **Cognitive Skill:** Recognizes Cues. **Test Taking Tip:** Drugs with generic names that end in "pril" are from the category ACE inhibitors which are antihypertensive.

2. **Ans: 3** After the first dose of any antihypertensive drug, the patient is at risk for dizziness due to decreased blood pressure and should be instructed to call for assistance until the effects of the drug are known. **Focus:** Prioritization; **QSEN:** EBP, PCC, S; **Concept:** Perfusion, Safety; **Cognitive Level:** Applying

3. **Ans: 1** Furosemide is a loop diuretic. When it is given in IV form, the drug works rapidly, so the patient will need to void very soon. The urinal should be easily available for use, and urine should be saved and measured to determine if the drug is having the expected effect. The patient does not need to be kept on bed rest. While checking vital signs is necessary, frequent checks are not needed unless the patient develops signs of dehydration. Encouraging extra fluids is not indicated for a patient receiving diuretic therapy. **Focus:** Delegation; Supervision; **QSEN:** PCC, TC; **Concept:** Elimination; **Cognitive Level:** Applying

4. **Ans: 3, 4, 5, 6** Atenolol is a beta-blocker drug with the action of slowing a patient's heart rate. A heart rate of 48/min is a bradycardia (slow rate). The nurse would recheck the heart rate by using the apical pulse and would also recheck the patient's blood pressure. If the nurse finds that the patient is experiencing bradycardia, the nurse would hold the atenolol and notify the HCP. Giving the scheduled dose would make the patient's slow heart rate worse. Waiting 30 minutes to recheck vital signs would be too long. Giving acetaminophen will not help the patient's heart rate. **Focus:** Prioritization, Delegation; **QSEN:** PCC, TC, S; **Concept:** Perfusion, Safety; **Cognitive Level:** Analyzing; **Cognitive Skill:** Analyzing Cues. **Test Taking Tip:** Drugs whose generic names end in "olol" are from the category of beta-blockers. They slow the heart rate and are used to treat hypertension, heart failure, and coronary artery disease.

5. **Ans: 4** A recent study revealed that the most common mistake with patients using an inhaler was not exhaling before using an inhaler. The second most common mistake was failure to shake the inhaler before use. **Focus:** Prioritization; **QSEN:** EBP, PCC, S; **Concept:** Gas Exchange; **Cognitive Level:** Applying

6. **Ans: 1, 2, 4** Administering medications and insertion of urinary catheters are within the scope of practice for an LPN/LVN. While the nurse could also check vital signs, feed patients, and assist with morning care, these tasks are better delegated to the AP. **Focus:** Assignment, Delegation; **QSEN:** TC, PCC; **Concept:** Care Coordination; **Cognitive Level:** Applying. **Test Taking Tip:** When assigning or delegating patient care, the nurse must be familiar with scope of practice for members of the health care team. Scope of practice may vary from state to state, so the nurse must review this for the state and facility where they practice.

7. **Ans: 4** The nurse must calculate the dosage. Have 1 mL/5000 units: need X mL/4000 units = 0.8 mL. **Focus:** Prioritization; **QSEN:** PCC, S; **Concept:** Safety; **Cognitive Level:** Analyzing

8. **Ans: 2** Beclomethasone is an antiinflammatory drug. Side effects of inhaled antiinflammatory drugs include leaving a bad taste in the mouth after use and increased risk for oral candidiasis (thrush). Rinsing with water or mouthwash helps remove the drug from the mouth and reduce the bad taste and oral infection risk and is within the scope of practice for APs. Teaching and assessing require additional skill and are appropriate to the scope of practice for professional nurses. **Focus:** Delegation; **Concept:** Care Coordination, Patient Care; **QSEN:** PCC, TC; **Cognitive Level:** Applying; **IPEC:** R/R

9. **Ans: 3** Promethazine is a phenothiazine drug commonly prescribed for nausea and vomiting. Common side effects include confusion, disorientation, dizziness, dry mouth, rash, and sedation. The nurse would monitor for sedation effects (e.g., drowsiness) and would be sure the call light was within reach and instruct the patient to call for help when getting out of bed. **Focus:** Prioritization; **QSEN:** PCC, S; **Concept:** Safety; **Cognitive Level:** Analyzing

10. **Ans: 4** Statins drugs can cause the adverse effect of rhabdomyolysis (muscle breakdown). Signs and symptoms include general muscle soreness, muscle pain and weakness, vomiting, stomach pain, and brown urine. The HCP must be notified immediately to stop the drug and prescribe another type of drug to control elevated cholesterol. **Focus:** Prioritization; **QSEN:** PCC, S, TC; **Concept:** Clinical Judgment, Safety; **Cognitive Level:** Analyzing; **IPEC:** IC

11. **Ans: 1, 3, 4, 5** A soft toothbrush should be provided to prevent bleeding from the gums. Removing extra or unused equipment from the room prevents trauma from accidentally colliding into the equipment while out of bed. The AP can remind patients about what

has already been taught, but the actual teaching must be done by the professional nurse. Options 1, 3, 4, and 5 are appropriate to the care of a patient receiving anticoagulant drugs and to the scope of practice for an AP. **Focus:** Delegation, Supervision; **QSEN:** PCC, S; **Concept:** Perfusion (Clotting); **Cognitive Level:** Analyzing

12. **Ans: 1**   An advantage of low-molecular weight heparins (e.g., enoxaparin) is that there is no need for repeated laboratory values to guide the therapy. Options 2, 3, and 4 are appropriate when a patient is prescribed this drug. **Focus:** Prioritization; **QSEN:** PCC, S; **Concept:** Perfusion (Clotting), Patient Education; **Cognitive Level:** Analyzing

13. **Ans: 3**   Loperamide is an antidiarrheal drug. Relief from diarrhea and no further diarrheal stools is the expected outcome for this drug. **Focus:** Prioritization; **QSEN:** PCC; **Concept:** Elimination, Clinical Judgment; **Cognitive Level:** Analyzing

14. **Ans: 2**   No drug has been developed that protects a patient's neurons from the changes that occur with Alzheimer's disease. Drug treatments have been developed that can temporarily slow the progression of symptoms in some patients (e.g., memantine, donepezil, galantamine, rivastigmine). **Focus:** Prioritization; **QSEN:** PCC, EBP; **Concept:** Cognition, Sensory Perception, Patient (Family) Education; **Cognitive Level:** Analyzing

15. **Ans: 3**   Amitriptyline is a tricyclic antidepressant (TCA). Smoking cigarettes may decrease the effectiveness of these drugs. The nurse would also ask about the use of St. John's wort, which is an herbal product used to treat depression. If the patient smokes or uses St. John's wort, the nurse would notify the HCP. Options 1 and 2 are not related to the action of amitriptyline. **Focus:** Prioritization; **QSEN:** PCC, S; **Concept:** Mood and Affect, Safety; **Cognitive Level:** Analyzing

16. **Ans: 4**   A common side effect of digoxin is bradycardia and a slow, irregular heart rate could be a sign of drug toxicity. This patient's situation is the most urgent and should be assessed first. **Focus:** Prioritization; **QSEN:** PCC, S; **Concept:** Perfusion, Clinical Judgment, Safety; **Cognitive Level:** Analyzing

17. **Ans: 2**   An AP's scope of practice includes weighing patients and the nurse would instruct the AP to report a weight gain, which could indicate fluid retention. The nurse would teach the patient to swallow the capsule whole for timed release of the drug. The nurse would also teach the patient to report any urinary difficulty. Assessing patients requires the skills of a professional nurse. **Focus:** Delegation; **QSEN:** PCC, TC; **Concept:** Elimination, Care Coordination; **Cognitive Level:** Applying; **IPEC:** IC

18. **Ans: 1, 3, 5**   The most common side effects of levothyroxine are symptoms of drug overdose, which are those of hyperthyroidism (e.g., difficulty sleeping, fine hand tremors, high blood pressure, irregular heartbeats, rapid heart rate, elevated body temperature). Lack of energy, slow heart rate, and feeling cold all the time are symptoms of hypothyroidism. **Focus:** Prioritization; **QSEN:** PCC, S; **Concept:** Hormonal Regulation, Clinical Judgment; **Cognitive Level:** Analyzing

19. **Ans:**   The nurse is providing care for a patient with erectile dysfunction. The patient will be discharged with a prescription for a **phosphodiesterase-5 inhibitor** drug for the treatment of this disorder. The nurse will instruct the patient about the **need for sexual stimulation for the drug to work**. A contraindication for the use of this drug would be **concurrent use of a nitrate drug**. The nurse will tell the patient to contact the HCP for an **erection that lasts more than 4 hours** and a **prolonged and painful erection** (priapism). **Focus:** Prioritization; **QSEN:** PCC, S; **Concept:** Sexuality; **Cognitive Level:** Analyzing; **Cognitive Skill:** Recognizes Cues

20. **Ans:**

> **Scenario:** The patient diagnosed with a bacterial pneumonia is prescribed amoxicillin 250 mg orally every 6 hours. On assessment, it is discovered that the patient is experiencing <u>nausea and vomiting and chills</u>. The AP reports that the patient's vital signs are <u>T 101.4°F (38.5°C)</u>, HR 88/min, RR 28/min, BP 132/84. A <u>rash is seen on the patient's face and chest</u> and the patient does not know his current location.

Instructions: Highlight or underline the findings that indicate the patient is experiencing a side effect of a penicillin drug.

Rationale: Common side effects of penicillin drugs (e.g., amoxicillin) include allergic reactions with signs and symptoms that include nausea and vomiting, fever, chills, and "red man syndrome" with rash and redness of the face, neck, upper chest, upper back, and arms. Other side effects can include reduced hearing and reduced kidney function. Central nervous system changes such as confusion and seizures are adverse effects that can occur with carbapenem antibacterial drugs (e.g., ertapenem, imipenem, meropenem). **Focus:** Prioritization; **QSEN:** PCC, EBP, S; **Concept:** Infection; **Cognitive Level:** Analyzing; **Cognitive Skill:** Analyzes Cues.

QSEN Key: PCC, Patient-Centered Care; **TC,** Teamwork & Collaboration; **EBP,** Evidence-Based Practice; **QI,** Quality Improvement; **S,** Safety; **I,** Informatics.

IPEC Key: Domain 1 Values/Ethics (**V/E**); Domain 2 Roles/Responsibilities (**R/R**); Domain 3 Interprofessional Communication (**IC**); Domain 4 Teams/Teamwork (**T/T**).

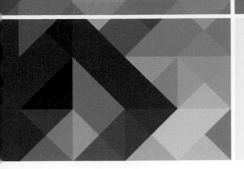

CHAPTER 19
Medication Administration

Questions

1. When a medication is to be given to a patient, which information must the nurse check before administering the drug? **Select all that apply.**
   1. Amount of drug per dose.
   2. Route of administration.
   3. Name of the drug.
   4. Expected action of the drug.
   5. Food allergies.
   6. Common side effects of the drug.

2. Which considerations are important whenever the nurse is preparing to administer medications? **Select all that apply.**
   1. Preparing to give medications in a distraction-free environment.
   2. Checking information on any unfamiliar drug before giving it.
   3. Opening the drug before taking it to the patient's bedside.
   4. Checking for the correct patient by using at least two identifiers.
   5. Questioning any excessive dosage with the health care provider.
   6. Understanding the reason why the patient is receiving the drug.

3. The health care provider prescribed acetaminophen 650 mg orally as needed for headache. Which type of drug order does the nurse recognize?
   1. Standing drug order.
   2. Emergency (stat) drug order.
   3. Single drug order.
   4. As-needed (PRN) drug order.

4. The nurse is administering a patient's prescribed morning medications. The patient tells the nurse to leave the drugs and she will take them in a few minutes. What is the nurse's **best** action?
   1. Leave the drugs at the bedside because the patient is alert and can be trusted to take her medications.

2. Ask another nurse to give the patient's medications at a later time.
   3. Instruct the patient that medications must be taken while the nurse is watching so that he or she can document that the drugs have been administered.
   4. Tell the assistive personnel (AP) to let the nurse know when the patient has taken the medications.

5. A 76-year-old patient with chronic emphysema is having difficulty using his metered-dose inhaler (MDI) after careful teaching and practice. What is the nurse's **best** action?
   1. Request that the pharmacy provide the patient with a spacer.
   2. In a distraction-free environment, go over the steps for MDI use again.
   3. Request that the respiratory therapist work with the patient.
   4. Ask the health care provider if the patient can take the medication in oral form.

6. The health care provider prescribes a throat lozenge to be given by the buccal route. What is the nurse's **best** action?
   1. Place the lozenge under the tongue.
   2. Place the lozenge over the tongue.
   3. Place the lozenge between the cheek and molar teeth.
   4. Instruct the patient to chew the lozenge and swallow.

7. Which self-protective measure will the nurse take before giving a drug by any parenteral route?
   1. Check the patient's heart rate and blood pressure.
   2. Put on a pair of clean gloves.
   3. Wear a disposable gown.
   4. Double check the written drug order.

8. A patient tells the nurse that she has not had a bowel movement for 6 days. The health care provider prescribes a bisacodyl suppository 10 mg by rectum. In which position does the nurse place the patient to give the drug?

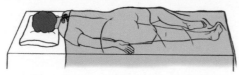

Figure from Williams P. (2022). *deWit's Fundamental Concepts and Skills for Nursing* (6th ed.), Elsevier.
1. Supine.
2. Prone.
3. Left dorsal recumbent.
4. Modified left lateral recumbent position.

9. The patient with asthma needs an injection for allergy testing given by the intradermal route. Which actions will the nurse use to provide this injection? **Select all that apply.**
1. Don clean gloves.
2. Clean the site using a circular motion.
3. Insert the needle at a 10- to 15-degree angle.
4. Aspirate with the syringe plunger.
5. Inject the fluid so that a little bump forms.
6. Massage the area after removing the needle.

10. The nurse is giving morning medications to a patient whose medical record states she has gender dysphoria. Which question will the nurse ask this patient?
1. "Have you been thinking about procedures for gender reassignment?"
2. "Would you like to discuss any issues related to your sexuality?"
3. "How do you prefer to be addressed?"
4. "Do you think of yourself as male or female?"

11. At his wellness check-up, the nurse is to give the 55-year-old patient a flu shot. What is the nurse's **best** response when the patient requests to have the shot given in his thigh instead of the arm?
1. "Your arm is the best place to give your shot because absorption is better there."
2. "It is a good idea to give the shot in your thigh because of the large muscle."
3. "We always give flu shots in the arm, so I will give your shot there."
4. "If your health care provider agrees, I will give it your shot in the thigh."

12. What is the nurse's **best** action when a patient states that he or she does not want to take the prescribed oral docusate 100 mg?
1. Instruct the patient that taking the drug is essential to prevent constipation.

2. Remind the patient that the health care provider's instructions must be followed.
3. Ask the patient why he or she does not want to take the docusate.
4. Document that the patient refused to take the drug.

13. The male patient with angina is prescribed a transdermal nitroglycerin patch (Nitro-Dur). Which actions will the nurse take when administering this drug? **Select all that apply.**
1. Shave the chest for better adherence of the patch to the skin.
2. Find and remove the patch from the previous day.
3. Firmly press the patch drug side down onto the skin.
4. Instruct the patient that he may shower with the patch in place.
5. Remove the patch at night.
6. Check blood pressure every 2 hours while the patch is in place.

14. Which strategies will the nurse use to prevent drug errors? **Select all that apply.**
1. Always follow the "rights" of medication administration.
2. Use a barcode scanner when available.
3. Limit interruptions and distractions.
4. Check the patient's identification wristband.
5. Ask the patient to state surname and age.
6. Always check the written drug order.

15. Which actions or interventions will the nurse take prior to giving a patient's medication through a feeding tube?
1. Make sure that the feeding tube is located in the stomach by withdrawing stomach contents or attaching an end-tidal carbon dioxide detector to the feeding tube.
2. Always hold tube feedings for an hour before giving medications and an hour after giving medications.
3. Suction the patient orally and nasally to remove any secretions and to check the patient's gag reflex.
4. Flush the feeding tube with at least 50 mL of sterile water to make sure that the tube is not clogged.

16. The patient with glaucoma is prescribed travoprost and timolol eye drops. Which important point will the nurse include when teaching the patient about the administration of eye drops?
1. Give the eye drops together to maximize their action.
2. Instruct the patient to expect blurry vision for several minutes after the administration of the eye drops.
3. Wait 5 to 10 minutes between eye drops to prevent drug interaction.
4. Give one eye drop in one eye and the other eye drop in the second eye.

Answer Key for this chapter begins on p. 130

Common Health Scenarios   PART 2

17. The patient with acid indigestion is prescribed magnesium hydroxide 1200 mg every 4 hours as needed. The pharmacy sends a bottle of magnesium hydroxide 400 mg/5 mL. How many mL will the nurse administer for each dose?
    1. 5 mL.
    2. 10 mL.
    3. 15 mL.
    4. 20 mL.

18. Which action or intervention would the nurse delegate to the AP when providing care for a patient before administering oral carbamazepine?
    1. Assess the patient's baseline level of consciousness.
    2. Ask the patient for a list of drugs he or she is currently taking.
    3. Document any seizure activity.
    4. Check and record baseline vital signs.

19. Nextgen (Drag and Drop)._____

Instructions: Choose the correct type of right from the left column for each nursing action in the right column and write the number for the correct right in the space next to the nursing action.

Type of Right	Nursing Action
1. Right person	_____ Confirm the drug had the desired effect
2. Right drug	_____ Check the last time the drug was given
3. Right dose	_____ Chart the time, route, and any other pertinent information
4. Right route	_____ Confirm the reason or need for the drug
5. Right time	_____ Check the drug order for frequency of administration
6. Right documentation	_____ Ask the patient why he or she does not want to take a drug
7. Right reason	_____ Check the patient's name using 2 identifiers
8. Right response	_____ Confirm that the patient can be given the drug as ordered
9. Right to refuse	_____ Check the drug order and drug label

20. Nextgen (Drag and Drop)._____

Instructions: Choose the correct route from Column 1 for each prescription in Column 2 and write the correct answer in Column 3.

Column 1	Column 2	Column 3
Routes for Drug Administration	**Prescription**	**Correct Route**
Oral	1. Regular insulin 5 units subcutaneously	
Parenteral	2. Nitroglycerin 0.3 mg sublingually	
Topical	3. Acetaminophen suppository 650 mg	
Mucous Membrane	4. Timolol 1 drop to each eye	
Transdermal	5. Normal saline 125 mL/h intravenously	
	6. Penicillin G 1.2 million units intramuscularly	
	7. Albuterol inhaler two puffs	
	8. Viscous lidocaine 15 mL swish in mouth and spit out	
	9. Nitroglycerin ointment 1 inch to chest	

 Answer Key for this chapter begins on p. 130

PART 2 Common Health Scenarios

Answers

1. **Ans: 1, 2, 3, 4, 6**   All of these options are important for the nurse to know before giving any prescribed drug, except for food allergies. The nurse would be sure to check for drug allergies. **Focus:** Prioritization; **QSEN:** PCC, S; **Concept:** Safety; **Cognitive Level:** Applying

2. **Ans: 1, 2, 4, 5, 6**   The nurse would keep the drug in its container until at the bedside when telling the patient which drugs they are to receive. All of the other options are important concerns when a nurse is preparing to administer patient medications. **Focus:** Prioritization; **QSEN:** PCC, S; **Concept:** Safety; **Cognitive Level:** Applying

3. **Ans: 4**   A PRN drug order is an "as-needed" order. The drug is given based on the nurse's clinical judgment of safety and the patient's need. Standing drug orders indicate that a drug is to be given until discontinued. Emergency drug orders are one-time orders that must be given immediately (stat). A single drug order is a one-time order to be given at a specified time. **Focus:** Prioritization; **QSEN:** PCC, S; **Concept:** Safety; **Cognitive Level:** Analyzing

4. **Ans: 3**   Medications should never be left at the patient's bedside and the nurse should not ask another nurse to give drugs he or she has not prepared. The AP's scope of practice does not include administration of drugs, nor is the AP responsible for ensuring that a patient takes her drugs. **Focus:** Prioritization, Delegation; **QSEN:** PCC, S; **Concept:** Clinical Judgment, Safety; **Cognitive Level:** Analyzing; **IPEC:** IC

5. **Ans: 1**   Older adults often have difficulty when using an MDI without a spacer. The spacer is attached to the MDI, then the medication is released into the spacer and the patient can then inhale the drug. **Focus:** Prioritization; **QSEN:** PCC; **Concept:** Gas Exchange, Patient Education; **Cognitive Level:** Analyzing

6. **Ans: 3**   When a drug is given by the buccal route, it is placed between the cheek and molar gums. Blood supply is very good in the mouth, so the lozenge will dissolve and be absorbed quickly. The nurse would instruct the patient not to eat or drink until the medication is dissolved and absorbed. **Focus:** Prioritization; **QSEN:** PCC; **Concept:** Perfusion; **Cognitive Level:** Applying

7. **Ans: 2**   When giving a drug by a parenteral route, the nurse's hands are at risk for contact with patient blood. Putting on clean gloves protects the nurse's hands. A disposable gown is not necessary. Checking vital signs and the drug order are protective measures for the patient. **Focus:** Prioritization; **QSEN:** S; **Concept:** Safety; **Cognitive Level:** Applying. **Test Taking Tip:** Whenever a member of the health care team is at risk for contact with patient fluids, always think of protective actions such as wearing gloves.

8. **Ans: 4**   When the patient is placed in the modified left lateral recumbent position, the patient lies on the side with the knee and thigh drawn upward toward the chest. This is the best position for giving rectal suppositories because of the anatomical position of the rectum and colon. **Focus:** Prioritization; **QSEN:** PCC, S; **Concept:** Elimination; **Cognitive Level:** Applying

9. **Ans: 1, 2, 3, 5**   When performing an intradermal injection, the nurse must not aspirate the syringe or massage the area after the injection. Options 1, 2, 3, and 5 are correct techniques for this type of injection. **Focus:** Prioritization; **QSEN:** PCC, S; **Concept:** Safety; **Cognitive Level:** Applying

10. **Ans: 3**   A patient with gender dysphoria experiences emotional or psychological distress caused by an incongruence between his or her natal (birth) sex and gender identity. The most appropriate question for the nurse to ask is how the client prefers to be addressed. **Focus:** Prioritization; **QSEN:** PCC; **Concept:** Sexuality; **Cognitive Level:** Analyzing

11. **Ans: 1**   The first option responds to the patient's question by telling him why the arm is the preferred site for the injection. Option 2 is not correct. Option 3 ignores the patient's request. Option 4 does not explain why the arm is the preferred site for flu shots. The arm site is readily available and useful for giving vaccinations for adolescents and adults. **Focus:** Prioritization; **QSEN:** PCC; **Concept:** Patient Teaching, Communication; **Cognitive Level:** Analyzing

12. **Ans: 3**   When a patient does not want to take a prescribed drug, the nurse must first gather additional information by asking the patient why the drug is being refused. There may be a good reason for the refusal (e.g., the patient is having diarrhea). Options 1 and 2 ignore the patient's concern. Option 4 is important but should not be done until after collecting more data. When the nurse documents a patient's refusal, the reason should be included. **Focus:** Prioritization; **QSEN:** PCC; **Concept:** Elimination, Communication; **Cognitive Level:** Analyzing. **Test Taking Tip:** Remember that a patient has the right to refuse to take any medication, but the nurse has an ethical responsibility to help the patient to make an informed choice. The nurse must discover why the patient is refusing before documenting the refused drug. This is sometimes called the ninth right of drug administration.

13. **Ans: 2, 3, 4, 5** Shaving the skin is not recommended. If hair needs to be removed, it should be clipped using scissors. The patch should be applied to a hairless area for best adherence and absorption. The previous patch must be removed to avoid giving too much of the drug. A Nitro-Dur patch may be left in place when showering. The patch should be removed at night because the drug loses effectiveness when used continuously. Checking blood pressure every 2 hours is not necessary. **Focus:** Prioritization; **QSEN:** PCC, S; **Concept:** Perfusion, Safety; **Cognitive Level:** Applying

14. **Ans: 1, 2, 3, 4, 6** All of these options are strategies the nurse would use to prevent medication errors except option 5. The nurse would ask the patient to state his or her full name and date of birth, which decreases the likelihood of mistaken identity. Drug errors are a leading cause of death and injury. Because nurses give most drugs to patients, nurses are the final defense for detecting and preventing drug errors. **Focus:** Prioritization; **QSEN:** PCC, S, EBP; **Concept:** Safety; **Cognitive Level:** Applying

15. **Ans: 1** The nurse must ensure that the feeding tube is correctly placed in the stomach before giving any drug through the tube. This is done by either aspirating (withdrawing) stomach contents or attaching an end-tidal carbon dioxide detector. The presence of carbon dioxide indicates that the tube is in the trachea instead of the stomach. For some drugs, if a patient is receiving tube feedings, it may be held for a period of time before and after the drugs. Other drugs are given with food to prevent stomach irritation. The patient does not need to be suctioned before giving drugs through a feeding tube. Flushing the tube is done after administering medications to prevent the tube from clogging. **Focus:** Prioritization; **QSEN:** PCC, S; **Concept:** Safety; **Cognitive Level:** Applying

16. **Ans: 3** The nurse will wait for 5 to 10 minutes between eye drops to prevent drug interactions. These eye drops must not be given together because of drug interactions and they should not cause blurry vision. When eye drops are prescribed, the health care provider indicates which eyes are affected and to which eyes the drops are to be applied (e.g., right eye, left eye, or both eyes). **Focus:** Prioritization; **QSEN:** PCC, S; **Concept:** Patient Education, Safety; **Cognitive Level:** Analyzing

17. **Ans: 3** The nurse must calculate the dosage. Have 400 mg/5 mL: need 1200 mg/X mL = 15 mL. **Focus:** Prioritization; **QSEN:** PCC, S; **Concept:** Safety; **Cognitive Level:** Analyzing

18. **Ans: 4** Carbamazepine is an antiseizure drug. Assessing, collecting data (e.g., current drugs), and documenting seizures require the additional skills and training of a professional nurse. Checking and recording vital signs are within the scope of practice of an AP. **Focus:** Delegation; **QSEN:** PCC, TC; **Concept:** Intracranial Regulation, Safety; **Cognitive Level:** Applying

19. **Ans:**

Type of Right		Nursing Action
1. Right person	8	Confirm the drug had the desired effect
2. Right drug	5	Check the last time the drug was given
3. Right dose	6	Chart the time, route, and any other pertinent information
4. Right route	7	Confirm the reason or need for the drug
5. Right time	3	Check the drug order for frequency of administration
6. Right documentation	9	Ask the patient why he or she does not want to take a drug
7. Right reason	1	Check the patient's name using two identifiers
8. Right response	4	Confirm that the patient can be given the drug as ordered
9. Right to refuse	2	Check the drug order and drug label

Focus: Prioritization; **QSEN:** PCC; **Concept:** Safety; **Cognitive Level:** Applying; **Cognitive Skill:** Generate Solutions. **Test Taking Tip:** Be sure to remember the "rights" of drug administration and use them whenever given medications to any patient.

20. Ans:

Column 1	Column 2	Column 3
Routes for Drug Administration	**Prescription**	**Correct Route**
Oral	1. Regular insulin 5 units subcutaneously	Parenteral
Parenteral	2. Nitroglycerin 0.3 mg sublingually	Oral
Topical	3. Acetaminophen suppository 650 mg	Mucous Membrane
Mucous Membrane	4. Timolol 1 drop to each eye	Topical
Transdermal	5. Normal saline 125 mL/h intravenously	Parenteral
	6. Penicillin G 1.2 million units intramuscularly	Parenteral
	7. Albuterol inhaler two puffs	Mucous Membrane
	8. Viscous lidocaine 15 mL swish in mouth and spit out	Oral
	9. Nitroglycerin ointment 1 inch to chest	Transdermal

Focus: Prioritization; **QSEN:** PCC, S; **Concept:** Safety; **Cognitive Level:** Applying; **Cognitive Skill:** Generate Solutions.

QSEN Key: PCC, Patient-Centered Care; **TC,** Teamwork & Collaboration; **EBP,** Evidence-Based Practice; **QI,** Quality Improvement; **S,** Safety; **I,** Informatics.

IPEC Key: Domain 1 Values/Ethics (**V/E**); Domain 2 Roles/Responsibilities (**R/R**); Domain 3 Interprofessional Communication (**IC**); Domain 4 Teams/Teamwork (**T/T**). Used only with appropriate questions.

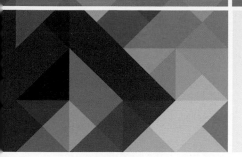

CHAPTER 20
Next-Generation NCLEX Questions

Questions

 1. Extended Multiple Response

Scenario: The nurse is caring for several patients on a busy medical surgical unit with an experienced assistive personnel (AP).

Question: Which duties can the nurse delegate to the AP?
Instruction: Highlight each duty that can be delegated to the AP. Select all that apply.
1. Observe the urine of a patient who has an indwelling catheter.
2. Assist a malnourished patient with finishing a protein supplement.
3. Observe the behavior of a patient who has a history of wandering.
4. Ensure the correct diet before delivering meals to all patients.
5. Turn and position a comatose patient every 2 hours.
6. Record the intake and output of a patient in renal failure.
7. Apply 2 L of oxygen by nasal cannula to a chronic obstructive pulmonary disease (COPD) patient.
8. Ambulate a patient with a recent hip fracture who is a fall risk.
9. Deliver postmortem care by placing the body in an anatomical position with waterproof padding underneath.
10. Administer a bisacodyl enema to a patient who is constipated.

 2. Cloze.

Instructions: Complete the sentences below by choosing the most probable option for the missing information that corresponds with the same numbered list of options provided.

Scenario: The nurse is caring for an unconscious 24-year-old male patient with multiple injuries sustained after a motor vehicle crash. The urinary catheter has drained 2 L of urine in the past 8 hours. The specific gravity of the urine is 1.002 and the serum osmolality is high. Based on the urine output and the laboratory results, it is probable that the injury sustained in the crash caused damage to the ___1___, which caused a decreased amount of ___2___ to be secreted. The nurse suspects the patient has ___3___. Nursing management includes meticulous intake and output ___4___ and administration of ___5___.

Option 1	Option 2
Kidneys	Adrenocorticotropic hormone (ACTH)
Autonomic nervous system	Antidiuretic hormone (ADH)
Adrenal medulla	Epinephrine
Pituitary gland	Cortisone
Option 3	Option 4
Syndrome of inappropriate antidiuretic hormone (SIADH)	Increased fluid intake
Diabetes insipidus (DI)	Decreased fluid intake
Cushing's syndrome	High-sodium diet
Diabetes mellitus	Low-carbohydrate diet

Option 5
Desmopressin acetate
Furosemide
Demeclocycline
Insulin

3. Enhanced Hot Spot.

Instructions: Underline or highlight the risk factors and symptoms that indicate the patient may have cardiovascular disease (CVD).

Scenario: Margaret is a 65-year-old obese female who presents to the clinic with complaints of feeling sluggish and short of breath for several weeks despite giving up her smoking habit 6 months ago. She states she used to be able to vacuum the house without stopping but now has to rest frequently. Vital signs: T 98.7°F (37°C), P 84, R 24, BP 176/98, O_2 Sat 95% room air.

4. Matrix.

Scenario: A 16-year-old African American male with sickle cell disease is being admitted from the emergency department (ED) to the medical unit for a sickle cell crisis.

Instructions: For each medical and/or nursing intervention, place an X to indicate which staff member would be best for each intervention.

Medical and/or Nursing Interventions	LPN/LVN	AP	RN
Administer hydroxyurea 15mg/kg by mouth			
Administer intravenous morphine sulfate every 15 minutes until pain under control			
Assess pain level			
Take and record vital signs every hour			
Application of gel heat packs to joints			
Monitor for excessive sedation			
Identify and treat an intravenous (IV) line infiltration			
Apply humidified oxygen at 2L nasal cannula			
Calculate and monitor intravenous (IV) flow rate			
Encourage use of incentive spirometer			
Ambulate as soon as possible			

5. Enhanced Hot Spot.

Scenario: The LPN/LVN is conducting a focused assessment on a 56-year-old female who is being seen in the clinic for symptoms of hearing loss. Place an X or highlight each aspect of data collection the nurse would perform when conducting a focused assessment on a patient with hearing loss. **Select all that apply.**

Instructions: Place an X or highlight each aspect of data collection the nurse would perform when conducting a focused assessment on a patient with hearing loss.

_____1. Observe the patient's gait.
_____2. Observe the level of the patient's voice.
_____3. Record all past and present prescribed, over-the-counter, and illicit drugs taken.
_____4. Ask about a history of high fevers.
_____5. Ask if the patient has had a trochlear nerve function test.
_____6. Prepare the opthalmoscope for use by the health care provider (HCP).
_____7. Ask the patient about any allergies.
_____8. Observe patient facial expressions.
_____9. Ask about exposure to loud noise.

Common Health Scenarios

PART 2

6. Cloze. _____

Scenario: A 17-year-old female patient sustained a burn to her right hand up to but not including her elbow when her hand slipped into the hot oil of a French fry-making machine at a local burger shop. The wound is wet and red, with blisters forming and the burn blanches when pressure is applied. The patient states that her pain level is 8/10. The nurse notes that this burn is a ___1___. The first action of the nurse is to ___2___. The estimated burn area using the rule of nines is ___3___. An intravenous saline lock was initiated and 0.5 mcg of fentanyl with 1 mg of midazolam administered prior to wound care. The nurse knows to assess for allergies to ___4___ prior to the application of mafenide acetate to the wound.

Instructions: Complete the sentences below by choosing the best option for the missing information that corresponds with the same numbered list of options provided.

Option 1	Option 2	Option 3	Option 4
Superficial	Apply oxygen	2%	Silver
Deep partial thickness	Take vital signs	9%	Chlorhexidine
Full thickness	Open the airway	6%	Sulfonamides
Superficial partial thickness	Remove rings	4.5%	Sodium sulfite

7. Enhanced Hot Spot. _____
Instructions: Underline or highlight the factors that increase the patient's risk for breast cancer.

Scenario: A woman, aged 57-years-old, comes to the clinic for an annual physical examination. She says, "I would like to schedule a mammogram. I've been avoiding this for a long time, but my mother died from breast cancer when she was in her 50s and last year, my sister had both breasts removed because of cancer and a *BRCA* mutation. I haven't noticed any problems or changes in my breasts, but as you can see, I am overweight and my breasts are quite large, so I am not sure if I could feel a small lump. The nurse asks additional focused questions and finds out that the woman had an early menarche and late menopause. She had one child at age 45 but was unable to breastfeed. She smoked cigarettes but quit at age 34. Currently, she has 1 to 2 servings of alcohol every day and is trying to lose weight.

8. Cloze. _____
Instructions: Complete the sentences below by choosing the best option for the missing information that corresponds with the same numbered list of options provided.

Scenario: The nurse is caring for a patient with borderline personality disorder (BPD). The patient is likely to display ___1___. One characteristic of BPD that is also common to other types of personality disorders (PDs) is ___2___. Impulsivity in at least two of the following areas is also a part of this disorder: ___3___, and ___4___. The priority interventions that the health care team must consistently use are ___5___.

Options for 1	Options for 2	Options for 3 & 4	Options for 5
Intense need for admiration	Feeling that others wish harm or evil	Reckless driving	Soliciting patient's feelings and controlling personal reactions
Emotional and mood instability	Concern for perfectionism	Attacking others	Responding with empathy and using active listening
Odd, eccentric behavior	Difficulty in interpersonal relationships	Impulsive spending	Encouraging medication compliance and participation in follow-up
Social inhibition	Obsessive need for control	Grandiose gestures	Monitoring for safety and securing the environment
Submissive behavior	Disregard for other's rights	Excessive cleaning	Establishing boundaries and setting limits

    Answer Key for this chapter begins on p. 138

9. Drag and Drop _____

Scenario: An experienced nurse was recently hired to work in a medical-surgical unit of a large urban hospital. The nurse's previous place of employment was very proactive about policies that addressed horizontal violence. The nurse recognizes that horizontal violence is occurring on the medical-surgical unit as evidenced by the aggression of staff members toward peer coworkers. The nurse decides to observe and record specific examples and then approach the nurse manager about the problem and possible solutions.

Instructions: Types of horizontal violence are listed in the left-hand column. In the right-hand column in the space provided write in the letter that matches each example of horizontal violence Note that all responses will be used only once.

Type of Horizontal Violence
a. Backstabbing
b. Bullying
c. Sabotage
d. Silent treatment
e. Verbal abuse
f. Workplace harassment
g. Unrealistic patient assignments

Examples
1. _____Newly graduated nurse is responsible for the five most critical and unstable patients on the weekend night shift.
2. _____Student Nurse A pretends to be friends with Student Nurse B but tells other students to shun her.
3. _____When a new nurse asks a question, the preceptor says, "A first-year nursing student would know the answer to that simple question."
4. _____A medical student asks where the gloves are located, and the nurse pretends not to hear.
5. _____Nurse threatens to get an AP fired for a minor mistake.
6. _____Unit secretary intentionally "forgets" to submit a new nurse's orientation checklist.
7. _____Nurse who is in a same-gender relationship has lewd notes taped to his locker every day.

10. Enhanced Multiple Response _____

Scenario: A patient who has myasthenia gravis is having trouble with chewing, swallowing, and talking. Consultation with a speech therapist is pending. The HCP has ordered thickened liquids and swallow precautions and has asked the nursing staff to vigilantly observe for signs and symptoms of aspiration. Which factors are signs and symptoms of dysphagia or aspiration?

Instructions: Place an X in the space provided, or highlight each sign or symptom of dysphagia or aspiration. Select all that apply.

1. _____Choking or coughing after eating or drinking
2. _____Repeated swallowing motions
3. _____Frequent throat clearing
4. _____Wet sounding or hoarse voice
5. _____Subjective sensation that something is in throat
6. _____Sneezing
7. _____Dryness of the mouth and lips
8. _____Food pocketing
9. _____Desaturation while eating
10. _____Coarse breath sounds on auscultation
11. _____Fever

11. Matrix._____

Scenario: The nurse is working with an AP to provide care for a bedridden patient admitted from a long-term care facility with a Stage 3 full skin thickness loss pressure injury in the sacral area. The wound is 3 cm by 6 cm. The patient is poorly nourished with a poor appetite and poor dentition; the entire body is very thin, with pale fragile skin. Level of consciousness is mildly confused but cooperative.

Instructions: For each potential HCP prescription, place an X in the box to indicate whether it is essential, nonessential, or contraindicated.

Potential Order	Essential	Nonessential	Contraindicated
Turn patient every 2 hours			
Insert a urinary catheter			
Consult with wound care specialist about best wound care and dressing			
Report changes in quantity, color, or odor of wound exudate to the HCP			
Consult with the registered dietician for a diet rich in carbohydrates and fats			
Massage reddened areas after each position change			
Culture the wound every other day using a sterile cotton-tipped swab			
Use pillows and padding devices to keep heels pressure free			
Insert a small-bore feeding tube for continuous tube feedings			
Measure depth of the wound			
Apply a thin layer of barrier cream to the injury site			
Review CBC and WBC counts			

PART 2   Common Health Scenarios

    Answer Key for this chapter begins on p. 138

Answers

1. **Ans: 1, 2, 3, 4, 5, 6, 9**   APs observe patient conditions and report their findings back to the nurse. APs are trained to meet the basic needs of patients, which include nutrition and basic hygiene and mobility needs. An AP can record the intake and output along with vital signs. An AP may not administer medications such as oxygen and a bisacodyl enema. Ambulating a patient with a hip fracture who is a fall risk is best left for the nurse, so they may observe for pain or increasing gait problems. Postmortem care can be performed by the AP. **Focus:** Delegation; **QSEN:** T/C; **IPEC:** R/R; **Concept:** Care Coordination; **Cognitive Level:** Analyzing; **Cognitive Skill:** Take Action

2. **Ans:** A 24-year-old male patient with a head injury sustained after a motor vehicle crash. The urinary catheter has drained 2 L of urine in the past 8 hours and the specific gravity of the urine is 1.002. The injury sustained in the crash caused damage to the **pituitary gland**, which caused a decreased amount of **ADH** to be secreted. The nurse suspects the patient has **diabetes insipidus** (DI). Nursing management and treatment includes meticulous intake and output, **increased fluid intake**, and administration of **desmopressin acetate**. The posterior portion of the pituitary gland releases ADH (vasopressin) in response to increased blood osmolarity (increased solutes), indicating that more water is needed. ADH then acts on the kidneys to regulate the amount of water in the body by decreasing urine. This is a continuous process. When there is less water available, as in the case of dehydration, the pituitary gland releases more ADH to conserve water, and when there is too much water, as in the case of overhydration, the pituitary gland releases less ADH. If ADH is not secreted due to pituitary damage (head trauma, hypovolemia, or tumors), DI occurs and water cannot be conserved, causing increased thirst and copious amounts of urine to be released. The kidneys cannot concentrate urine and the specific gravity is very low (1.001–1.003). Management of DI includes increasing both oral and intravenous fluids and administration of desmopressin (synthetic ADH or vasopressin). SIADH occurs when too much ADH is secreted also in response to pituitary damage. Too much water is conserved, resulting in increased blood volume, hyponatremia from the dilution, and decreased urine output. Fluids must be restricted and sodium chloride and diuretics, along with demeclocycline, are given to increase water excretion. **Focus:** Prioritization; **QSEN:** EBP; **Concept:** Hormonal Regulation; **Cognitive Level:** Analyzing; **Cognitive Skill:** Recognize Cues; Analyze Cues; Prioritize Hypotheses, Generate Solutions, Take Action. **Test Taking Tip:** So to not confuse DI with diabetes mellitus, the word diabetes comes from the Greek word meaning passing through or siphoning. The word insipidus means tasteless (like water). The word mellitus means sweet or sugary. Both conditions cause increased urine but are completely different processes. So to not confuse DI with SIADH, think of the words diabetes insipidus (passing through tasteless water). In SIADH no water is passed.

3. **Ans:** Margaret is a **65-year-old obese female** with a history of **diabetes** who presents to the clinic with complaints of feeling **sluggish** and **short of breath** for several weeks despite giving up her **smoking** habit 6 months ago. She states she used to be able to vacuum the house without stopping but now has to **rest frequently**. Vital signs: T 98.7°F (37°C), P 100, R 24, **BP 176/98**, O_2 Sat 95% room air. Women are more likely to have a heart attack after the age of 50 because of the cardioprotective loss of estrogen during menopause. Diabetes increases the risk of CVD because high blood sugar over time damages arteries and nerves. Diabetics and women are at risk for silent heart attacks and typically have either no symptoms or symptoms of shortness of breath, fatigue, nausea, and back or jaw pain. Risk factors for CVD include smoking, high blood pressure, high cholesterol, family history, obesity, and diabetes. Focus: Prioritization; QSEN: EBP; Concept: Perfusion; Cognitive Level: Analyzing; Cognitive Skill: Recognize Cues

4. Ans:

Medical and/or Nursing Interventions	LPN/LVN	AP	RN
Administer hydroxyurea 15mg/kg by mouth	X		
Administer intravenous morphine sulfate every 15 minutes until pain under control			X
Assess pain level			X
Take and record vital signs every hour		X	
Application of gel heat packs to joints		X	
Monitor for excessive sedation	X		
Identify and treat an intravenous (IV) line infiltration	X		
Apply humidified oxygen at 2L nasal cannula	X		
Calculate and monitor intravenous (IV) flow rate	X		
Encourage use of incentive spirometer		X	
Ambulate as soon as possible	X		

The LPN is licensed to administer oral medications and respiratory medications and identify and treat an IV infiltration. The LPN/LVN has knowledge regarding the effects of opiates that the AP may not be aware of, so the LPN/LVN should monitor for excessive sedation as well as ambulate the patient as soon as possible to reduce the risk of acute chest syndrome (sickling in the small pulmonary blood vessels). The LPN/LVN can calculate and monitor the IV flow rate. The RN must assess the pain level as part of a comprehensive pain assessment because vasoocclusion may cause infection, stroke, renal dysfunction, or acute coronary syndrome. The RN must also administer intravenous morphine and reassess the effects accordingly. Under the direction of the LPN/LVN or RN, it is within the scope of AP practice to take and record vital signs every hour and apply gel heat packs to joints. **Clinical Tip:** IV access in a sickle cell patient is difficult because of vein closure due to frequent cannulation. Rapid hydration must occur because deterioration, infarction, and infection occur quickly in a sickle cell crisis. **Focus:** Assignment/Delegation; **QSEN:** EBP, S; **Concept:** Care Coordination; **Cognitive Level:** Analyzing; **Cognitive Skill:** Take Action

5. **Ans: 1, 2, 3, 4, 7, 8, 9** Observing the patient's gait alerts the nurse of any balance issues caused by damage to the inner ear. If the patient speaks in a loud voice, they may not be able to hear themselves and this could indicate sensorineural hearing loss. High doses of broad-spectrum antibiotics, some chemotherapy agents, loop diuretics, and aspirin and aspirin-containing products are ototoxic. High fevers and exposure to loud noise can damage the cochlea and cause hearing loss. Seasonal allergies cause fluid buildup in the inner ear eustachian tube and congestion may affect hearing. A trochlear nerve function test is used to assess a portion of ocular mobility and would not be used to assess hearing loss. The vestibulocochlear nerve transmits sound and information about balance from the inner ear to the brain. An opthalmoscope is used to examine the eye and is not needed for an assessment of hearing. **Focus:** Prioritization; **QSEN:** EBP; **Concept:** Sensory Perception, Communication; **Cognitive Level:** Analyzing; **Cognitive Skill:** Analyze Cues. **Test Taking Tip:** When considering ototoxic drugs, think of the mnemonic CALM: Chemotherapy, Aspirin, Loop diuretics, Microbial-macrolides, aminoglycosides, vancomycin.

6. **Ans:** A 17-year-old female patient sustained a burn to her right hand up to but not including her elbow when her hand slipped into the hot oil of a French fry-making machine at a local burger shop. The wound is wet and red, with blisters forming and the burn blanches when pressure is applied. The patient states that her pain level is 8/10. The nurse notes that this burn is a **superficial partial thickness**. The first action of the nurse is to **remove rings**. The estimated burn area using the rule of nines is **2%**. An intravenous saline lock was initiated and 0.5 mcg of fentanyl with 1 mg of midazolam administered prior to wound care. The nurse knows to assess for allergies to **sulfonamides** prior to the application of mafenide acetate to the wound. Burns to the hand are considered major. Hands present a high risk of infection because they are used constantly. Superficial partial-thickness burns blanche on pressure, but deep partial-thickness burns do not. They both form blisters but superficial partial-thickness burns can be more sensitive and painful than

deep partial-thickness burns because they are not deep enough to destroy nerve endings. This patient has an airway because she is speaking about her pain. There is no evidence the patient would need oxygen. The rings must be removed immediately to prevent constriction of the fingers. The entire arm accounts for 4.5% surface area, so the hand and arm up to the elbow would make up approximately 2% of the surface area. Mafenide acetate contains sulfa and would not be applied if the patient is allergic. Silver nitrate can be used if a sulfa allergy exists. **Focus:** Prioritization; **QSEN:** PCC, EBP; **Concept:** Infection, Tissue Integrity; **Cognitive Level:** Analyzing; **Cognitive Skill:** Take Action

7. **Ans:** A **woman**, aged **57-years-old**, comes to the clinic for an annual physical examination. She says, "I would like to schedule a mammogram. I've been avoiding this for a long time, but my **mother died from breast cancer when she was in her 50s** and last year, my **sister had both breasts removed because of cancer and a *BRCA* mutation**. I haven't noticed any problems or changes in my breasts, but as you can see, I am **overweight** and my breasts are quite large, so I am not sure if I could feel a small lump. The nurse asks additional focused questions and finds out that the woman had an **early menarche and late menopause.** She had **one child at age 45** but was **unable to breastfeed.** She **smoked cigarettes** but quit at age 34. Currently, she has **1 to 2 servings of alcohol every day** and is trying to lose weight. Risk factors for breast cancer include female gender, age over 50, family or personal history for breast cancer; history of some types of breast biopsy or certain benign breast conditions; certain forms of contraceptive or hormonal replacement therapy or history of exposure to diethylstilbestrol; and history of chest radiation. Women who had early menarche or late menopause, those who had no children or late-in-life pregnancy, and those who did not breastfeed have a greater risk. Obesity, alcohol consumption, and higher educational and socioeconomic status are also contributing factors. A woman's risk of breast cancer remains increased for at least 20 years after smoking cessation. **Focus:** Prioritization; **QSEN:** PCC; **Concept:** Cellular Regulation; **Cognitive Level:** Analyzing; **Cognitive Skill:** Recognize Cues

8. **Ans:** The nurse is caring for a patient with borderline personality disorder (BPD). The patient is likely to display **emotional and mood instability.** One characteristic of BPD that is also common to other types of personality disorders (PDs) is **difficulty in interpersonal relationships.** Impulsivity in at least two of the following areas is also a part of this disorder: **reckless driving** and **impulsive spending.** The priority interventions that the health care team must consistently use are **establishing boundaries and setting limits.** BPD is characterized by emotional and mood instability, marked impulsivity, and problems with self-image. According to the American Psychiatric Association,

a diagnosis of BPD is supported by impulsivity in at least two of the following areas: gambling, overeating, impulsive spending, abusing substances, unsafe sex, binge eating, and reckless driving. There are four characteristics that are associated with PDs: maladaptive response to life, difficulty with relationships, tendency to evoke conflict, and tendency to evoke negative emotion in others. Patients with BPD often attempt to manipulate the staff; therefore all health care staff must maintain boundaries and consistently set limits. In addition, the staff helps the patient to learn healthy ways to interact with other people; this decreases the need to use manipulative behaviors. The long-term goal for the patient is to learn how to maintain their own boundaries and set limits for themselves. An intense need for admiration and grandiosity is characteristic of narcissistic personality disorder (NPD). Odd eccentric behavior is characteristic of schizotypal PD. Feeling that others wish harm or evil is characteristic of paranoid PD; paranoid individuals may attack others if they feel threatened. Social inhibition is characteristic of avoidant PD. Submissive behavior is characteristic of dependent PD. Perfectionism, obsessive need for control, and excessive cleaning are characteristic of obsessive-compulsive PD. Disregard for other's rights is seen in antisocial PD. In the care of patients with mental health disorders all of the following interventions are used at the appropriate time and prioritized according to the patient's needs: soliciting feelings, using empathy, active listening, controlling personal reactions, encouraging medication compliance and participation in follow-up, and monitoring for safety in the environment. **Focus:** Prioritization; **QSEN:** PCC; **Concept:** Mood and Affect; **Cognitive Level:** Analyzing; **Cognitive Skill:** Recognizes Cues, Analyze Cues. **Test Taking Tip:** PDs are organized under three clusters. Cluster A is described as odd and eccentric. Cluster B is characterized by behaviors that are dramatic, erratic, and emotional. Cluster C is characterized by anxious and fearful behaviors.

9. **Ans: 1g, 2a, 3e, 4d, 5b, 6c, 7f** Horizontal violence is considered aggression toward or bullying of coworkers who are at the same level within a workplace or organization. This type of behavior results in an increased risk for errors, problems with retention and recruitment, negative effect on patient outcomes, and adverse effects on the emotional and physical health of coworkers who are targeted. There is overlap in the types of horizontal violence and some actions will be more obvious, while other behaviors will be subtle and may even seem to be normal for the circumstances. Backstabbing occurs when one person makes a negative comment and the "victim" is not present. Bullying comes in many forms, but the underlying intent is to make the victim feel threatened or helpless. Sabotage includes actions that prevent a coworker

from succeeding. Verbal abuse is similar to bullying, but the words are meant to embarrass, humiliate, and cause stress. Workplace harassment could also take many forms, but repetitive actions, words, or behaviors are intended to make the coworker feel unwelcome. Unrealistic patient assignments can be viewed as part of the job, a rite of passage, or needing to prove oneself, but unrealistic patient assignments can yield poor patient outcomes. **Focus:** Prioritization; **QSEN:** N/A; **Concept:** Ethics; **Cognitive Level:** Analyzing; **Cognitive Skill:** Analyze Cues; **IPEC:** V/E

10. **Ans: 1, 2, 3, 4, 5, 6, 8, 9, 10, 11** Dysphagia is defined as difficulty with swallowing. Aspiration is inhaling foreign matter into the airways (e.g., food, fluids, saliva, vomit). Recurring pneumonia and weight loss are additional signs of chronic dysphagia and aspiration. Fever is a sign of silent aspiration. In silent aspiration, coughing or choking are not observed and the person may be unaware that food or fluids have entered the airways. Risk for silent aspiration increases with cognitive or sensory impairment in older people. Infants are also at risk. Dryness of the mouth and lips are not associated with aspiration, because drooling or increased salivation are more likely to occur. **Focus:** Prioritization; **QSEN:** S; **Concept:** Gas Exchange; **Cognitive Level:** Analyzing; **Cognitive Skill:** Recognize Cues. **Test Taking Tip:** Disorders that increase the risk for aspiration include muscular dystrophies (e.g., myasthenia gravis is a neuromuscular disorder that causes weakness in the skeletal muscles, including face and throat), stroke, severe dental problems or mouth sores, acid reflux, Parkinson disease or other nervous system disorders, obstructions from esophageal cancer, or cancer treatments to the throat or neck.

11. Ans:

Potential Order	Essential	Nonessential	Contraindicated
Turn patient every 2 hours	X		
Insert a urinary catheter			X
Consult with wound care specialist about best wound care and dressing	X		
Report changes in quantity, color or odor of wound exudate to the HCP	X		
Consult with the registered dietician for a diet rich in carbohydrates and fats			X
Massage reddened areas after each position change			X
Culture the wound every other day using a sterile cotton-tipped swab		X	
Use pillows and padding devices to keep heels pressure free	X		
Insert a small-bore feeding tube for continuous tube feedings		X	
Measure the depth of the wound	X		
Apply a thin layer of barrier cream to the injury site			X
Review CBC and WBC counts	X		

Turning the patient and using pillow and padding devices help to decrease pressure, prevent further injury, and facilitate healing. Reporting changes in the wound exudate to the HCP is essential because of potential infection. A urinary catheter may be contraindicated because it is another potential source of infection. Culturing the wound every other day is nonessential because wound infections are based on clinical indicators of infection (e.g., cellulitis, exudate changes, increase in injury size or depth) and systemic signs of bacteremia (e.g., fever, elevated white blood cell [WBC] count). Before inserting a feeding tube, the nurse would find out if the client can self-feed or be fed. A thin, mildly confused patient with poor dentition just needs an assessment of how much help is needed for eating, not a feeding tube. The dietician should be consulted but for a diet rich in protein to facilitate healing. Reddened areas should not be massaged because this increases the risk for skin breakdown. Measuring the depth of the wound would be essential because the size and depth will impact the type of dressing that would be recommended by the wound care specialist. Barrier cream would be appropriate for the patient's healthy skin, but not for the pressure injury site, which would have a special dressing to facilitate healing. The nurse would review the complete blood count (CBC) and WBC count for potential infection. **Focus:** Prioritization; **QSEN:** S; **Concept:**

Tissue Integrity; **Cognitive Level:** Analyzing; **Cognitive Skill:** Analyze Cues

QSEN Key: PCC, Patient-Centered Care; **TC,** Teamwork & Collaboration; **EBP,** Evidence-Based Practice; **QI,** Quality Improvement; **S,** Safety; **I,** Informatics.

IPEC Key: Domain 1 Values/Ethics (**V/E**); Domain 2 Roles/Responsibilities (**R/R**); Domain 3 Interprofessional Communication (**IC**); Domain 4 Teams/Teamwork (**T/T**).

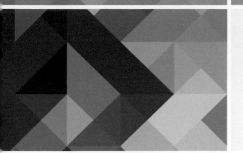

CASE STUDY 1

Patient With a Urinary Tract Infection

Questions

Mrs. A is a 74-year-old who has been visiting her primary health care provider (HCP) for diarrhea over the past 3 days. She has a 10-lb unintentional weight loss and states that she feels dizzy and not quite herself. Her past medical history includes hypercholesterolemia, glaucoma, arthritis, and anemia.

Vital signs are T 98.8°F (37.1°C), RR 20/min, HR 82/min, BP 124/78.

Current medications are multivitamin each morning; ferrous sulfate 324 mg each morning, atorvastatin 40 mg each evening; timolol eye drops one drop each eye twice a day, brimonidine eye drops one drop each eye twice a day, travoprost eye drops one drop each eye at bedtime, and naproxen 200 mg as needed.

The HCP prescribes loperamide 2 mg after each diarrheal stool until diarrhea stops.

1. Which assessment indicates that loperamide is producing the expected action?
   1. Normal vital signs.
   2. Ability to stand without dizziness.
   3. Absence of electrolyte abnormalities.
   4. Normal bowel sounds.

After 3 doses of loperamide, Mrs. A's diarrhea improves; however, she is still feeling dizzy and her husband notices that she has become confused. The HCP instructs her husband to take her to the hospital, where she is admitted and IV fluids are started.

2. Mrs. A's symptoms on admission include dizziness, painful urination, fatigue, decreased appetite, and confusion. Her urine is cloudy and has a strong odor. What does the admitting nurse suspect?
   1. Cystitis
   2. Acute renal failure.
   3. Pyelonephritis.
   4. Urethral obstruction.

Laboratory tests ordered by the HCP include: complete blood count (CBC) with differential, metabolic panel, urinalysis (UA), urine culture and sensitivity, and stool for bacteria and parasites.

3. Which actions or interventions would the nurse delegate to the assistive personnel (AP) when collecting samples for the lab tests? **Select all that apply.**
   1. Performing a venipuncture to draw blood for CBC and metabolic panel.
   2. Placing a container under the toilet seat to obtain a stool sample.
   3. Providing a urine cup and wipes to clean the urinary meatus.
   4. Instructing the patient about how to collect the urine sample.
   5. Having the patient take a shower or bath before collecting stool and urine samples.
   6. Taking the samples to the laboratory as soon as possible.

4. Which instruction will the nurse provide for the AP regarding Mrs. A's dizziness?
   1. "Assess her for dizziness before allowing her to get out of bed."
   2. "Assist Mrs. A whenever she needs to go to the bathroom."
   3. "Provide her with a complete bath and mouth care."
   4. "Include periods of rest between activities in her plan of care."

5. The HCP prescribes trimethoprim/sulfamethoxazole orally every 12 hours. For which common side effects will the nurse be sure to monitor while the patient is taking this drug? **Select all that apply.**
   1. Loss of appetite.
   2. Nausea and vomiting.
   3. Ringing in the ears.
   4. Constipation.
   5. Fatigue.
   6. Muscle aches.

6. Which patient teaching will the nurse reinforce while the patient is taking trimethoprim/sulfamethoxazole?
   1. "Continue taking the medication until your urine is clear."
   2. "If you miss a dose, take two pills when your next dose is due."

3. "Drinks a full glass of water with this medication."
4. "If you have any nausea, take the medication on an empty stomach."

Laboratory tests reveal the following: blood urea nitrogen (BUN): 24; creatinine: 2.39; urine culture positive for E. coli; UA positive for protein and blood; Hct: 25; Hgb: 8.1; WBC 11.8; stool positive for E. coli.

7. The AP reports that Mrs. A's temperature is now 103°F (39°C). What is the nurse's **first** action?
1. Assessing the patient.
2. Notifying the HCP.
3. Placing the patient on a cooling blanket.
4. Administering acetaminophen 650 mg.

8. On assessment, the nurse finds that the patient has a fever, chills, nausea, flank pain, and BP 120/80. Which condition does the nurse suspect?
1. Ureter obstruction.
2. Acute glomerulonephritis.
3. Acute pyelonephritis.
4. Hydronephrosis.

9. Which diagnostic test will the nurse anticipate that the HCP will order for Mrs. A's condition?
1. Kidney, ureter, and bladder (KUB) radiograph.
2. Abdominal computed tomography (CT) with contrast.
3. Intravenous pyelogram.
4. Bedside bladder scan.

10. Nextgen Matrix.
Instructions: For each potential HCP prescription, place an X in the box to indicate which health care team would be **best** to assign or delegate the action.

Potential Order	RN	LPN/LVN	AP
Administer acetaminophen 650 mg orally for discomfort			
Remind the patient to wipe from front to back after bowel movements			
Teach the patient to remain in bed and call for assistance getting out of bed			
Administer first dose of IV ciprofloxacin to treat infection			
Assist the patient with ambulating to the bathroom for a bowel movement			
Assess the patient for relief of symptoms after treatment with ciprofloxacin			
Collect urine sample for culture and sensitivity and deliver to the laboratory			
Complete a bedside bladder scan for urine retention			
Check and record vital signs, and report any changes			

11. The HCP prescribes 1 L of IV normal saline for the patient to run over 8 hours. How fast will the nurse set the IV pump to safely complete this action?
1. 100 mL/h.
2. 125 mL/h.
3. 150 mL/h.
4. 175 mL/h.

12. Which nursing care actions or interventions will the nurse include when caring for a patient with pyelonephritis such as Mrs. A? **Select all that apply.**
1. Encourage fluid intake.
2. Place a urinary catheter.
3. Monitor for changes in urine.
4. Restrict fluid intake.
5. Record intake and output.
6. Teach how to prevent urinary tract infection (UTI).

Mrs. A is now alert and oriented and feeling much better. The HCP states that she is ready for discharge. Her IV fluids have been discontinued and she is taking oral antibiotics.

13. Which action would the nurse delegate to the AP to help Mrs. A prepare for discharge to home?
1. Discontinuing Mrs. A's saline lock.
2. Discussing the HCP's instructions with Mrs. A.
3. Assisting Mrs. A with packing her belongings.
4. Giving the final oral dose oral antibiotic to Mrs. A.

14. The nurse is preparing Mrs. A for discharge. Which teaching points will be included for the prevention of UTI ? **Select all that apply.**
1. Always wipe from front to back after a bowel movement.
2. Wash underclothes with strong detergent and bleach.
3. Wear undergarments that do not retain moisture.
4. Drink at least eight full glasses of water every day.
5. Regularly use over-the-counter vaginal douche products.
6. Empty your bladder by urinating promptly after sexual intercourse.

Answers

1. **Ans: 4** When a patient has diarrhea, bowel sounds are likely to be hyperactive. Normal bowel sounds would indicate that loperamide is working as expected by slowing intestinal motility. **Focus:** Prioritization; **QSEN:** PCC; **Concept:** Elimination; **Cognitive Level:** Applying. **Test Taking Tip:** Nurses must know the expected effect of medications to be able to assess whether any drug is working.

2. **Ans: 1** Cystitis is an inflammation of the urinary bladder that is common in women and is commonly caused by *Escherichia coli* bacteria. When caused by bacteria, cystitis is also called a UTI. One of the earliest signs of cystitis in older adults is confusion in a patient who is usually alert. Signs and symptoms include painful urination, frequent and urgent urination, fatigue, anorexia, and feeling of pressure in the bladder area. **Focus:** Prioritization; **QSEN:** PCC; **Concept:** Elimination, Infection, Clinical Judgment; **Cognitive Level:** Analyzing; **Cognitive Skill:** Recognizing Cues

3. **Ans: 2, 3, 6** The scope of practice for an AP does not routinely include performing venipuncture or providing patient instructions, which require additional training and skill and are more appropriately completed by nurses or specially trained phlebotomists. Bathing before samples are collected is not necessary. APs can provide equipment to patients for collecting specimens and take the samples to the lab as soon as possible. Urine samples that stand for longer than 15 to 30 minutes change characteristics and the urinalysis may not be accurate. **Focus:** Delegation, Supervision; **QSEN:** PCC, TC, S; **Concept:** Safety; **Cognitive Level:** Applying; **IPEC:** IC

4. **Ans: 2** The AP's scope of practice includes assisting with ambulation. Assessing and preparing care plans should be completed by the nurse and not delegated. The AP would assist with morning care as needed but allow the patient to complete what she is able to do. **Focus:** Delegation, Supervision; **QSEN:** PCC, S, TC; **Concept:** Safety; **Cognitive Level:** Applying; **IPEC:** IC

5. **Ans: 1, 2, 3, 5** Common side effects of trimethoprim/sulfamethoxazole include loss of appetite, nausea and vomiting, painful or swollen tongue, dizziness, spinning sensation, ringing in ears, tiredness, and sleep problems (insomnia). **Focus:** Prioritization; **QSEN:** PCC, S; **Concept:** Safety; **Cognitive Level:** Analyzing

6. **Ans: 3** It is recommended that a patient takes trimethoprim/sulfamethoxazole with a full glass of water (8 oz). The drug must be taken for as long as the HCP prescribes. Patients should never take a double dose when a dose of medication is missed because of the risk for overdose and adverse effects. If a patient experiences nausea, taking the medication with food is recommended. **Focus:** Prioritization; **QSEN:** PCC, S; **Concept:** Safety; **Cognitive Level:** Applying

7. **Ans: 1** The first action the nurse would take is to assess the patient for any other signs or symptoms to collect more information before taking any other action. The HCP would need to write prescriptions for a cooling blanket or acetaminophen. **Focus:** Prioritization; **QSEN:** PCC, S; **Concept:** Infection; **Cognitive Level:** Analyzing. **Test Taking Tip:** Before giving acetaminophen for fever, it is essential to discover the cause in order to treat an infection appropriately; **Test Taking Tip.** *E. Coli* is a bacterium that normally lives in the gastrointestinal tract. Diarrhea increases the risk for UTI, especially in older women because of changes associated with urogenital aging.

8. **Ans: 3** Signs and symptoms of acute pyelonephritis includes fever, chills, headache, malaise, nausea and vomiting, and flank pain. This condition is an infection of the kidneys that occurs when bacteria such as *E. coli* from a bladder infection travels up the ureters to infect the kidneys. Urethra obstruction causing stasis of urine can lead to acute pyelonephritis. **Focus:** Prioritization; **QSEN:** PCC, S; **Concept:** Infection; Clinical Judgment; **Cognitive Level:** Analyzing; **Cognitive Skill:** Recognizing Cues

9. **Ans: 2** The imagining study of choice for acute pyelonephritis is abdominal/pelvic CT with contrast. IV pyelograms and KUB radiographs are rarely used now. A bedside bladder scan will not provide information about the kidneys. **Focus:** Prioritization; **QSEN:** PCC; **Concept:** Elimination; **Cognitive Level:** Applying

PART 3 Complex Health Scenarios

10. **Ans:**

Potential Order	RN	LPN/LVN	AP
Administer acetaminophen 650 mg orally for discomfort		X	
Remind the patient to wipe from front to back after bowel movements			X
Teach the patient to remain in bed and call for assistance getting out of bed	X		
Administer first dose of IV ciprofloxacin to treat infection	X		
Assist the patient with ambulating to the bathroom to urinate			X
Assess the patient for relief of symptoms after treatment with ciprofloxacin	X		
Collect urine sample for culture and sensitivity by intermittent catheterization		X	
Complete a bedside bladder scan for urine retention		X	
Check and record vital signs, and report any changes			X

The registered nurse (RN) would provide teaching instructions and in-depth assessment. The RN would be best to administer the first dose of any IV antibiotic and monitor for any adverse reaction. In some states an LPN/PVN with additional training may administer IV antibiotics. Be sure to check the scope of practice for your state and institution. An LPN/LVN can administer oral drugs and perform intermittent catheterizations and bedside bladder scans. The AP's scope of practice includes reminding patients about what has already been taught and assisting with ambulation. **Focus:** Assignment, Delegation; **QSEN:** PCC, TC; **Concept:** Safety, Care Coordination; **Cognitive Level:** Analyzing; **IPEC:** R/R; **Cognitive Skill:** Taking Action. **Test Taking Tip:** Review and be familiar with the scope of practice for all members of the health care team to safely assign and delegate patient care.

11. **Ans: 2** A liter of saline contains 1000 mL of fluid. Divide 1000 by 8 to come up with the correct setting for the IV pump (1000/8 = 125 mL/h). **Focus:** Prioritization; **QSEN:** PCC, S; **Concept:** Safety; **Cognitive Level:** Applying

12. **Ans: 1, 3, 5, 6** Nursing management of a patient with pyelonephritis includes encouraging oral fluids (IV fluids would be given if the patient experiences nausea and vomiting), monitoring for any changes in urine, recording intake and output, and keeping the patient comfortable. The nurse would also teach a patient how to avoid a UTI. Placement of a urinary catheter is not usual. **Focus:** Prioritization; **QSEN:** PCC; **Concept:** Elimination, Infection; **Cognitive Level:** Applying

13. **Ans: 3** The AP would assist Mrs. A with gathering and packing her belongings before discharge. Discontinuing a saline lock, discussing discharge instructions, and giving oral medications require additional knowledge, training, and skills of professional nurses. In some states an experienced AP may discontinue a saline lock. Be sure to know the scope of practice for your state or institution. **Focus:** Delegation, Assignment; **QSEN:** S; **Concept:** Care Coordination; **Cognitive Level:** Analyzing

14. **Ans: 1, 3, 4, 6** Teaching how to prevent UTIs is essential before a patient is discharged. Options 3, 4, and 6 are appropriate for UTI prevention. Women would also be taught that showering is preferred over taking a bath and that prolonged sitting can contribute to the development of cystitis. Underclothes should be washed in a mild detergent and over-the-counter douche products, bubble bath, perfumed soap, and feminine hygiene sprays should be avoided. **Focus:** Prioritization; **QSEN:** PCC, S; **Concept:** Patient Education; **Cognitive Level:** Applying

QSEN Key: PCC, Patient-Centered Care; **TC,** Teamwork & Collaboration; **EBP,** Evidence-Based Practice; **QI,** Quality Improvement; **S,** Safety; **I,** Informatics.

IPEC Key: Domain 1 Values/Ethics (**V/E**); Domain 2 Roles/Responsibilities (**R/R**); Domain 3 Interprofessional Communication (**IC**); Domain 4 Teams/Teamwork (**T/T**).

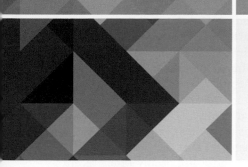

CASE STUDY 2
Nutritional Problems

Questions

The nurse is working in a long-term care facility with 20 patients. The most common problems related to nutrition in the facility are weight loss and protein energy undernutrition. The unit is staffed with a registered nurse (RN) nurse manager, one LPN/LVN and four assistive personnel (AP) during the day. The facility also employs a dietician and food service staff, a pharmacist, housekeeping staff, and a recreational therapist.

1. The AP is rushing to get her assigned residents to the breakfast table on time. She tells the nurse that she is delayed because Mrs. V is refusing to get out of bed. What is the **first** action of the nurse?
   1. Tell the AP to leave the resident in bed.
   2. Take Mrs. V's vital signs and evaluate her condition.
   3. Tell the AP to bring a breakfast tray to Mrs. V's room.
   4. Tell Mrs. V that if she can't come to the dining room her breakfast will be cold.

2. The nurse overhears Mrs. C, who is blind, scold the AP who is trying to feed her: "Leave me alone, I can do it myself." How should the nurse intervene?
   1. Tell the AP it's okay for Mrs. C to feed herself.
   2. Ask Mrs. C if she would guide the AP on the best way to assist her.
   3. Instruct the AP on the best way to assist a blind resident with meals.
   4. Help feed Mrs. C herself.

3. Mr. M has a stage 3 pressure ulcer on the sacral area. Which nursing interventions can the nurse delegate to the AP? **Select all that apply.**
   1. Order Mr. M a protein shake twice a day.
   2. Reposition Mr. M every 2 hours.
   3. Assist Mr. M with eating at least 75% of each meal.
   4. Take Mr. M to the bathroom after every meal and every 2 hours in between.
   5. Take Mr. M's temperature every shift.
   6. Reapply Mr. M's alginate dressing when it becomes soiled.

4. The nurse has assigned an AP to care for Ms. P who has a diagnosis of folate deficiency. Which food on the dinner plate will the nurse instruct the AP is most important for Ms. P to finish?
   1. Mashed potato.
   2. Asparagus.
   3. Tomato.
   4. Chicken.

5. Several of the residents on the unit have chronic constipation. Which interventions must be assigned to a nurse? **Select all that apply.**
   1. Offer the residents extra fluid intake during the day.
   2. Give the resident fresh fruit daily.
   3. Ask the recreational therapist to increase movement therapies.
   4. Administer saline enemas as delegated by the nurse.
   5. Offer the residents a cup of senna tea at bedtime.
   6. Check residents for impaction as symptoms dictate.

6. Extended Multiple Response _____

   The nurse is conducting a class of newly hired APs on safe and correct methods to feed residents. **Highlight each item that the nurse will include in her lecture.**

   1. Offer foods that the resident prefers first.
   2. Feed small portions using a 1/3 full teaspoon.
   3. Offer a prayer of thanks with the residents before the meal.
   4. Offer fluids only at the end of the meal so the patient will eat more.
   5. Do not let residents hold hot liquids
   6. Tell visually impaired residents what foods are on their plate and where, using a clock to describe position.
   7. Seat the resident in a 45-degree position for meals.
   8. Keep conversation quiet to allow the resident to eat without interruption.
   9. Sit facing the person you are feeding.

7. Mr. J tells the nurse that he has a flare-up of his gout. The nurse notes that he has redness and swelling at the base of his right big toe. Which food will the nurse ask the AP to take off Mr. J's breakfast plate?
   1. Fresh fruit.
   2. Coffee.
   3. Bacon.
   4. Eggs.

8. The AP is filling all the water pitchers at the beginning of the shift. Which action by the AP causes the nurse to stop and reeducate the AP per proper procedure?
   1. The AP labeled each pitcher with the patient's name and room number.
   2. The AP filled the pitcher directly from the ice machine before filling it with water.
   3. The AP checked the chart for fluid orders.
   4. The AP provided straws at the request of the nurse.

9. The daughter of one of the residents with renal failure tells the nurse she doesn't think her mother is receiving enough protein in her diet. What is the **best** response of the nurse?
   1. "I will ask the health care provider (HCP) to call you so she can explain the order."
   2. "I will ask the dietician if more protein foods can be given to your mom."
   3. "I will recheck the order to make sure she is on the correct diet."
   4. "A high-protein diet can make your mom's kidney failure worsen."

10. Mr. M has a stage 3 pressure sore that is slow to heal. Which food item will the nurse encourage Mr. M to eat in order to increase his intake of zinc?
    1. Whole grain bread.
    2. Avocado.
    3. Corn.
    4. Dates.

11. Mrs. B, a resident who was recently admitted to the unit, has been on a vegan diet for several years. Mrs. B tells the nurse she is too tired to enjoy arts and crafts and would rather take a nap every day instead. Which vitamin deficiency initiated by a vegan diet would lead the nurse to discuss Mrs. B's diet needs with the dietician and HCP?
    1. Vitamin E.
    2. Vitamin B12.
    3. Vitamin C.
    4. Vitamin D.

12. Mr. C has lost 2 pounds this week and the nurse notes that the APs have charted that he has been eating only 50% of his meals. Mr. C tells the nurse that for the last couple of weeks his mouth has been dry and everything tastes like metal. What data should the nurse gather before speaking with the HCP at the weekly rounds? **Select all that apply.**
    1. List of medications the patient is taking.
    2. List of medical diagnoses that the patient has.
    3. Current vital signs and a list of any other recent symptoms.
    4. Body mass index (BMI).
    5. Social history.
    6. Diet information.

13. Mr. W is a comatose resident on continuous tube feedings. The AP tells the nurse that she thinks something is wrong because Mr. W is agitated and his respiratory rate and heart rate are elevated. What is the first action of the nurse?
    1. Call the HCP.
    2. Check for placement of the feeding tube.
    3. Stop the tube feeding.
    4. Ask the AP to get a full set of vital signs.

14. The nurse is preparing to administer a continuous enteral feeding bag to Mrs. S, who has a percutaneous endoscopic gastrostomy (PEG) tube with the formula running at 50 mL/h. The residual returns 250 mL of stomach contents. What is the **first** nursing intervention?
    1. Discard the residual, hold the feeding, and notify the RN.
    2. Decrease the amount of formula feeding to 30 mL/h.
    3. Wait for 6 hours and recheck the residual.
    4. Replace the residual, hold the feeding, and notify the HCP.

15. The nurse is delegating some nursing interventions for Mrs. S, who has a PEG tube. Which interventions can the nurse safely delegate to the experienced AP? **Select all that apply.**
    1. Perform oral care every 2 hours.
    2. Perform fingerstick blood glucose every 6 hours.
    3. Maintain an intake and output.
    4. Listen for bowel sounds every 8 hours.
    5. Keep the head of the bed at 30 degrees.
    6. Examine for abdominal distention.

Answers

1. **Ans: 2** The first step in the nursing process is to collect data and find out information about the patient. Based on the findings, the nurse can decide the next course of action. If the patient is sick, the nurse should consult with either the nurse manager or the HCP for further assessment. Leaving Mrs. V in bed without finding out the reason she doesn't want to get up is not good nursing care. Bringing the tray to the resident's room may be indicated if that is her preference but she needs to be assessed first. Telling the resident her breakfast will be cold if she doesn't come to the dining room is unkind. **Focus:** Prioritization; **QSEN:** PCC; **Concept:** Communication; **Cognitive Level:** Analyzing

2. **Ans: 2** Mrs. C may well be able to feed herself properly. A person who is blind may find it offensive when someone trying to help intervenes with their independence. The nurse should intervene by asking Mrs. C for guidance on how she needs assistance. By allowing Mrs. C self-determine, her independence is maintained and the staff shows respect for her. **Focus:** Prioritization; **QSEN:** PCC; **Concept:** Nutrition, Communication; **Cognitive Level:** Analyzing

3. **Ans: 2, 3, 4, 5** Protein is necessary for wound healing but the nurse or nurse manager in consultation with the dietician is responsible for ordering the protein shake. Good nutrition and preventing incontinence assist with wound healing. A below-normal or above-normal temperature can indicate an infection and should be reported to the nurse. Reapplying the alginate dressing is the responsibility of the nurse. **Focus:** Delegation; **QSEN:** PCC, T/C; **Concept:** Tissue Integrity; **Cognitive Level:** Analyzing; **IPEC:** R/R

4. **Ans: 2** Asparagus has 100 mcg of folate. Dark green, leafy vegetables are the best sources of folate. Potatoes, tomatoes, and chicken are not good sources of folate. **Focus:** Prioritization; **QSEN:** PCC; **Concept:** Nutrition; **Cognitive Level:** Application

5. **Ans: 3, 5, 6** Chronic constipation is a problem for many residents due to illness, aging, medications, and diet. The nurse should consult with other professional caregivers for modalities they provide that might improve resident health care. Senna tea is an herbal tea that also comes in pill form. Side effects of abdominal discomfort, cramps, and hypokalemia can occur, so it is considered a medication to be given by a nurse. A nurse must check the patient for an impaction and perform digital removal if necessary. Bradycardia and syncope can occur during the digital removal of stool due to stimulation of the vagal nerve. An AP can administer a saline enema in many states if delegated by the nurse. **Focus:** Assignment; **QSEN:** PCC, S; **Concept:** Nutrition, Elimination; **Cognitive Level:** Analyzing

6. **Ans: 1, 2, 5, 6, 9** If the resident prays before eating a meal, it is appropriate to pray with them; however, prayer should be initiated by the patient and not by the AP or nurse unless institution policy dictates differently. Fluids should be offered during the meal to make chewing easier. Residents should sit at a 90-degree angle or Fowler's position to prevent choking. Eating is a social occasion and pleasant conversation provides much-needed social contact for residents. Facing the person allows the AP to be alert for chewing and swallowing difficulties. **Focus:** Prioritization; **QSEN:** PCC, S; **Concept:** Nutrition, Safety; **Cognitive Level:** Analyzing

7. **Ans: 3** Some meats have high purine levels. The body breaks down purines into uric acid, which then gets into the bloodstream to cause gout symptoms. Meats such as bacon, turkey, veal, and lamb and organ meats like liver should be avoided. Shellfish, anchovies, and sardines are some fish that should be avoided as well. There are many foods that have high purine levels and the patient can be put on a low purine diet, which can help him avoid gout attacks in the future. **Focus:** Delegate; **QSEN:** PCC; **Concept:** Nutrition; **Cognitive Level:** Analyzing

8. **Ans: 2** A used water pitcher placed directly inside an ice machine could transmit pathogens into the ice. The proper procedure is to use a scoop to place ice into the pitcher from the ice machine, being careful not to touch the inside of the pitcher with the scoop. The scoop should then be placed on a towel or a scoop holder and not inside the ice machine. **Focus:** Priority; **QSEN:** PCC, S; **Concept:** Fluid and Electrolytes, Safety; **Cognitive Level:** Analyzing

9. **Ans: 4** Healthy kidneys are able to filter the end products of protein metabolism but in people with kidney disease and kidney failure the kidneys cannot keep up with the workload and kidney function worsens. **Focus:** Prioritization; **QSEN:** PCC, S, EBP; **Concept:** Nutrition, Elimination, Patient Education; **Cognitive Level:** Analyzing

10. **Ans: 1** Whole grains, dairy products, meat, shellfish, and eggs all have high zinc content. Zinc is involved in every stage of wound healing. It is necessary for DNA synthesis, immune function, collagen, and protein formation. These processes are necessary for wound healing. **Focus:** Prioritization; **QSEN:** PCC, EBP; **Concept:** Nutrition, Immunity; **Cognitive Level:** Analyzing

PART 3 Complex Health Scenarios

11. **Ans: 2**   Vegans do not eat animal products that contain vitamin B12 such as fish, chicken, meat, milk products, or eggs. Vitamin B12 is nearly never found in vegetables. The nurse can discuss the diet and the patient's condition as they may warrant further testing and/or vitamin B12 supplementation. **Focus:** Prioritization; **QSEN:** PCC, EBP; **Concept:** Nutrition; **Cognitive Level:** Analyzing

12. **Ans: 1, 2, 3, 4, 6**   Medications can cause impaired taste and dry mouth. This is especially true for someone on multiple medications. Chronic illnesses such as autoimmune disease or periodontal disease can alter taste as well as a recent cold or sinus infection. Aging itself can cause problems with taste. A BMI reading will alert the HCP regarding undernourishment. Any change in diet or the introduction of new foods should also be investigated. A social history is always important to know about a new resident but it is not pertinent to impaired taste. **Focus:** Prioritization; **QSEN:** PCC T/C, EBP; **Concept:** Nutrition; **Cognitive Level:** Analyzing; **IPEC:** R/R, IC

13. **Ans: 3**   Increased heart and respiratory rate and decreased oxygen saturation are all signs of aspiration from a tube feeding. On auscultation, audible rhonchi and wheezes can be heard. The first action is to stop the tube feeding. Placement can be checked but not before stopping the tube feeding, getting a full set of vital signs, and calling the HCP. **Focus:** Prioritization; **QSEN:** PCC; **Concept:** Oxygenation; **Cognitive Level:** Analyzing

14. **Ans: 4**   Large residuals (100–500 mL) are thought to result in vomiting and aspiration. Replacing the residual is thought to be necessary to avoid inadequate nutrition. The HCP should be notified of the large residual as the feeding may need to be slowed or medication to increase bowel motility may be ordered. It is recommended to check residuals every 4 hours. **Focus:** Prioritization; **QSEN:** PCC; **Concept:** Nutrition; **Cognitive Level:** Analyzing

15. **Ans: 1, 2, 3, 5**   The nurse should listen for bowel sounds and observe for abdominal distention. The nurse is responsible for the safe care of the patient. Abdominal distention or absent bowel sounds could indicate an ileus, infection, obstruction, or displacement of the tube. The AP can perform oral care. An AP who has been trained can perform fingerstick glucose. Maintaining intake and output and adjusting the head of the bed is a basic function of the AP. **Focus:** Delegation; **QSEN:** PCC; **Concept:** Nutrition; **Cognitive Level:** Analyzing

QSEN Key: PCC, Patient-Centered Care; **TC,** Teamwork & Collaboration; **EBP,** Evidence-Based Practice; **QI,** Quality Improvement; **S,** Safety; **I,** Informatics.

IPEC Key: Domain 1 Values/Ethics (**V/E**); Domain 2 Roles/Responsibilities (**R/R**); Domain 3 Interprofessional Communication (**IC**); Domain 4 Teams/Teamwork (**T/T**).

Complex Health Scenarios   PART 3

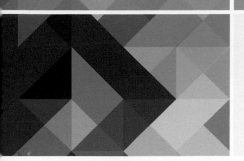

CASE STUDY 3
Patient With Immobility

Questions

Ms. D is a 52-year-old woman who has rheumatoid arthritis (RA). An acute exacerbation (flare) started several weeks ago; this caused her to have increased pain and decreased ability to perform self-care. Additionally, Ms. D lives alone and struggles with depression and social isolation. Obesity, lack of exercise, and chronic obstructive pulmonary disease (COPD) also contribute to Ms. D's difficulties with self-care and management of the RA. The home health team was contacted to assist during the flare. The long-term goal is to improve Ms. D's self-management.

1. Drag and Drop.

Scenario: The home health team includes the registered nurse (RN), LPN/LVN, physical therapist, home health aide, respiratory therapist and a dietitian.

Which team member is **best** for each task?

a. RN
b. LPN/LVN
c. Home health aide
d. Physical therapist
e. Respiratory therapist
f. Dietician

The list below includes some of the admission assessments that are necessary for Ms. D.

Instructions: The left-hand column includes all of the members of the home health team. In the right-hand column, in the space provided, write in the letter to indicate which staff member is best to assign or delegate to each task. Note that letters will be used only once.

1. _____Assess understanding of and motivation to achieve goals of the treatment plan
2. _____Assess strength, mobility, and balance
3. _____Check functionality of oxygen tank and quantity of respiratory supplies
4. _____Assess pain and use of non-pharmacological pain methods
5. _____Evaluate typical 24-hour food and fluid intake
6. _____Obtain weight and height measurements

2. Enhanced Multiple Response._____

Scenario: The nurse uses her knowledge of the pathophysiology of RA to observe for expected signs and symptoms. This knowledge is used as a guideline to perform assessments and to anticipate the patient's needs.

Which signs and symptoms are characteristic of RA? **Select all that apply.**

Instructions: Place an X in the space provided or highlight each sign/symptom that is characteristic of RA.

1. _____Reports of stiffness in multiple joints, especially in the morning.
2. _____Bilateral soft tissue swelling, warmth, and edema in the hands and wrists.
3. _____Muscle atrophy with reports of muscular weakness and aching.
4. _____Single-sided involvement of a weight-bearing joint, such as the hip.
5. _____Systemic involvement, such as low-grade fever, malaise, and anorexia.
6. _____Well-nourished appearance and usually overweight.
7. _____Low red blood cell (RBC) count with iron-deficient anemia.
8. _____Joint stiffness, which increases during cold, wet weather.
9. _____Onset usually around 50–60 years old.

3. The LPN/LVN and the RN collaborate to complete the comprehensive intake assessment for Ms. D. Which portion of the assessment must be completed by the RN?
1. Auscultating breath sounds and assessing respiratory effort.
2. Evaluating the potential effect of depression and isolation on the plan of care.
3. Assessing and comparing vital signs and pulse oximetry trends.
4. Observing the patient's abilities to walk to the bathroom and use the toilet.

4. Which question is the nurse **most** likely to ask when performing a focused assessment of Ms. D's RA?
1. Have you ever had an injury that damaged one of your joints?
2. When was the last time you had bone density testing?
3. Do you smoke? If so, how much and for how long?
4. Do you have a personal or family history of cancer?

5. Which tasks related to the admission assessment would be **best** to delegate to the home health aide? **Select all that apply.**
1. Obtain equipment required for the Timed Get up and Go Test (TUG).
2. Obtain and clean the goniometer prior to measuring joint motion.
3. Prepare the equipment to draw blood for calcium and phosphorus levels.
4. Gather medication containers, with permission, from storage areas.

5. Observe for pitting edema and skin changes in the lower extremities.
6. Inspect the environment for safety, such as stairs or hard-to-reach shelves.

Members of the home health team have completed their assessments of Ms. D and have summarized their findings as follows: Ms. D's primary worries are pain and difficulty with accomplishing activities of daily living (ADLs). She reports pain and stiffness in hands, wrists, and knees in the morning. She independently walks short distances (around the house) and she occasionally uses supplemental oxygen after exertion. Her gait is unsteady and she grimaces when shifting her weight. Hygiene has become difficult because she has trouble with maintaining balance, bending, and reaching in the shower. Ms. D states, "I know that smoking and overeating are not good for me, but that's how I cope with depression and my health problems."

- *Medications: hydroxychloroquine 400 mg PO every day, etanercept 50 mg intramuscular once a week, ibuprofen 300 mg PO QID, prednisone 5 mg PO every day; taper as soon as symptoms improve (prescribed for flare), fluticasone inhaler two puffs BID, albuterol inhaler two puffs every 4 to 6 hours as needed for rescue breathing, oxygen per nasal cannula as needed to maintain an oxygen saturation of 93%.*

Objective data:
- *5'5", 180 pounds*

Vital signs on admission are:
- *T 99.7°F (37.6°C)*
- *HR 85*
- *Respirations 30 breaths/min*
- *BP 130/82*
- *Oxygen saturation (O$_2$ Sat) 93% on room air*

Complex Health Scenarios   PART 3

6. What are the two **priority** nursing concerns based on the summarized findings of the home health team?
   1. Mobility and nutrition.
   2. Functional ability and pain.
   3. Pain and stress and coping.
   4. Gas exchange and mood and affect.

7. Which action will the nurse take **first** after reviewing the admission vital signs: T 99.7°F (37.6°C), HR 85, R 30 breaths/min, BP 130/82, O_2 Sat 93% on room air?
   1. Assist Ms. D to don the nasal cannula and check pulse oximeter.
   2. Assess Ms. D for signs and symptoms of infection.
   3. Monitor pulse, respirations, and O_2 Sat after minor exertion.
   4. Ask the home health aide to take vital signs every 4 hours.

8. Which class of medications is considered the first-line choice for treatment of RA?
   1. Nonsteroidal antiinflammatory drugs (NSAIDs).
   2. Corticosteroids.
   3. Disease-modifying antirheumatic drugs (DMARDs).
   4. Tumor necrosis factor (TNF) inhibitors.

9. Which laboratory test is the **most** important to verify when a patient is prescribed etanercept?
   1. Negative results for human immunodeficiency virus (HIV).
   2. Negative result for tuberculosis (TB).
   3. Negative results for human papillomavirus (HPV).
   4. Negative results for a pregnancy test.

10. Under which circumstances would the nurse expect the health care provider (HCP) to prescribe morphine for Ms. D?
    1. Daily low dose for long-term pain management.
    2. As needed (PRN) for pain not controlled by ibuprofen.
    3. Short-term use during acute phase of flare-up.
    4. Rarely prescribed because morphine worsens RA.

11. Which instruction will the nurse give to the home health aide about positioning Ms. D during the acute flare?
    1. Assist Ms. D with sitting with good body alignment in a firm, straight back chair for several hours each day.
    2. Put Ms. D in a supine position with the body aligned and use several pillows to support the head and neck.
    3. Advise Ms. D to protect joints and frequently turn and reposition herself while in bed.
    4. Assist Ms. D with resting during acute pain and avoid positioning joints in a flexed position.

12. Which laboratory result **best** supports the nurse's supposition that Ms. D's fatigue is related to anemia?
    1. Albumin: 3.5 g/dL (35 g/L).
    2. Platelets: 170,000/mm³ (170 × 10⁹).
    3. RBCs: 3.2 million/mm³ (3.2 × 10¹²).
    4. Partial thromboplastin time: 25 seconds (25 seconds).

13. Which instruction would the nurse give to the home health aide about assisting Ms. D with ADLs?
    1. Assist Ms. D with any activity that she is unable to accomplish herself.
    2. Have her sit down before starting the activity whenever possible.
    3. Be available to assist with activities but wait until she asks for help.
    4. Do most of the activities in the late afternoon when she feels better.

14. Which task related to a cold application would be delegated to the home health aide?
    1. Ask Ms. D about past problems with circulation or disorders that affect sensation.
    2. Check circulation and appearance of skin before and after the application.
    3. Determine if the treatment relieved the pain or whether to reapply the application.
    4. Reinforce to report sensation of numbness so that application can be removed.

15. What are important teaching points to reinforce about joint protection? **Select all that apply.**
    1. Exercise just past the point of pain and expect joints to feel sore for the rest of the day.
    2. Conserve your energy for things you really want to do.
    3. Choose exercise activities, such as water aerobics, that are less stressful to joints.
    4. Avoid jerky rapid movements; move slowly and smoothly.
    5. Avoid lifting weights and, when necessary, pick up heavier items using two hands.
    6. Change body position frequently, alternating between standing, sitting, and lying down.

16. Which action by Ms. D indicates that she is applying the principle of joint protection: "use the biggest muscles and the strongest joints"?
    1. Uses her fingers to push up from a chair when standing.
    2. Uses a small comb to style and untangle her hair.
    3. Carries a purse with a short handle rather than a shoulder bag.
    4. Pushes the door open using the arm rather than the hand.

Answer Key for this chapter begins on p. 155

17. Which statement by Ms. D **most** strongly suggests a barrier to addressing the long-term goals of therapy?
    1. "This flare seems worse and is lasting longer than some of the previous episodes."
    2. "Could you help me stand up? My legs feel weak and my knees are painful."
    3. "I'm so glad the team is available. I don't know what I would do without you."
    4. "Could you call the physical therapist? I want advice on bathroom safety bars."

18. **Enhanced Multiple Response.** _____

Scenario: The nurse is preparing an end-of-the-month summary. This information will be included in a report to the supervising RN. The report is important for continuity of care and allows the home health team to review Ms. D's progress and revise the plan of care as needed.

Which information is the **most** important for the nurse to include in the monthly summary? **Select all that apply.**

Instructions: Place an X in the space provided or highlight each item that should be included in the monthly summary for this patient.

1. _____Vital signs recorded at each visit.
2. _____Any safety or unexpected issues that occurred, such as falls or trips to the emergency department (ED).
3. _____Topics of patient education sessions and Ms. D's receptiveness.
4. _____Types of routine medication and schedule of administration.
5. _____Number of times and reasons that the HCP had to be notified.
6. _____Number of extra or unscheduled visits that the nurse had to make.
7. _____Indication of readiness or barriers to meeting long-term goal of self-management.
8. _____Repetitive occurrences where Ms. D was unable or refused to participate in the treatment plan.
9. _____Indication that Ms. D is having low self-esteem or problems with body image related to weight or joint deformity.

Complex Health Scenarios   PART 3

Answers

1. **Ans: 1 a, 2 d, 3 e, 4 b, 5 f, 6 c**   The entire team is involved in the initial assessment of the home health patient. Each member uses skills and knowledge in their area of expertise to assess the patient's needs. **Focus:** Assignment, Delegation; **QSEN:** TC; **Concept:** Care Coordination; **Cognitive Level:** Applying; **Cognitive Skill:** Generate Solutions; **IPEC:** R/R

2. **Ans: 1, 2, 3, 5, 7**   Many of the same nursing interventions are used for RA and osteoarthritis (OA). However, RA is a systemic autoimmune inflammatory disease that bilaterally affects multiple joints. Stiffness in the morning is common and the joints in the hands, wrists, and feet have soft tissue swelling, warmth, and edema. Muscle atrophy with weakness and aching occurs in the later stages. Systemic involvement includes, fever, anorexia with weight loss, malaise, and iron-deficient anemia with a low RBC count. OA is a degenerative joint disease that is characterized by single-sided involvement of weight-bearing joints and a well-nourished, overweight appearance; symptoms manifest at around age 50-60 years With OA, joint stiffness is more likely to increase during cold, wet weather. **Focus:** Prioritization; **QSEN:** N/A; **Concept:** Mobility, Inflammation; **Cognitive Level:** Applying; **Cognitive Skill:** Recognize Cues. **Test Taking Tip:** Notice that RA and OA are typically grouped together, and many nursing interventions apply to both. However, pay attention to the differences in the underlying pathology and clinical manifestations, as this will help you to perform focused assessments and individualized care when the patient tells you, "I have arthritis."

3. **Ans: 2**   Depression and isolation create complex emotional states, which may affect motivation to participate or outcomes of the treatment plan. The RN would assess for baseline behaviors and feelings and conduct periodic formative evaluations and revise the care plan accordingly. The LPN/LVN who is more likely to be making the routine home visits can perform the other assessments and monitor for changes. **Focus:** Assignment; **QSEN:** TC; **Concept:** Care Coordination; **Cognitive Level:** Applying; **IPEC:** T/T

4. **Ans: 3**   Smoking for more than 20 years increases the risk for developing RA. Smoking also worsens symptoms and reduces the chance for remission. Smoking cessation may help to relieve pain, stiffness, and some of the other symptoms. Previous injury to joints is more associated with OA. Bone density testing is used to diagnose osteoporosis. The nurse would ask about family or personal history of cancer to assist the HCP in diagnosing bone malignancies (or other cancers). **Focus:** Prioritization; **QSEN:** EBP; **Concept:** Mobility; **Cognitive Level:** Applying

5. **Ans: 1, 4**   The home health aide can obtain a stable straight back chair with armrests, which is used for TUG. The test measures balance, mobility, walking, and risk for falls. The patient sits in a chair; when the nurse says, "Go" (timer begins) the patient rises, walks 10 feet, returns, and sits back down (timer ends). Times ≥12 seconds are considered a fall risk. The home health aide can also assist in medication reconciliation by gathering medication containers from areas where Ms. D stores them. The physical therapist is the most likely team member to carry, maintain, and use the goniometer. Collecting blood is a sterile, invasive procedure and specimens are collected in specific containers. The person (RN, LPN/LVN, or phlebotomist) drawing the blood usually prepares the equipment. The home health aide would be expected to report any observed skin changes or swelling; however, the baseline assessment would be performed by the RN. Initial assessment of the environment would be performed by the RN. The LPN/LVN would observe for and report any safety issues that are observed during the routine home visits. **Focus:** Delegation; **QSEN:** S; **Concept:** Mobility, Care Coordination; **Cognitive Level:** Applying

6. **Ans: 2**   Ms. D has several chronic health problems and health maintenance issues, but the flare of the RA has caused pain and the impact of pain is affecting her ability to perform self-care. This situation prompted the initial referral to the home health team. All of the nursing concerns are relevant to Ms. D's comprehensive care plan. While gas exchange is frequently the priority, Ms. D is managing her COPD by using medication and supplemental oxygen as needed. An O_2 Sat of 93% on room air is an acceptable finding for patients with COPD. Smoking cessation, weight loss, and moderate exercise would be encouraged to improve tissue oxygenation. **Focus:** Prioritization; **QSEN:** PCC; **Concept:** Pain, Functional Ability; **Cognitive Level:** Applying. **Test Taking Tip:** To answer this type of question, you have to consider all of the information that you have been given. (*"Ms. D's primary worries are pain and difficulty with accomplishing activities of daily living."*) This may seem very difficult at first, to remember everything or to go back and reread the excerpts from the case study; however, the ability to identify salient information and to "connect the dots" mimics what you must do when you care for patients in the clinical setting.

7. **Ans: 3**   The nurse would monitor for changes in vital signs after minor exertion, especially pulse, respiratory

rate, and O_2 Sat. Low-grade fever is a systemic sign that often accompanies RA. Respirations and blood pressure that are slightly above the normal range would be expected findings for patients who are overweight or those with COPD. An O_2 Sat of 93% on room air is an acceptable level for patients with COPD. If Ms. D shows signs of increased respiratory effort, pulse oximetry would be checked and oxygen would be administered via nasal cannula as needed. An increase in temperature would signal need to observe for signs/symptoms of infection (increases in pulse and respiratory rate are likely to accompany a fever). If vital signs are ordered every 4 hours by the HCP, the nurse would consult with the supervising RN about advocating for transfer to a facility with around-the-clock staff. **Focus:** Prioritization; **QSEN:** PCC; **Concept:** Clinical Judgment; **Cognitive Level:** Analyzing

8. **Ans: 1**   NSAIDs are prescribed for pain relief and to decrease inflammation and are considered first-line medications for RA. DMARDs can prevent joint deterioration if administered in the early stages. TNF inhibitors have serious side effects and must be administered by IV or by subcutaneous injection. Corticosteroids are usually used for controlling flare-ups. **Focus:** Prioritization; **QSEN:** EBP; **Concept:** Pain, Inflammation; **Cognitive Level:** Applying

9. **Ans: 2**   Etanercept is a TNF inhibitor and has a "black box warning" for exacerbation of TB. Patients should be advised to inform the HCP about conditions that affect immunity, such as HIV or diabetes. Patients should discuss the use of contraception with the HCP before starting etanercept. If the patient is pregnant, the benefits of taking etanercept would be weighed against the possible risk to the fetus (birth defects). HPV is a sexually transmitted disease; some types of HPV increase the risk for cervical cancer or genital warts. **Focus:** Prioritization; **QSEN:** S; **Concept:** Immunity, Infection; **Cognitive Level:** Applying. **Test Taking Tip:** A "black box warning" is the strongest warning issued by the Food and Drug Administration. It alerts the public and the health care staff that the drug has serious side effects that could result in injury or death. If you must administer a medication with a "black box warning" during your clinical rotations, consult the charge nurse or your instructor as needed.

10. **Ans: 3**   Morphine is used to relieve the pain that occurs during an acute exacerbation of RA. Morphine is not recommended for long-term management as a daily dose or PRN for pain. Decreasing inflammation that causes the pain is considered a better approach. **Focus:** Prioritization; **QSEN:** EBP; **Concept:** Pain; **Cognitive Level:** Applying

11. **Ans: 4**   During the flare, extra rest will help Ms. D to deal with the pain. Joints should not be positioned in flexion. In RA, joints have a tendency for flexion contractures that decrease mobility. At this point,

sitting for several hours may be too much for Ms. D. In the supine position, one pillow is used to support the head and neck. The nurse would advise Ms. D about how to protect joints and explain the rationale for frequent repositioning. The nurse must periodically assess Ms. D's ability to reposition herself. In the acute phase, she may need more assistance because of the pain and her weight. **Focus:** Prioritization, Supervision; **QSEN:** PCC; **Concept:** Fatigue, Inflammation; **Cognitive Level:** Applying

12. **Ans: 3**   Iron deficiency anemia is a common problem for patients with RA. Low levels of RBCs decrease the oxygen-carrying capacity of the blood and the patient experiences fatigue, which worsens with exertion. The normal range for RBCs: 4.2–5.4 million/mm^3 (4.2–5.4×10^{12}). In iron deficiency anemia, platelet levels would increase. The normal range for platelets is 150,000–400,000/mm^3 (150–400×10^9). Albumin and globulin are blood proteins that reflect nutritional status. Decreased levels of either indicate malnutrition; an increased level of beta globulin is associated with iron deficiency anemia. The normal range of albumin is 3.5–5 g/dL (35–50 g/L). Partial thromboplastin time is a coagulation test that measures blood clotting times. The normal range is 25–35 seconds. **Focus:** Prioritization; **QSEN:** EBP; **Concept:** Fatigue, Perfusion; **Cognitive Level:** Analyzing

13. **Ans: 2**   During a flare, rest helps to reduce pain and workload on the joints. Sitting is a way to conserve energy (as opposed to standing or walking around). The nurse would avoid giving instructions that are vague or instructions that require the home health aide to make judgments that exceed the scope of practice. The nurse must assess and determine the types of activities that would include "any activity that she is unable to accomplish." An example of an unsafe and incorrect instruction is, "Wait until she asks for help." The team has already identified key times when Ms. D requires help: in the morning when joints are stiff and painful; during showering; and whenever bending, reaching, or balancing are required. Ms. D is likely to feel better in the afternoon compared to the morning; however, activities must be interspersed with periods of rest. During the acute phase, the nurse would assess Ms. D's energy and pain levels throughout the day and instruct the aide accordingly. **Focus:** Prioritization, Supervision; **QSEN:** PCC; **Concept:** Pain, Functional Ability; **Cognitive Level:** Analyzing **IPEC:** IC

14. **Ans: 4**   The home health aide can reinforce instructions that are given by the nurse. Applications should be removed if the patient notes a sensation of numbness. The other interventions are used for cold and heat applications, but these should be performed by the nurse. **Focus:** Delegation, Supervision; **QSEN:** S; **Concept:** Pain, Sensory Perception; **Cognitive Level:** Applying; **IPEC:** R/R

15. **Ans: 2, 3, 4, 5, 6** Exercising past the point of pain is incorrect. Patients should be advised to stop at the point of pain. If joints are still sore 1 to 2 hours postexercise, this indicates that the workout was excessive and should be scaled back. The other points are important for joint protection. **Focus:** Prioritization; **QSEN:** S; **Concept:** Mobility, Patient Education; **Cognitive Level:** Applying

16. **Ans: 4** The muscles and joints in the arm are larger and stronger than those in the hand. Ms. D would be reminded to push up using the palmar surface of the hands, not the fingers. A small comb requires fine motor finger manipulation, whereas using with a long-handled brush activates the elbow and shoulder joints. Likewise, a shoulder bag rests on the shoulder, while a purse with a short handle must be held by the hand and the fingers. **Focus:** Prioritization; **QSEN:** PCC; **Concept:** Patient Education; **Cognitive Level:** Analyzing

17. **Ans: 3** In option 3, Ms. D is expressing thankfulness for the presence of the team and doubt about self-management of care. Self-doubt and fear of abandonment are barriers that prevent Ms. D from progressing. The home health team is currently fulfilling several needs for Ms. D: pain management, help with ADLs, and socialization. As she progresses toward the long-term goal of self-management, the home health team would begin to reduce the frequency of visits. Ms. D might be anxious about the potential loss of support. The nurse would consult with the other team members so that the plan of care can be evaluated and updated. Revisions could include interventions to meet the needs that the home health team is currently fulfilling, such as identifying support groups and offering outpatient visits or follow-up phone calls. Options 1 and 2 reflect feelings and needs related to the acute flare. Option 4 suggests a readiness to work toward the long-term goal of self-management. **Focus:** Prioritization; **QSEN:** PCC; **Concept:** Self-Management, Anxiety; **Cognitive Level:** Analyzing

18. **Ans: 2, 3, 5, 6, 7, 8, 9** The nurse and the home health aide are the team members who will spend most of the time with Ms. D in the home setting, so the other members of the health care team must be informed about events that are unexpected, such as falls, trips to the ED, calls to the HCP, and extra or unscheduled visits. Occurrences that indicate that the care plan needs to be revised (receptiveness to patient education, readiness or barriers to meeting goals, inability or refusal to participate, and indications of low self-esteem) should be discussed and the plan should be revised accordingly. Routine information, such as vital signs and scheduled medication, does not need to be discussed unless there is a problem. **Focus:** Prioritization; **QSEN:** PCC; **Concept:** Care Coordination, Self-Management; **Cognitive Level:** Analyzing; **IPEC:** IC

QSEN Key: PCC, Patient-Centered Care; **TC,** Teamwork & Collaboration; **EBP,** Evidence-Based Practice; **QI,** Quality Improvement; **S,** Safety; **I,** Informatics.
IPEC Key: Domain 1 Values/Ethics (**V/E**); Domain 2 Roles/Responsibilities (**R/R**); Domain 3 Interprofessional Communication (**IC**); Domain 4 Teams/Teamwork (**T/T**).

PART 3 Complex Health Scenarios

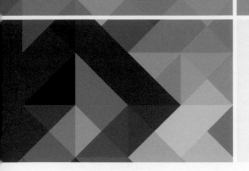

Patient With Pneumonia

Questions

Ms. S is a 69-year-old living at home with her daughter's family, which includes two school-age children. Her past medical history includes smoking cigarettes (one pack/day) for 48 years (she quit a year ago when she moved in with her daughter). She received a flu shot 1 month ago during her annual check-up. Her medical history includes hypertension and chronic obstructive pulmonary disease (COPD) with a cough, but she has not required supplemental oxygen. She is alert and oriented. After caring for her 13-year-old granddaughter, who was off from school for 3 days with cold-like symptoms and a sore throat, Ms. S developed a fever, chills, productive cough, and muscle aches. Her daughter makes an appointment with the primary health care provider (HCP) for an evaluation.

1. What does the nurse at the HCP's office suspect is the **most** likely cause of Ms. S's symptoms?
   1. Hospital-acquired pneumonia (HAP).
   2. Influenza (flu).
   3. Health care–associated pneumonia (HCAP).
   4. Community-acquired pneumonia (CAP).

2. Which factors does the nurse recognize increase a patient's risk for the development of CAP? **Select all that apply.**
   1. Frequent use of gastrointestinal (GI) acid-suppressive therapy.
   2. Immunosuppressive therapy.
   3. Living in a long-term care facility.
   4. Aging with decreased immune system function.
   5. Exposure to pneumonia-causing bacteria.
   6. Chemotherapy.

3. Which actions or interventions will the nurse delegate to the assistive personnel (AP)? **Select all that apply.**
   1. Checking and recording the patient's current weight.
   2. Assisting the patient up on to the exam table.
   3. Collecting and recording the patient's current medications.
   4. Checking and recording the patient's vital signs.
   5. Asking the patient about current symptoms.
   6. Auscultating the patient's lung sounds.

Ms. S's vital signs are: T 101.8°F (38.8°C), HR 98/min, RR 26/min, BP 164/86. Her weight is 188 lb. (85.3 kg). Oxygen saturation by pulse oximetry is 92% on room air.

4. Which diagnostic tests will the nurse expect to be prescribed by the HCP?
   1. Chest x-ray (radiograph) and streptococcal throat swab.
   2. Chest computed tomography (CT) and tuberculin skin test.
   3. Chest magnetic resonance imaging (MRI) and pulmonary function tests.
   4. Alpha-1 antitrypsin and complete blood count.

5. After assessment, the HCP diagnoses Ms. S with typical CAP. Which medication will the nurse expect the HCP to prescribe?
   1. Trimethoprim-sulfamethoxazole.
   2. Erythromycin.
   3. Acyclovir.
   4. Pyrazinamide.

6. Which types of interventions will be included in the nursing care plan for Ms. S? **Select all that apply.**
   1. Promoting oxygenation.
   2. Controlling elevated temperature.
   3. Providing adequate rest.
   4. Monitoring vital signs and respiratory status.
   5. Decreasing fluid intake.
   6. Providing good oral hygiene.

7. Which interventions that help promote oxygenation can be delegated to the AP? **Select all that apply.**
   1. Teaching the patient the use of incentive spirometry.
   2. Reminding the patient to take deep breaths every 2 hours.
   3. Increasing the oxygen flow rate from 1 to 3 L by nasal cannula.
   4. Elevating the patient's head of bed to 30 degrees.
   5. Assessing the patient's ability to perform incentive spirometry.
   6. Administering acetaminophen 650 mg orally as needed.

Ms. S is discharged to home with instructions to take her prescribed medication, use acetaminophen for fever, rest, and drink extra fluids. After a day has passed, she becomes confused, is short of breath, and continues to run a low-grade fever (100.2°F [37.9°C]) and experience cough and chills. The HCP has her admitted to the hospital stepdown unit with a diagnosis of pneumonia.

8. Which actions or interventions will the admitting nurse delegate to the experienced AP? **Select all that apply.**
   1. Checking the patient's oxygen saturation.
   2. Placing the patient on a telemetry monitor.
   3. Taking and recording vital signs every 4 hours.
   4. Placing an intravenous (IV) catheter for fluid administration.
   5. Completing the patient's initial assessment.
   6. Reminding the patient to call for assistance to get out of bed.

9. Which action related to Ms. S's confusion will be **best** to protect Ms. S's safety?
   1. Raising all four bed rails.
   2. Applying soft restraints.
   3. Instituting fall precautions.
   4. Placing the call light within reach.

10. The HCP prescribes IV ciprofloxacin 50 mg every 8 hours. What is the nurse's **best** response when Ms. S's daughter asks about the purpose of this drug?
    1. "Ciprofloxacin is an antibacterial drug and is given to kill the bacteria that are causing your mother's pneumonia."
    2. "Ciprofloxacin is an antiacid drug given to prevent stomach ulcers that are common in older hospitalized patients."
    3. "The ciprofloxacin is being given intravenously because your mother is confused and cannot take the oral form of the drug."
    4. "We think your mother may have a viral pneumonia and ciprofloxacin will help destroy the virus that is causing her pneumonia."

11. Nextgen Drag and Drop

Instructions: The admitting nurse's assessment of Ms. S demonstrates these findings. Place an X beside the assessment findings that require immediate follow-up by the nurse.

Assessment Finding	Assessment Finding That Requires Immediate Follow-up
Confused as to place, date, and time.	
Temperature 101.4°F (38.6°C).	
Heart rate 92/min, irregular.	
RR 26/min.	
BP 160/68.	
Active bowel sounds.	
Crackles bilaterally in lung bases.	
Productive cough thick blood-specked sputum.	
Muscle aches.	
Oxygen saturation 89%.	
Chills.	

Ms. S is placed on supplemental oxygen at 3 L per nasal cannula. Her respiratory rate increases to 32/min and SaO$_2$ decreases to 87%. Crackles are heard bilaterally from the bases to halfway up the lungs.

12. What is the **first** action for the nurse to take at this time?
    1. Increasing the oxygen flow rate to 8 L/min.
    2. Initiating a rapid response or notifying the HCP.
    3. Changing the nasal cannula to a simple face mask.
    4. Requesting the respiratory therapist to provide incentive spirometry.

13. Ms. S is placed on oxygen with a nonrebreather mask. Which action will the nurse take to ensure a high concentration of oxygen?
    1. Making sure that the reservoir bag deflates during inspiration.
    2. Teaching the patient how to provide oral suctioning.
    3. Checking to make sure that the mask fits snugly.
    4. Washing and drying the mask twice each shift.

14. Which medication does the nurse prepare to administer to the patient to help improve the abnormal breath sounds?
    1. Furosemide.
    2. Dexamethasone.
    3. Spironolactone.
    4. Acetaminophen.

After 4 hours on a nonrebreather mask, Ms. S's respiratory rate is 22/min, SaO$_2$ is 93%, and crackles are heard in the lung bases.

15. Which assessment findings indicate to the nurse that Ms. S's respiratory status has improved after 4 hours on the nonrebreather mask? **Select all that apply.**
    1. RR is 22/min.
    2. Inspirational wheezes are auscultated.
    3. SaO$_2$ is 92%.
    4. Heart rate is 88 and irregular.
    5. Urine output is decreased.
    6. Crackles occur in lung bases.

Answers

1. **Ans: 4** CAP is defined as pneumonia that is acquired outside of the hospital. It can be spread from person to person and may be caused by bacteria, viruses, or fungi. Signs and symptoms include high fever, chills, productive cough, sweating, chest pain, malaise, and aching muscles. HAP and HCAP are acquired in a hospital or an other health care setting. Since the patient had a flu shot 1 month ago, the cause of her symptoms is not likely to be influenza. **Focus:** Prioritization; **QSEN:** PCC; **Concept:** Gas Exchange, Infection; **Cognitive Level:** Analyzing; **Cognitive Skill:** Recognizing Cues

2. **Ans: 1, 4, 5** Research has demonstrated that GI acid-suppressive therapy makes people in the community more susceptible to CAP. Decreased immune system function associated with age and exposure to pneumonia-causing bacteria also increase the risk of CAP. Immunosuppressive therapy, chemotherapy, and living in a long-term care facility are risk factors for the development of HCAP. **Focus:** Prioritization; **QSEN:** PCC, S; **Concept:** Infection; **Cognitive Level:** Analyzing

3. **Ans: 1, 2, 4** Checking a patient's weight and vital signs, as well as assisting a patient with getting up on the exam table, is within the scope of practice for an AP. Collecting information about current medication and symptoms, as well as listening to a patient's lung sounds, requires the additional training and skills of a professional nurse. **Focus:** Delegation, Supervision; **QSEN:** PCC, TC, S; **Concept:** Gas Exchange, Care Coordination; **Cognitive Level:** Applying; **IPEC:** R/R, IC

4. **Ans: 1** A diagnosis of pneumonia is confirmed by chest radiograph, which reveals densities in the affected lung(s). The HCP may also order a streptococcal throat swab because Ms. S was exposed to cold-like symptoms and had a sore throat while caring for her granddaughter. **Focus:** Prioritization; **QSEN:** PCC; **Concept:** Gas Exchange, Infection; **Cognitive Level:** Analyzing

5. **Ans: 2** Typical pneumonia is treated with antibiotic drugs such as erythromycin, macrolides such as clarithromycin, cephalosporins such as cefazolin, aminoglycosides such as amikacin, and fluoroquinolones such as ciprofloxacin. Trimethoprim is used to treat *P. jirovecii* associated with acquired immunodeficiency syndrome (AIDS). Acyclovir is an antiviral drug, and pyrazinamide is used to treat tuberculosis. **Focus:** Prioritization; **QSEN:** PCC, EBP; **Concept:** Infection; **Cognitive Level:** Analyzing

6. **Ans: 1, 2, 3, 4, 6** All of these types of interventions are important when caring for a patient with pneumonia except decreasing fluids. Maintaining adequate nutrition and fluid intake are essential for Ms. S. **Focus:** Prioritization; **QSEN:** PCC; **Concept:** Gas Exchange, Infection; **Cognitive Level:** Analyzing; **Cognitive Skill:** Generating Solutions

7. **Ans: 2, 4** APs can remind the patient what has already been taught and elevate the head of the patient's bed. The nurse would be responsible for supervision. Teaching about or assessing the use of incentive spirometry and making changes in the patient's oxygen flow rate require additional knowledge and skills and should be done by the professional nurse or physical therapist. Giving acetaminophen will not promote oxygenation. **Focus:** Delegation, Supervision; **QSEN:** PCC, TC, S; **Concept:** Gas Exchange; **Cognitive Level:** Analyzing

8. **Ans: 1, 2, 3, 6** The experienced AP would have been trained on how to measure oxygen saturation using a pulse oximeter and correct placement of leads for telemetry monitoring. The nurse would be responsible for assuring that the AP is proficient in these skills. Checking and recording vital signs is within an AP's scope of practice, as well as reminding the patient about what has already been taught by the nurse. Placing an IV catheter and completing the patient's initial assessment requires the skills and training of the nurse. **Focus:** Delegation; Supervision; **QSEN:** PCC, TC; **Concept:** Care Coordination; **Cognitive Level:** Applying; **Cognitive Skill:** Generating Solutions

9. **Ans: 3** When an older adult is confused, the risk for falls increases, so instituting fall precautions is the best way to protect the patient. The application of restraints must not be used until other strategies have been tried and requires an order from the HCP. Raising all siderails is not recommended and will likely increase the risk of falls for a patient who is confused and is also considered a form of restraint. Because of her confusion, Ms. S does not understand that she is in the hospital and may not remember how to use the call light. **Focus:** Prioritization; **QSEN:** PCC, S; **Concept:** Safety; **Cognitive Level:** Analyzing

10. **Ans: 1** Ciprofloxacin is a DNA synthesis inhibitor antibacterial drug used to kill the bacteria causing the pneumonia. The second and fourth options are not correct. The third option may be accurate but does not answer the daughter's question. **Focus:** Prioritization; **QSEN:** PCC; **Concept:** Infection, Patient Education; **Cognitive Level:** Analyzing

PART 3 Complex Health Scenarios

11. **Ans:**

Assessment Finding	Assessment Finding That Requires Immediate Follow-up
Confused as to place, date, and time.	
Temperature 101.4°F (38.6°C).	X
Heart rate 92/min, irregular.	X
RR 26/min.	
BP 160/68.	
Active bowel sounds.	
Crackles bilaterally in lung bases.	X
Productive cough thick blood-specked sputum.	
Muscle aches.	
Oxygen saturation 89%.	X
Chills.	

While all of these findings are important, some were noted on admission and so do not require immediate follow-up (e.g., confusion, BP) and some are expected findings for pneumonia (e.g., muscle aches, chills, productive cough). Some are normal findings (e.g., RR, active bowel sounds). Increased temperature may indicate worsening fever. Wheezes and crackles on auscultation of the lungs and decreased SaO_2 indicate worsening or lung status with fluid-filled alveoli and decreased gas exchange. An irregular heart rate may indicate atrial fibrillation with the risk of pulmonary emboli. These changes require immediate follow-up. **Focus:** Prioritization; **QSEN:** PCC, S; **Concept:** Gas Exchange, Clinical Judgment; **Cognitive Level:** Analyzing; **Cognitive Skill:** Analyzing Cues. **Test Taking Tip:** When the assessment of a patient demonstrates changes that indicate a worsening condition, follow-up is needed immediately.

12. **Ans: 2**   The changes in Ms. S's respiratory status indicate worsening of the pneumonia and immediate follow-up is necessary to prevent a life-threatening event such as a respiratory arrest. She will require changes in the plan of care to treat her pneumonia and may need to be transferred to the intensive care unit. Increasing oxygen flow rate is contraindicated for a patient with COPD without an order from the HCP. Incentive spirometry alone will not treat the patient's worsening symptoms. **Focus:** Prioritization; **QSEN:** PCC, S; **Concept:** Gas Exchange, Clinical Judgment, Safety; **Cognitive Level:** Analyzing; **Cognitive Skill:** Recognizing Cues. **Test Taking Tip:** When a question asks what the nurse should do first, think about ABCs and what may be life-threatening when a patient's condition is worsening.

13. **Ans: 3**   To ensure that the patient receives a high concentration of oxygen (80%–95%), the nonrebreather mask must sit snugly on the face. A reservoir should not be allowed to deflate during inspiration because oxygen delivery is decreased and rebreathing of exhaled air is increased. Oral suctioning as well as washing and drying the mask requires that the patient remove the mask, which will decrease oxygen delivery. **Focus:** Prioritization; **QSEN:** PCC; **Concept:** Gas Exchange; **Cognitive Level:** Applying

14. **Ans: 1**   Ms. S's crackles increased from the base to halfway up the lungs, indicating fluid-filled alveoli. Furosemide is a loop diuretic that will help to decrease the fluid in her lungs. Dexamethasone is a corticosteroid that will decrease inflammation. Spironolactone is a potassium-sparing diuretic. Acetaminophen will help to bring down the patient's temperature. **Focus:** Prioritization; **QSEN:** PCC, EBP; **Concept:** Gas Exchange; **Cognitive Level:** Analyzing

15. **Ans: 1, 3, 6**   Improved respiratory status is indicated by decreased respiratory rate, increased oxygen saturation (87%–92%), and decreased presence of crackles. Wheezes might be an indication of worsening respiratory status. Since the patient received furosemide, increased urine output would indicate improvement. The heart rate and rhythm are essentially unchanged. **Focus:** Prioritization; **QSEN:** PCC, EBP; **Concept:** Gas Exchange, Clinical Judgment; **Cognitive Level:** Analyzing; **Cognitive Skill:** Recognizing Cues

QSEN Key: PCC, Patient-Centered Care; **TC,** Teamwork & Collaboration; **EBP,** Evidence-Based Practice; **QI,** Quality Improvement; **S,** Safety; **I,** Informatics.

IPEC Key: Domain 1 Values/Ethics (**V/E**); Domain 2 Roles/Responsibilities (**R/R**); Domain 3 Interprofessional Communication (**IC**); Domain 4 Teams/Teamwork (**T/T**).

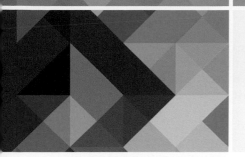

CASE STUDY 5

Patient With a Brain Attack (Stroke)

Questions

Mr. S is an 80-year-old man who had a brain attack (stroke or cerebral vascular accident [CVA]) 4 weeks ago and is being transferred from a rehabilitation center to a long-term care facility. The transfer report indicates that he sustained left-sided brain damage and has residual weakness and paralysis. Dysphagia has created problems with eating. He is aphasic and is having difficulty following commands or performing simple tasks. He is depressed and withdrawn. His wife and daughter want to be involved in his care. He has a history of high blood pressure, atrial fibrillation, and diabetes. Prescribed medications include furosemide, lisinopril, nimodipine, warfarin, and metformin.

 1. Enhanced Drag and Drop.

Scenario: The health care team includes the registered nurse (RN), LPN/LVN, physical therapist, occupational therapist, assistive personnel (AP), speech therapist, social worker, dietitian, and health care provider (HCP). Each will contribute to the admission assessment by performing tasks within their area of expertise

Which tasks are **best** to assign or delegate to each team member?

Instructions: Team members are listed in the left column. In the right-hand column, in the space provided, write in the letter for the best staff member to delegate or assign each task. Note that all responses will be used only once.

Team members

a. RN
b. LPN/LVN
c. AP
d. Physical therapist
e. Speech therapist
f. Occupational therapist
g. Social worker
h. Dietician
i. HCP

Admission Tasks

1. _____ Measure weight and height
2. _____ Assess understanding and use of community-based resources
3. _____ Assess level of consciousness and level of cognitive function
4. _____ Assess use of strategies for medication adherence
5. _____ Evaluate diagnostic and physical findings; make treatment plan
6. _____ Assess strength, mobility, and balance
7. _____ Evaluate ability to swallow and speak
8. _____ Assess ability to perform fine motor tasks with unaffected hand
9. _____ Evaluate understanding and compliance with diabetic and heart-healthy dietary recommendations

2. Cloze. _____

Scenario: Based on knowledge of the pathophysiology of brain attack, the nurse is able to anticipate problems that Mr. S is likely to experience.

Instructions: Complete the sentences below by choosing the best option for the missing information that corresponds with the same numbered list of options provided.

With left-sided brain damage, Mr. S is likely to have _____1_____. With left-sided brain damage, there are typical patterns of behavior. Mr. S is likely to act _____2_____ For sensory information, Mr. S is most likely to have problems with _____3_____

Options for 1

a. global quadriplegia

b. generalized hemiparesis

c. bilateral paraplegia

d. right-sided hemiplegia

e. left-sided hemiplegia

Options for 2

a. slowly and cautiously

b. quickly and impulsively

c. childlike and regressive

d. agitated and belligerent

e. fearful and paranoid

Options for 3

a. smelling subtle odors

b. losses in visual field

c. hearing high frequencies

d. generalized pain perception

e. tasting difference between salt and sour

3. The LPN/LVN is assigned to care for Mr. S and is assisting the RN to complete the comprehensive admission assessment. Which portion of the assessment would be the **most** appropriate for the LPN/LVN to perform?
   1. Assessment of family's level of involvement in care.
   2. Focused assessment of Mr. S's skin to establish baseline.
   3. Assessment of Mr. S's understanding of therapeutic goals.
   4. Obtaining and reporting vital signs and pulse oximeter reading.

4. The nurse is reviewing the hospital documentation and a rhythm strip is included in the record. Which cardiac arrythmia increases the risk for a brain attack secondary to emboli?
   1. Atrial fibrillation.
   2. Sinus tachycardia.
   3. Sinus rhythm with premature ventricular contractions.
   4. Ventricular tachycardia.

5. Mr. S received IV heparin in the hospital; warfarin is currently prescribed. Which instruction would the nurse give to the AP?
   1. "Use bleeding precautions."
   2. "Handle Mr. S very gently."
   3. "Use a disposable safety razor for shaving."
   4. "Avoid brushing Mr. S's teeth."

6. Which instruction would the nurse give to the AP regarding receptive aphasia for Mr. S?
   1. Keep the environment interesting and stimulating.
   2. Give reminders, as needed, about the purpose of a spoon or fork.
   3. Ask one question at a time and repeat using the exact words.
   4. Keep bed flat and frequently help him to turn or reposition.

7. Because Mr. S has dysphagia, the nurse instructs the AP to immediately report which signs or symptoms that may indicate aspiration?
   1. Difficulty with chewing.
   2. Pain or discomfort in the mouth.
   3. Coughing or wheezing after eating.
   4. Dryness of mucous membranes.

8. Which instruction would the nurse give to the AP to prevent aspiration when assisting Mr. S to eat or drink?
   1. Suggest that he eat breakfast toast first and then drink plenty of liquids afterward.
   2. Offer him a straw to drink cool fluids and encourage small frequent servings.
   3. Help him into an upright position and tilt his head slightly forward before eating.
   4. Serve lukewarm foods first and then serve the cold foods and liquids.

Complex Health Scenarios   PART 3

9. Social isolation is a nursing concern that is included in the care plan for Mr. S because of depression and withdrawal. Which response is the **most** therapeutic?
   1. "I think you would enjoy the company and conversation in the dining room."
   2. "Some children are giving a performance today. You like children, don't you?"
   3. "I'll take you to the dayroom so that you can see that everyone is friendly."
   4. "Would you like to see the schedule of activities for this week?"

10. The nurse takes vital signs, as ordered, immediately before administering the prescribed dose of nimodipine. The BP is 88/60 mm Hg and the P is 80 beats/min. Which action would the nurse take **first**?
    1. Hold the dose and notify the supervising RN.
    2. Perform a complete neurological assessment.
    3. Wait 15–20 minutes and then recheck the vital signs.
    4. Give nimodipine, but hold BP medications.

11. Which instruction would the nurse give to the AP about assisting Mr. S to dress because of the hemiplegia?
    1. Watch Mr. S and see what he will do for himself, before you offer to help him.
    2. Select clothes that are loose and easy to pull over the head, shoulders, and arms.
    3. Put clothing on the weak side first and remove clothing from the strong side first.
    4. Have Mr. S use the affected side as much as possible for range-of-motion exercise.

12. Mr. S is having problems with ataxia. Which member of the health care team would be **best** to assess deficits and suggest interventions?
    1. HCP.
    2. Speech therapist.
    3. Occupational therapist.
    4. Physical therapist.

After several weeks, the nurse notices that Mr. S is slowly progressing, but he is increasingly irritable and impatient toward his family and the staff. He has refused physical therapy several times and has expressed disinterest in using assistive devices that would safely increase his mobility and self-care. The AP reports that he rarely uses the call bell. He has made several attempts to get out of bed by himself and refuses help when it is offered.

13. The nurse confers with the supervising RN who advises the nurse to gather more data related to the **priority** nursing concern. On which area does the nurse focus?
    1. Mobility.
    2. Mood and affect.
    3. Safety.
    4. Stress and coping.

14. The nurse is assessing and supervising Mr. S as he tries to grasp and use an assistive device for self-feeding. He is not able to manipulate the device; he gets frustrated and uses profanity. Which response is the **most** therapeutic?
    1. "Mr. S, I'm sorry, I didn't quite understand what you were saying."
    2. "I understand your frustration, but please don't use that language."
    3. "You had a firm hold on the handle and that is a good place to start."
    4. "You seem upset; let me do this for you, I am here to help you."

15. Mr. S tells the nurse, "I just want to do things my own way." Which action would the nurse use **first**?
    1. Respect his wishes and allow him to do what he wants.
    2. Call the wife and daughter and tell them about his wishes.
    3. Ask the HCP to prescribe a safety reminder device (restraint).
    4. Inform the supervising RN and assist in developing a revised care plan.

Answers

1. **Ans: 1 c, 2 g, 3 a, 4 b, 5 i, 6 d, 7 e, 8 f, 9 h**   The nursing staff anchors the daily care, but including the expertise of other team members is the best way to accomplish the complex process of rehabilitation. The RN is responsible for the initial intake assessments. The LPN/LVN routinely performs focused assessments and is the team member who is likely to give daily care. The AP can collect basic information, such as weight, height, and vital signs, and performs most of the tasks associated with activities of daily living. Physical, occupational, and speech therapists and the dietician assess and help with problems that are related to their specialized knowledge. The social worker links the patient and family to community resources. The HCP uses physical and diagnostic findings to make a treatment plan. **Focus:** Assignment, Delegation; **QSEN:** TC; **Concept:** Care Coordination; **Cognitive Level:** Applying; **Cognitive Skill:** Recognize Cues; **IPEC:** R/R

2. **Ans: 1d, 2 a, 3 b**   With left-sided brain damage, Mr. S is likely to have **right-sided hemiplegia.** With left-sided brain damage, there are typical patterns of behavior. Mr. S is likely to act **slowly and cautiously.** For sensory information, Mr. S is most likely to have problems with **losses in visual field.** Left-sided brain damage causes right-sided weakness or hemiplegia (paralysis) and is associated with slow, cautious behavior; speech problems, such as aphasia; difficulty in following verbal commands; apraxia (difficulty with certain movements that can affect speech or other types of movement such as controlling extremities); and difficulty performing simple tasks. For sensory perception, visual disturbances are common. Paresthesia or loss of sensation to touch can occur on the affected side. **Focus:** Prioritization; **QSEN:** N/A; **Concept:** Intracranial Regulation; **Cognitive Level:** Analyzing; **Cognitive Skill:** Recognize Cues. **Test Taking Tip:** A working knowledge of common prefixes (para, quad, hemi) and suffixes (plegia, paresis) allows you to rapidly read the questions and understand patient conditions.

3. **Ans: 2**   The LPN/LVN can perform a focused assessment on the skin. Baseline and periodic skin assessment are required for facilities that receive Medicare funding. The RN is responsible for assessing family involvement and understanding therapeutic goals. These are complex issues and there are likely to be many questions, obstacles, and negotiations. The AP can obtain and report vital signs and pulse oximeter reading. **Focus:** Assignment; **QSEN:** TC; **Concept:** Care Coordination; **Cognitive Level:** Applying

4. **Ans: 1**   In atrial fibrillation, the atrium is not completely emptied; flow is abnormal, and blood tends to pool and form emboli. These emboli are then ejected into the circulation. Brain attack occurs when emboli are lodged in a blood vessel and blood flow is obstructed to a portion of the brain. **Focus:** Prioritization; **QSEN:** N/A; **Concept:** Perfusion, Clotting; **Cognitive Level:** Analyzing

5. **Ans: 2**   The AP is instructed to handle Mr. S very gently. Warfarin is an anticoagulant and this increases the risk for bleeding and bruising. Using bleeding precautions is correct; however, instructions should include specific details (e.g., use a soft toothbrush, avoid bumping into hard surfaces, avoid use of sharp objects such as scissors); the AP is not expected to know the pathophysiology of blood clotting or to determine which routine activities would be harmful to Mr. S. Electric razors are used rather than disposable safety razors and the teeth are brushed very gently with a soft bristle brush. **Focus:** Delegation, Supervision; **QSEN:** S; **Concept:** Perfusion, Clotting; **Cognitive Level:** Applying. **Test Taking Tip:** Pay extra attention to high-alert medications, such as anticoagulants. High-alert medications are identified because patient harm can occur if there are errors in administration. Safety issues and actions that prevent patient harm are likely to be tested during NCLEX. For list see: https://www.ismp.org/recommendations/high-alert-medications-acute-list.

6. **Ans: 3**   Receptive aphasia manifests as trouble understanding written or verbal communication. The nurse would instruct the AP to ask one question (or make one statement) at a time and, if necessary, repeat the phase using the exact wording. Additional instructions would include reducing environmental distractors, facing the person when speaking, and allowing extra time for communication. Gestures, hand signals, or picture boards may also be useful. Agnosia may cause troubles in recognizing common objects, such as a spoon or fork. Following a brain attack, some patients may need help to turn or reposition in bed, but keeping the bed flat increases the risk for aspiration. **Focus:** Delegation, Supervision; **QSEN:** TC; **Concept:** Cognition, Communication; **Cognitive Level:** Analyzing; **IPEC:** IC

7. **Ans: 3**   Aspiration occurs when food, fluid, or a foreign object is inhaled into the airway. Coughing is the body's attempt to expel the foreign material. Wheezing occurs when the airway is narrowed or partially obstructed. Difficulty chewing, uncomfortable sensations in the throat (pain or sensation that

something is in the back of the throat), and drooling can occur with dysphagia. **Focus:** Delegation, Supervision; **QSEN:** S; **Concept:** Gas Exchange, Safety; **Cognitive Level:** Analyzing

8. **Ans: 3** Positioning in an upright position during and after eating helps to prevent aspiration and facilitates the peristaltic action of the esophagus in moving the food down into the stomach. Toast, crackers, and other dry foods and lukewarm foods are difficult to swallow and are poor choices for patients with dysphagia. Straws are avoided; muscle control is required for simultaneous sucking and swallowing and can be difficult for patients with dysphagia. **Focus:** Delegation, Supervision; **QSEN:** S; **Concept:** Gas Exchange, Safety; **Cognitive Level:** Applying. **Test Taking Tip:** The risk for aspiration increases with dysphagia (difficulty swallowing), supine position, unconscious states, poor dentition, or laughing or talking while eating. Can you name other causes? Aspiration is dangerous and largely preventable through vigilant nursing interventions. Such topics are likely to be tested by NCLEX.

9. **Ans: 4** This is a closed question that requires a yes or no answer, but it is the only option that offers Mr. S the freedom of choice. "I think you would" is an example of giving unsolicited advice. "You like children, don't you?" is phrased so that "yes" is the only correct response. "I'll take you" indicates that the decision is made for Mr. S and "Everyone is friendly" indicates the expected social norm. **Focus:** Prioritization; **QSEN:** PCC; **Concept:** Communication; **Cognitive Level:** Analyzing

10. **Ans: 1** Nimodipine, a calcium channel blocker, is one of the commonly prescribed medications after a brain attack. Vital signs should be obtained immediately before administration and the dose is held for a systolic BP of <90 mm Hg or a P <60 beats/min. After notifying the supervising RN, a complete neurological assessment, rechecking the vital signs, and holding BP medications would be appropriate. **Focus:** Prioritization; **QSEN:** S; **Concept:** Perfusion, Safety; **Cognitive Level:** Analyzing

11. **Ans: 3** Putting clothing on the weak side first and removing clothing from the strong side first allows the AP and Mr. S to maximize the use of the stronger side in accomplishing this task. Assessing what Mr. S can and cannot do for himself is the nurse's responsibility. This cannot be delegated to the AP. Selecting clothes for Mr. S is not appropriate; he should be allowed to choose his own clothes. The physical therapist or RN may have Mr. S use his weak side to evaluate

function and progress; this is not an appropriate task to delegate to the AP. **Focus:** Delegation, Supervision; **QSEN:** TC; **Concept:** Mobility; **Cognitive Level:** Analyzing; **IPEC:** IC

12. **Ans: 4** Ataxia is loss of balance or poor coordination. The physical therapist would be the best team member to evaluate Mr. S and to suggest exercises and assistive devices that increase strength and improve balance. **Focus:** Assignment; **QSEN:** TC; **Concept:** Mobility; **Cognitive Level:** Applying; **IPEC:** R/R

13. **Ans: 3** The priority issue is Mr. S's safety. He is at risk for falls and refusal or reluctance to ask for or receive help is an obstacle to safety and to achieving short-term and long-term goals. All of these nursing concerns must eventually be addressed. **Focus:** Prioritization; **QSEN:** Safety; **Concept:** Safety; **Cognitive Level:** Applying

14. **Ans: 3** The nurse gives positive feedback on the portion of the task that was successfully completed (firm hold). Frustration is expected and the use of profanity is not uncommon. Rather than denying (did not understand) or chastising (do not use that language), the nurse focuses on giving positive reinforcement. Acknowledging feelings (you seem upset) is therapeutic and performing a task for Mr. S is appropriate if he is fatigued or unable to accomplish it ("I'll do this for you"), but the nurse must also foster expectations for future success (you can try later). **Focus:** Prioritization; **QSEN:** PCC; **Concept:** Communication; **Cognitive Level:** Analyzing

15. **Ans: 4** The nursing staff must evaluate and revise the care plan. Recovering from a brain attack is a long process and the patient and family may experience episodic discouragement and frustration. Conveying respect is always important, but the staff is responsible for maintaining safety. The patient and family should be involved in revising the plan and reevaluating the goals. Least restrictive measures are used first; safety reminder devices are always used as a last resort. **Focus:** Prioritization; **QSEN:** PCC; **Concept:** Communication; **Cognitive Level:** Analyzing; **IPEC:** T/T

QSEN Key: PCC, Patient-Centered Care; **TC,** Teamwork & Collaboration; **EBP,** Evidence-Based Practice; **QI,** Quality Improvement; **S,** Safety; **I,** Informatics.

IPEC Key: Domain 1 Values/Ethics (**V/E**); Domain 2 Roles/Responsibilities (**R/R**); Domain 3 Interprofessional Communication (**IC**); Domain 4 Teams/Teamwork (**T/T**).

PART 3 Complex Health Scenarios

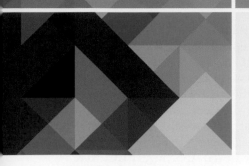

Patient With Chronic Obstructive Pulmonary Disease

Questions

Mr. K is a 74-year-old retired coal miner who is brought to the emergency department (ED) with reports of increased shortness of breath on exertion. He states that he has a cold that started with a dry cough but for the last 2 weeks, the cough has become productive of thick, green sputum. He is short of breath and reports chest discomfort. He has crackles in the bases of his lungs with an occasional expiratory wheeze. He is wearing a simple face mask and the triage nurse has placed him in an isolation room.

History: chronic obstructive pulmonary disease (COPD) for 10 years after a 25-year history of smoking two packs of cigarettes a day, left cerebrovascular accident (CVA) with right-sided weakness 2 months ago, for which he wears an arm splint. Medications: fluticasone/salmeterol two puffs twice a day, albuterol inhaler two puffs every 8 hours and prn. He has an allergy to penicillin. A chest x-ray, complete blood count (CBC), electrolytes, arterial blood gases (ABGs), 12-lead EKG, peak flow, sputum specimen for culture and sensitivity, a rapid diagnostic COVID-19 antigen test, and a venturi mask at 28% oxygen were prescribed.

Vital signs on admission are:
T 102°F (38.9°C)
HR 108
R 30 breaths/min
BP 154/92
O_2 Sat 85% on 1 L of oxygen.

1. What is the **priority** action for the nurse?
   1. Place the patient on the venturi mask at 28% oxygen.
   2. Perform a 12-lead EKG.
   3. Place the patient on the monitor.
   4. Apply personal protective equipment (PPE).

2. Which nursing actions can the nurse delegate to the assistive personnel (AP) in the ED? **Select all that apply.**
   1. Increase the oxygen level of the venturi mask to 31%.
   2. Record vital signs every 15 minutes.
   3. Assist the patient to the bathroom.
   4. Give an update to Mr. K's wife in the waiting room.
   5. Assist the respiratory therapist (RT) with collecting the ABGs.
   6. Place an airborne precaution sign on Mr. K's door.

3. When is the **best** time for the nurse to collect the sputum specimen on Mr. K?
   1. In the morning to get a fresh specimen.
   2. Before the nebulizer treatment in the ED.
   3. After the nebulizer treatment in the ED.
   4. After the antibiotics have been given.

4. Which position is **best** for the nurse to instruct the AP to place Mr. K in?
   1. A 45-degree Fowler's position.
   2. A 90-degree Fowler's position.
   3. Tripod position.
   4. Supine position.

5. Mr. K is in a compensated respiratory alkalosis according to his blood gases:
   pH = 7.45
   $PaCO_2$ = 29
   HCO_3 = 24
   PaO_2 = 58

   Which intervention by the nurse would be beneficial to improve Mr. K's gas exchange?
   1. Sit with the patient and encourage him to take slow, deep breaths.
   2. Have the patient cough and deep breathe three times.
   3. Request the registered nurse (RN) administer an order for Solu-Medrol 125 mg IV
   4. Have the patient breathe in a paper bag for 2 minutes.

6. The health care provider (HCP) has told Mr. K his rapid COVID-19 test is negative. Which statement made by Mr. K indicates he needs further instruction on public health practices for the prevention of COVID-19?
   1. "Thank goodness I am negative, now my pastor can visit."
   2. "Even though I have breathing problems, I always wear a mask when I leave the house."
   3. "My wife is making hand sanitizer with rubbing alcohol and aloe vera gel."
   4. "I am taking vitamin D and zinc to boost my immunity."

7. The HCP has ordered the antibiotic piperacillin-tazobactam intravenously. What is the **first** action the nurse should take?
   1. Ask the RN to start a saline lock.
   2. Make sure that the RT has collected and sent the sputum specimen to the lab.
   3. Review Mr. K's allergy status.
   4. Conduct a baseline hearing test.

8. Mr. K's potassium level is 3.4 mEq/L (3.4 mmol/L). He asks if he can have something to eat because he is hungry and hasn't had anything to eat since last night. The nurse asks the AP to retrieve some food from the dietary department. Which food items should the nurse ask the AP to look for? **Select all that apply**.
   1. Tuna sandwich.
   2. Potatoes.
   3. Tomato juice.
   4. Herbal iced tea.
   5. Chicken sandwich.
   6. Carrots.

9. Mr. K was transferred from the ED to the medical unit. Which nursing actions or interventions can the nurse safely delegate to the experienced AP? **Select all that apply.**
   1. Place the patient on telemetry.
   2. Check vital signs.
   3. Apply the splint to Mr. K's right arm.
   4. Obtain a peak flow meter reading.
   5. Assist Mr. K with filling out his food menu.
   6. List all Mr. K's valuables and call security for safe storage.

10. The AP reports to the nurse that Mr. K's left arm is red and swollen where the normal saline IV is infusing. What is the **first** action of the nurse?
    1. Ask the AP to discontinue the IV.
    2. Place a moist, warm pack on the red and swollen area.
    3. Fill out an incident report and document assessment of the site.
    4. Turn off the IV pump.

11. The nurse hears the oxygen saturation alarm go off in Mr. K's room. His O$_2$ Sat is 92%. He is alert and oriented and eating breakfast with a venturi mask on, which he removes momentarily when he places food in his mouth. Which is the first nursing action that the nurse should take?
    1. Tell the patient to keep the venturi mask on his face.
    2. Check the placement of the oxygen saturation finger pulse oximeter.
    3. Request the HCP to prescribe oxygen with a nasal cannula during meals.
    4. Turn off the alarm during meals.

12. The AP tells the nurse that Mr. K has a reddened area on his right elbow. Which action should the nurse take **first?**
    1. Request the AP to place a transparent dressing over the site.
    2. Request the AP to keep pressure off the elbow.
    3. Notify the wound care nurse.
    4. Inspect the area on the right elbow.

13. Mr. K tells the nurse his mouth is sore. The nurse notes that Mr. K's mouth is red with white patches on his tongue and inside his cheek. Which nursing interventions will the nurse take? **Select all that apply.**
    1. Encourage Mr. K to eat more fruits and dairy products.
    2. Ask the AP to brush Mr. K's dentures with toothpaste.
    3. Increase the frequency of Mr. K's mouth care using a soft toothbrush.
    4. Remind Mr. K to rinse his mouth after using his fluticasone/salmeterol inhaler.
    5. Encourage Mr. K to drink plenty of water throughout the day.
    6. Notify the HCP.

14. The AP tells the nurse that Mr. K is becoming agitated and disoriented, particularly toward the evening hours. Which interventions can be delegated to the AP? **Select all that apply.**
    1. Close the curtains before dusk.
    2. Keep the room clean and uncluttered.
    3. Limit caffeine and sugar from the diet.
    4. Collect a urine specimen.
    5. Ambulate Mr. K during the day.
    6. Use therapeutic communication to decrease feelings of anxiety and fear.

15. The hospital staff is planning for Mr. K's discharge. The nurse is reviewing the elements of a healthy diet. Which recommendations related to healthy eating should be added to the instruction page?
    1. Wash hands often.
    2. Eat protein twice a day.
    3. Exercise 30 minutes a day.
    4. Weigh yourself daily.
    5. Get an annual influenza shot.
    6. Eat four to six small meals a day.

Answer Key for this chapter begins on p. 171

16. Mr. K asks the nurse if he is more vulnerable to COVID-19 because he has COPD. Which response from the nurse is correct?
1. "You are not vulnerable to getting the virus because your immune system is not compromised."
2. "You are not more vulnerable to getting the virus, but you are at greater risk for getting seriously ill if you get COVID-19."
3. "Smoking or vaping cigarettes increases the risk of severe COVID-19."
4. "If you wear a mask, wash your hands, and practice social distancing you will not get COVID-19."

Answer Key for this chapter begins on p. 171

Answers

1. **Ans: 4** The first action of the nurse before applying oxygen is to perform safety measures. The patient has symptoms of COVID-19 and until the rapid antigen test is a confirmed negative, the staff must wear full PPE: National Institute for Occupational Safety and Health (NIOSH)-approved N95 filtering facepiece respirator or higher (use a facemask if a respirator is not available), isolation gown, and face shield or goggles, and gloves are the appropriate PPE for COVID-19. **Focus:** Prioritization; **QSEN:** S; **Concept:** Safety, Gas Exchange, Infection; **Cognitive Level:** Analyzing. **Teaching Tip:** Airway, Breathing, and Circulation are the priority concerns in all clinical emergencies for immediate assessment and treatment but only when personal safety is met **first**.

2. **Ans: 2, 3, 5, 6** Oxygen is considered a medication, so the nurse or the RT must change the setting on the venturi mask. The RN or the HCP should give an update to explain the treatment modalities, results of lab work, prognosis, etc. The AP is able to assist an HCP as needed as long as it is within the AP's scope of practice. The Centers for Disease Control and Prevention (CDC) recommends airborne precautions for suspected or infected COVID-19 patients. **Focus:** Delegation; **QSEN:** PCC; **Concept:** Care Coordination; **Cognitive Level:** Applying

3. **Ans: 3** Sputum specimens are best collected first thing in the morning after the patient wakes up. Mr. K's sputum should be collected after the nebulizer treatment because sputum is easier to cough up. Mr. K's fever is elevated and he has a productive cough with chest discomfort, so a culture and sensitivity should be done ASAP in the ED so that broad-spectrum antibiotic treatment can begin for a suspected pneumonia. Sputum specimens are also best when collected first thing in the morning after the patient wakes up; however, waiting until first thing the next morning could be detrimental to Mr. K's recovery. **Focus:** Prioritization; **QSEN:** PCC, EBP; **Concept:** Gas Exchange; **Cognitive Level:** Applying

4. **Ans: 3** The best position for a patient in respiratory distress is the tripod position (sitting, bent forward with elbows on the knees or bedside table). This position gives the patient maximum expansion of the chest, allowing for better gas exchange. **Focus:** Prioritization, Assignment; **QSEN:** EBP; **Concept:** Gas Exchange; **Cognitive Level:** Applying

5. **Ans: 2** The patient's respiratory rate is 30 breaths/minute which is why his $PaCO_2$ is low (normal $PaCO_2$ 35–45) and his oxygen is low (normal PaO_2 75–100). Coughing and deep breathing will clear the airways of the excess mucous and allow for more oxygen to enter the lungs as well as carbon dioxide to exit the lungs. Solu-Medrol IV will begin to decrease inflammation in 1 hour, during which time gas exchange could worsen. Slowing the breathing may return the $PaCO_2$ back to normal but does not relieve the reason why the $PaCO_2$ and PaO_2 are low. Mr. K's $PaCO_2$ and PaO_2 are low because his lower airway is obstructed with inflammation and mucous. Unless authorized by an HCP, patients should never breathe in a paper bag to correct an alkalosis. **Focus:** Prioritization; **QSEN:** EBP; **Concept:** Gas Exchange; **Cognitive Level:** Analyzing

6. **Ans: 1** Patients at high risk for COVID-19 should limit interactions with people outside of the home. Mr. K should be cautioned to stay home and visitors should be limited to his wife and home health professionals. **Focus:** Prioritization; **QSEN:** PCC, EBP; **Concept:** Patient Education; **Cognitive Level:** Analyzing

7. **Ans: 3** Piperacillin-tazobactam is a beta-lactam antibiotic like penicillin. It is possible to have a cross-reactive allergic reaction and the HCP should be reminded of Mr. K's allergy status to penicillin before giving the drug. **Focus:** Prioritization; **QSEN:** PCC, S; **Concept:** Infection, Immunity; **Cognitive Level:** Analyzing

8. **Ans: 1, 2, 3** Mr. K's potassium is low (normal range 3.5–5.0 mEq/L [3.5–5.0 mmol/L]). Fish and beef, along with green vegetables and potatoes and most juices, are high in potassium. Chicken, carrots, and herbal iced tea are poor sources of potassium. **Focus:** Assignment; **QSEN:** PCC; **Concept:** Nutrition, Fluids and Electrolytes; **Cognitive Level:** Analyzing

9. **Ans: 1, 2, 5** Although it is reasonable for the AP to apply the splint to Mr. K's right arm, the admitting nurse should apply the splint to the right arm so that she can perform a focused assessment on circulation, sensation, and level of weakness. A peak flow meter reading is obtained by either the nurse or the RT. The AP can assist Mr. K in filling out his menu and check vital signs, and an experienced AP would have been taught how to place a patient on telemetry. The nurse is ultimately responsible for the patient's valuables that are placed in the safe. The nurse should collect all the valuables and place them in the appropriately filled out and signed envelope and give the envelope to security for safe-keeping. **Focus:** Delegation; **QSEN:** PCC; **Concept:** Care Coordination; **Cognitive Level:** Applying

10. **Ans. 4** The first action is to turn off the fluid running into the site, then discontinue the IV, place a moist warm pack to the area, and document assessment of the site and the nursing actions taken. **Focus:**

PART 3 Complex Health Scenarios

Prioritization; **QSEN:** PCC; **Concept:** Inflammation; **Cognitive Level:** Applying. **Test Taking Tip:** An incident report records includes the details of an unexpected event and should be completed whenever there is a patient complaint, a medication error, a mechanical error, or when anyone is injured or involved in a situation with the potential for injury. A normal saline IV would not cause an injury but if the IV had a medication that caused real injury to the tissue, an incident report would be necessary. Always check with the nurse manager and the institution policy for when an incident report should be made out.

11. **Ans: 2. The first action the nurse should take is to check the pulse oximeter to make sure it is correctly applied. The patient's** O$_2$ Sat is 92% and within normal limits, leading the nurse to think the finger placement may be compromised. The next best intervention is to call the HCP and request a change in oxygen delivery during meals. The patient won't be able to finish eating with the venturi mask in place. It is never appropriate to turn off alarms for any reason. Continue to monitor the patient because a hypoxic episode can cause residual damage. **Focus:** Prioritization; **QSEN:** PCC, S; **Concept:** Gas Exchange; **Cognitive Level:** Applying

12. **Ans: 4** The first step in the nursing process is to inspect and collect data. The nurse should inspect the area, take measurements, and document the findings. Then a transparent dressing can be applied, and the AP can be asked to position the patient's arm so that there is little to no pressure on the elbow. The wound care nurse can be notified of the area, but the wound care nurse does not need to see the patient at this time. **Focus:** Prioritization; **QSEN:** PCC; **Concept:** Inflammation; **Cognitive Level:** Applying

13. **Ans: 3, 4, 5, 6** Fruit has a high sugar content and dairy products have lactose, also a sugar, which can worsen thrush. Dentures should be cleaned with a nonabrasive denture cleanser and not abrasive toothpaste that can ruin dentures. Increasing the frequency of mouth care with a soft toothbrush will not create further soreness and help decrease the thrush. Dehydration can worsen thrush, so increasing fluids, especially water, will help flush out toxins. When using a steroid inhaler, it is necessary to rinse the mouth out afterward to prevent thrush. The HCP should be notified as an antifungal agent such as nystatin may be necessary. **Focus:** Prioritization; **QSEN:** PCC, EBP; **Concept:** Infection; **Cognitive Level:** Analyzing

14. **Ans: 1, 2, 4** Mr. K may be sundowning or experiencing a delirium. Sundowning is common in the elderly patient who is away from home. The AP can close the curtains before dusk and keep the room uncluttered to alleviate shadows and unfamiliar items that could cause confusion. The nurse needs to contact the HCP and the dietary department for a diet change to limit caffeine and sugar that could cause sleep problems. The AP can collect a urine specimen and the nurse can contact the HCP for an order to check for a urinary tract infection, which is a common cause of confusion and delirium in older patients. Increasing daytime exercise will help Mr. K sleep better at night but the nurse should ambulate Mr. K during the day to assess for decreased gas exchange during exercise and right-sided weakness. The nurse is trained in therapeutic communication and should try and alleviate anxiety and fear that could be causing his evening confusion. **Focus:** Delegation; **QSEN:** PCC, EBP; **Concept:** Mood and Affect; **Cognitive Level:** Analyzing

15. **Ans: 1, 2, 3, 4, 6** Washing hands often decreases the chance for infection, especially during food preparation. Protein will support respiratory muscle function. Exercising improves appetite by burning calories and also supports healthy respiratory muscles. Daily weights establish weight loss or weight gain. Eating four to six small meals a day is best for COPD patients. Eating large meals requires oxygen consumption, which causes fatigue and leads to incomplete consumption of calories. Getting an annual flu shot is important for continued health but is not related to healthy eating. **Focus:** Prioritization; **QSEN:** EBP; **Concept:** Patient Education, Nutrition; **Cognitive Level:** Analyzing

16. **Ans: 2** People with chronic underlying medical problems are not more vulnerable to contracting COVID-19, but they are more likely to get a serious illness if they do get COVID-19. People who are more vulnerable to getting COVID-19 are people who are immunosuppressed. The chronic lung inflammation in COPD leads to extensive lung damage and impaired immunity. There is no clear evidence that smoking or vaping increases the risk for severe illness from COVID-19; however, some studies have suggested it may be so. Masks, frequent good handwashing, and social distancing can greatly reduce the risk of infection with COVID-19, but they will not prevent infection. **Focus:** Prioritization; **QSEN:** PCC; **Concept:** Patient Education, Infection; **Cognitive Level:** Analyzing

QSEN Key: PCC, Patient-Centered Care; **TC,** Teamwork & Collaboration; **EBP,** Evidence-Based Practice; **QI,** Quality Improvement; **S,** Safety; **I,** Informatics.
IPEC Key: Domain 1 Values/Ethics (**V/E**); Domain 2 Roles/Responsibilities (**R/R**); Domain 3 Interprofessional Communication (**IC**); Domain 4 Teams/Teamwork (**T/T**).

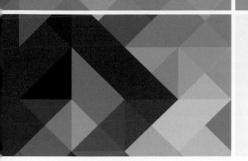

Patient With Heart Failure

Questions

Mr. RC, a 72-year-old male, was admitted to the cardiac care stepdown unit in the hospital accompanied by his wife. He reports shortness of breath for the last 2 weeks that is worsening. He states that he is so tired he can barely walk to the bathroom and back.

Medical Diagnoses: hypertension, heart failure, hypercholesterolemia. Medications: furosemide 40 mg every day, aspirin 160 mg every day, sacubitril/valsartan 41 mg/59 mg twice a day, simvastatin 40 mg every day. No known drug allergies (NKDA). Social history: smoked 10 cigarettes a day for 35 years (quit 20 years ago). He states he drinks five beers per week. Mr. RC is alert and oriented. Vital signs: T 98.7°F (37°C), P 94 irregular, R 18, BP 150/90, O_2 Sat 90% on room air. Lung sounds: crackles in both bases, 3+ pedal edema both lower extremities. Orders: Complete blood count (CBC), liver function studies, 12-lead EKG, cardiac enzymes, urinalysis, chest x-ray. Oxygen via nasal cannula 3 L, furosemide 40 mg intravenously.

1. Which nursing actions must be performed before the furosemide is administered? **Select all that apply**
   1. Place the patient on intake and output.
   2. Record vital signs.
   3. Obtain electrolyte levels.
   4. Record weight.
   5. Obtain a urinalysis.
   6. Ask the patient about any allergies.

2. Which evaluation is **most** important to determine if the furosemide had the desired effect?
   1. Urine output of 100 mL.
   2. Clear lung sounds.
   3. Blood pressure 150/74.
   4. Potassium level of 3.5 mmol/L.

3. Mr. RC's vital signs: T 98.7°F (37°C), P 90 irregular, R 16, BP 140/76, O_2 Sat 95% on 3 L oxygen. How will the nurse ask the assistive personnel (AP) to position Mr. RC?
   1. Right lateral position.
   2. Supine position.
   3. Prone position.
   4. Left lateral position.

4. Mr. RC's *urinalysis shows there is blood and protein with granular casts present.* Which order will the nurse anticipate from the health care provider (HCP) **next**?
   1. Urine culture and sensitivity.
   2. Glomerular filtration rate (GFR).
   3. Increase fluids to 2000 mL a day.
   4. Insertion of an indwelling bladder catheter.

5. Mr. RC's rhythm on the telemetry monitor shows an irregularly irregular cardiac rhythm with no visible P waves at a variable rate between 70 and 130 per minute. Which signs and symptoms will the nurse be **most** concerned about?

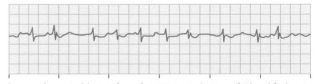

(Figure from Aehlert B. [2018]. *ECGss Made Easy.* [6th ed.] Elsevier.)

   1. Numbness, weakness, difficulty speaking.
   2. Pain, redness in the joints.
   3. Stomach pain, nausea, vomiting.
   4. Respiratory rate of 16 and palpitations.

6. *Vital signs are now: T 37°C (98.7°F), P 86 irregular, R 20, BP 140/82, O_2 Sat 95% on 3 L oxygen. Mr. RC's sacubitril/valsartan dosage was increased to 97 mg/103 mg twice a day. He is reporting nasal stuffiness and asking to get out of bed to have a bowel movement.* Which nursing interventions can the nurse delegate to the AP? **Select all that apply.**
   1. Take blood pressure every 4 hours during the day.
   2. Attach a humidification bottle to the wall oxygen.
   3. Ambulate Mr. RC to the bathroom.
   4. Measure both mid calves and check degree of edema.
   5. Assist Mr. RC with menu choices.
   6. Observe for jugular vein distention.

7. Mr. RC reports chest palpitations and discomfort. Vital signs are T 98.7°F (37°C), P 156 irregular, R 22, BP 110/64, O₂ Sat 92% on 3 L oxygen. The HCP is on the unit and is going to perform a carotid massage. How will the nurse assist the HCP and the registered nurse (RN) team member with the procedure? **Select all that apply.**
1. Place the code cart outside Mr. RC's room.
2. Place Mr. RC on the portable monitor.
3. Take vital signs before, during, and after carotid massage.
4. Tell Mr. RC how and why the procedure is being done.
5. Place the patient in a supine position.
6. Assure saline lock patency.

8. The carotid massage successfully decreased Mr. RC's heartrate. Vital signs are T 98.7°F (37°C), P 89 irregular, R 18, BP 140/84, O₂ Sat 95% on 3 L oxygen. The HCP has ordered digoxin 0.25 mg intravenously. What information is **most** important to inform the HCP about before the injection is administered?
1. The patient's apical pulse is 89.
2. The potassium level is 3.2 mEq/L.
3. The patient's GFR is 80.
4. The magnesium level is 2.4 mEq/L.

9. The physical therapist was walking with Mr. RC when he suddenly became dyspneic and reported chest pain. As he is placed back in bed, the patient becomes unresponsive. His color is ashen and his carotid pulse is rapid and weak. What is the **first** nursing action?
1. Begin cardiopulmonary compressions.
2. Call for the rapid response team (RRT).
3. Ask the physical therapist to bring the crash (code) cart to the room.
4. Notify the HCP immediately.

10. Nextgen Matrix. _____

Scenario: *The RRT initiates advanced cardiac life support measures to successfully resuscitate Mr. RC. Vital signs are T.37.2°C (99°F), P 90 irregular, R 18, BP 104/64, O₂ Sat 96% on 100% oxygen nonrebreather mask and he responds to verbal stimuli. The HCP arrives to assess and speak with the patient and his wife. For each potential prescription listed below, check to specify whether the prescription is anticipated, nonessential, or contraindicated.*

Potential Prescriptions	Anticipated	Nonessential	Contraindicated
Oxygen via nasal cannula 4 L/minute			
Digoxin level			
Pulmonary function studies			
Cardiac isoenzymes and troponin level			
12-Lead EKG			
Normal saline intravenously at 250 mL/h			
Indwelling urinary catheter			
Electrolytes			
Chest x-ray			
Intake and output			

11. Mr. RC's cardiac enzymes, troponin level, electrolyte levels, and digoxin level were normal. His 12-lead EKG showed atrial fibrillation with a rapid ventricular rate. Chest x-ray showed an enlarged heart. The HCP prescribed carvedilol 10 mg extended release once a day. Mr. RC asks the nurse why he is on this new medication. Which statement given by the nurse is **most** correct?
1. "Carvedilol is an antihypertensive."
2. "Carvedilol protects your heart from a heart attack."
3. "Carvedilol decreases the force of heart muscle contractions."
4. "Carvedilol will slow and stabilize your heart rate."

12. Mr. RC was placed on Coumadin 5 mg every day. Which instructions will the nurse give the AP taking care of him?
1. Make sure he is wearing shoes when out of bed.
2. Keep his room clear of obstacles.
3. Make sure he is using his electric razor.
4. Have him use soft oral swabs for mouth care.
5. Observe his bowel movements for blood or dark color stools.
6. Do not give him cranberry juice.

13. Mr. RC's vital signs are now T 98.7°F (37°C), P 66 regular, R 18, BP 120/82, O₂ Sat 95% on 3 L oxygen. The telemetry monitor shows a normal sinus rhythm. Medications: furosemide 40 mg every day, aspirin 162 mg every day, sacubitril/valsartan 41 mg/59 mg twice a day, simvastatin 80 mg every day (increased from 40 mg), carvedilol 10 mg once a day, digoxin 0.125 mg every day. He was transferred out of the cardiac care step-down unit and has been on the rehab unit for 3 days.

Mr. RC tells the nurse that he thinks the physical therapist is working him too hard because he has muscle pain and weakness. Which nursing intervention should the nurse take?

1. Discuss the complaint with the director of the physical therapy department.
2. Tell Mr. RC to talk to the physical therapist about lessening the exercise workload.
3. Review Mr. RC's medications and possible side effects with the HCP.
4. Ask the nurse manager if it is okay for Mr. RC to skip his physical therapy session today.

14. Nextgen Drag and Drop. _____

Scenario: *The HCP has explained to Mr. RC and his family that heart failure is an incurable chronic condition that will worsen in time.*

Select the member of the team that would be **best** to assign or delegate to each task. **(Letters may be used only once.)**

1. ___Ensure accurate and effective communication between the patient, family, and health care team.
2. ___Assist with activities of daily living (ADLs).
3. ___Monitor and report changes in signs and symptoms.
4. ___Teach use of a shower chair to conserve energy.
5. ___Begin progressive indoor walking.
6. ___Assure continued access to health care, palliative care, and/or hospice.
7. ___Optimize continued medical therapies.
8. ___Nutritional counseling.

a. LPN/LVN
b. RN
c. AP
d. Physical therapist
e. Occupational therapist
f. Social worker
g. Dietician
h. HCP

15. Mr. RC tells the nurse that if he is going to die, he might as well start smoking cigarettes again. Which response by the nurse is **most** therapeutic?
1. "Smoking increases your heart rate and blood pressure and will make you sicker."
2. "Your heart will work even harder when you smoke and you could have a heart attack."
3. "You worked so hard to quit, so why waste all that hard work now?"
4. "Tell me more about how you are feeling about your prognosis."

16. Mr. RC is going home. Which instructions will the nurse make sure he and his wife understand prior to discharge? **Select all that apply.**
1. Walk and continue physical activity every day.
2. Call your HCP if you gain more than 2 pounds in one day.
3. Call 911 for extreme shortness of breath or chest pain.
4. Follow your low-sodium diet and limit water intake to 8 cups a day.
5. Limit eating dark green leafy vegetables.
6. Call your HCP if you have nausea, vomiting, loss of appetite, or have vision changes.

PART 3 · Complex Health Scenarios

     Answer Key for this chapter begins on p. 176

Answers

1. **Ans: 1, 2, 3, 4, 6** Furosemide is a potent diuretic. The patient should be on intake and output to gauge fluid balance. Vital signs should be taken before the injection because furosemide can lower the blood pressure, which in turn increases the heart rate and can place added stress on the failing heart. Furosemide lowers potassium levels and since the patient has been taking furosemide at home, his potassium level may already be low. Giving this drug intravenously may lead to an even lower potassium level. Hypokalemia is associated with lethal cardiac dysrhythmias. The patient's base weight and daily weights should be measured to determine fluid loss and gain. A urinalysis is not necessary for furosemide to be administered. Before administering any drug, an allergy history must be taken. **Focus:** Prioritization, Assignment; **QSEN:** S; **Concept:** Perfusion, Elimination, Fluid and Electrolytes; **Cognitive Level:** Analyzing

2. **Ans: 2** Furosemide causes increased urine output by blocking salt and water absorption in the kidneys. It is a diuretic that will lower blood pressure and potassium levels. However, the reason the furosemide was given to Mr. RC was to clear the fluid from his lungs in order to improve gas exchange and decrease preload and cardiac output in order to decrease demand on the failing heart. **Focus:** Prioritization; **QSEN:** EBP; **Concept:** Fluid and Electrolytes, Perfusion, Gas Exchange; **Cognitive Level:** Analyzing. **Test Taking Tip:** Remember to establish priorities using the mnemonic ABC: airway, breathing, and circulation.

3. **Ans: 1** The right lateral position decreases sympathetic tone. Two functions of the sympathetic nervous system are increasing heart rate and constricting blood vessels. Both of these functions are detrimental to a failing heart by increasing workload. **Focus:** Delegation; **QSEN:** EBP; **Concept:** Perfusion; **Cognitive Level:** Analyzing

4. **Ans: 2** Blood, protein, and granular casts can indicate the beginning of kidney disease. Kidney disease is not uncommon in patients with heart failure because the failing heart cannot supply the kidneys with the necessary blood supply. GFR would be ordered because it estimates the amount of blood that gets filtered through the kidneys. A GFR of 90 or higher indicates healthy kidneys. Kidney function declines with age, so for Mr. RC's age, his GFR should be greater than 75. There are no nitrites or leukocyte esterase present, so a culture and sensitivity would not be indicated. Increasing fluids will worsen the heart failure and an indwelling catheter would be contraindicated due to risk for infection. **Focus:** Prioritization; **QSEN:** EBP; **Concept:** Fluid and Electrolytes, Perfusion; **Cognitive Level:** Analyzing

5. **Ans: 1** The patient's rhythm is atrial fibrillation, which greatly increases the risk for stroke because the atria do not contract effectively with this dysrhythmia. Blood pools in the upper atria because and blood clots form. Parts of the clots (emboli) can break off and can be carried through the bloodstream to the brain causing a stroke. Pain and redness in the joints can be signs of arthritis or gout. Stomach pain, nausea, and vomiting can be signs of gastrointestinal distress. A patient with heart failure is expected to have varying levels of dyspnea. Atrial fibrillation sometimes causes the patient to feel palpitations that are not serious and a respiratory rate of 16 is normal for adults. **Focus:** Prioritization; **QSEN:** PCC, EBP; **Concept:** Clotting, Perfusion; **Cognitive Level:** Analyzing

6. **Ans: 1, 2** Mr. RC's medication was just changed to a higher dose and he is receiving furosemide, which leaves him at risk for hypotension and falls. The AP can take serial blood pressures and attach the humidification bottle to the wall oxygen, which will help the nasal stuffiness. The nurse should ambulate Mr. RC to the bathroom to assess his degree of weakness and fatigue. The nurse should mark and measure the mid calves and record the degree of edema. The nurse should assist Mr. RC with his menu choices the first time so that she can take the opportunity to instruct him on a low-salt diet and discover his likes and dislikes regarding food choices. Although APs can observe patient conditions, observing and measuring for jugular vein distention is not within the AP scope of practice and should be done by the nurse. **Focus:** Delegation; **QSEN:** PCC; **Concept:** Clinical Judgment; **Cognitive Level:** Analyzing

7. **Ans: 1, 2, 3, 5** The RN or HCP should explain the procedure and any adverse effects that could occur. The RN should assure that the saline lock is patent in the event that intravenous cardiac medications need to be given. **Focus:** Assignment; **QSEN:** TC; **Concept:** Care Coordination, Perfusion; **Cognitive Level:** Analyzing; **IPEC:** T/T, R/R

8. **Ans: 2** The HCP should be informed of the low potassium level. Potassium transport from the blood into cells is impaired by digoxin and hypokalemia increases the risk of digoxin toxicity. Digoxin is excreted by the kidneys and a GFR of 80 is considered normal for Mr. RC. The magnesium level is within normal limits, as is the apical pulse. **Focus:** Prioritization; **QSEN:** PCC, S; **Concept:** Fluids and Electrolytes; **Cognitive Level:** Analyzing

9. **Ans: 2** The RRT should be initiated first because it will take time for them to respond to the emergency. While waiting for the RRT the nurse should stay with the patient, placing him back on oxygen and attaching him to the portable EKG monitor with defibrillator pads. Vital signs should be continually assessed and cardiopulmonary resuscitation (CPR) started if the patient becomes apneic or pulseless. The HCP should then be notified. **Focus:** Prioritization; **QSEN:** S; **Concept:** Perfusion; **Cognitive Level:** Analyzing

10. **Ans:**

Potential Prescriptions	Anticipated	Nonessential	Contraindicated
Oxygen via nasal cannula 4 L/minute	X		
Digoxin level	X		
Pulmonary function studies		X	
Cardiac isoenzymes and troponin level	X		
12-Lead EKG	X		
Normal saline intravenously at 250 mL/h			X
Indwelling urinary catheter			X
Electrolytes	X		
Chest x-ray	X		
Intake and output	X		

Pulmonary function studies are not a useful diagnostic test for congestive heart failure unless the patient has dyspnea from chronic obstructive pulmonary disease. A 12-lead EKG, cardiac isoenzymes, troponin level, electrolytes, and a chest x-ray would all be anticipated to diagnose a myocardial infarction if it had occurred. Normal saline at 250 mL/h is contraindicated because it could cause fluid overload in this patient with an adequate blood pressure. An indwelling urinary catheter is contraindicated as there is no evidence the patient is incontinent and it could lead to sepsis. Recording intake and output is anticipated to monitor for hypo- and hypervolemia. **Focus:** Prioritization; **QSEN:** EBP, S; **Concept:** Perfusion; **Cognitive Level:** Analyzing

11. **Ans: 4** Carvedilol is both a beta$_{1 \& 2}$ blocker as well as an alpha-blocker. Heart rate and contractility are decreased through beta-blocking activity and blood pressure is decreased by decreasing arterial vascular resistance by alpha-blocking (constriction) activity. Carvedilol also has been shown to have antidysrhythmic properties against atrial fibrillation. **Focus:** Prioritization; **QSEN:** EBP; **Concept:** Patient Education; **Cognitive Level:** Analyzing. **Test Taking Tip:** The sympathetic nervous system consists of beta$_{1\&2}$ receptors stimulated by epinephrine. Beta$_1$ (one heart) increases heart rate, increases force of contraction, and increases conductivity. Beta$_2$ (two lungs) dilates vascular and bronchial passages. Alpha receptors are stimulated by norepinephrine and constrict vasculature. Beta- and alpha-blockers would have the opposite effect.

12. **Ans: 1, 2, 3, 5** Coumadin inhibits an enzyme necessary for vitamin K activation and synthesis. This action reduces clotting factors dependent on vitamin K. Mr. RC is at risk for bleeding, so he should be wearing shoes when out of bed and his room should be clear of obstacles that could cause an injury that produces cuts and bruising. He should use an electric razor to prevent razor cuts. Oral swabs do not provide adequate oral care, so he should be using a soft toothbrush and waxed dental floss. Blood and or dark stools should be reported to the nurse immediately. At one time it was thought that cranberry juice interfered with liver enzymes that metabolized Coumadin but research shows that a moderate amount of cranberry juice is probably safe. **Focus:** Delegation; **QSEN:** EBP, S; **Concept:** Clotting; **Cognitive Level:** Analyzing

13. **Ans: 3** Simvastatin, particularly at higher doses, can cause myositis and rhabdomyolysis. The myositis is dose dependent and usually subsides within 2 to 3 months of discontinuing the drug. The HCP should be notified so that either the dose can be reduced or the drug discontinued and another drug prescribed if necessary. **Focus:** Prioritization; **QSEN:** PCC, EBP, S; **Concept:** Pain; **Cognitive Level:** Analyzing

14. **Ans: 1 b, 2 c, 3 a, 4 e, 5 d, 6 f, 7 h, 8 g** The RN functions as the gatekeeper for the health care team with regard to education, coordination, and communication to ensure safe, quality care. The LPN/LVN assists the RN by continuingly assessing and reporting patient conditions so that they can be addressed appropriately. The AP's role is to assist that patient with all forms of ADLs. The occupational therapist teaches patients

how to improve and maintain ADLs such as how to use a shower chair and handheld shower head. The physical therapist restores physical functioning and mobility through conditioning exercises such as walking. The social worker provides access to health care services such as home care, palliative, and hospice care. Nutritional counseling is done by the dietician and the HCP is responsible for optimizing Mr. RC's wellbeing by directing medications and medical therapies. **Focus:** Assignment, Delegation; **QSEN:** PCC, TC, S; **Concept:** Care Coordination; **Cognitive Level:** Analyzing; **IPEC:** T/T

15. **Ans: 4**   By asking Mr. RC to share more information about how he is feeling, the nurse exhibits a caring attitude that can lead to more open conversations about dying. **Focus:** Prioritization; **QSEN:** PCC; **Concept:** Communication; **Cognitive Level:** Analyzing

16. **Ans: 1, 2, 3, 4, 6**   Physical activity strengthens muscles, including the heart muscle, and helps the patient become aware of increasing shortness of breath that could indicate worsening heart failure. Gaining more than 2 pounds of weight per day indicates water retention and worsening heart failure. A low-sodium diet and limited fluid intake will help decrease fluid retention and decrease the workload of the heart. Patients on Coumadin should not change the foods they were eating when they start taking Coumadin. If vitamin K–rich foods were eaten before, patients should not increase or decrease consumption. Loss of appetite, vision changes, nausea, vomiting, and diarrhea are signs of digoxin toxicity. **Focus:** Prioritization; **QSEN:** PCC; **Concept:** Communication, Patient Education; **Cognitive Level:** Analyzing

QSEN Key: PCC, Patient-Centered Care; **TC,** Teamwork & Collaboration; **EBP,** Evidence-Based Practice; **QI,** Quality Improvement; **S,** Safety; **I,** Informatics.
IPEC Key: Domain 1 Values/Ethics (**V/E**); Domain 2 Roles/Responsibilities (**R/R**); Domain 3 Interprofessional Communication (**IC**); Domain 4 Teams/Teamwork (**T/T**).

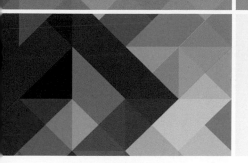

Patient in a Memory Care Unit

Questions

Daughter reports that Mrs. D, 86-years-old, has been mildly confused and forgetful for several years. "Last year, Mom needed more support, so she moved in with us. Within the past few months, she has become more restless and has started wandering outside, once at 2:00 a.m. We are struggling to get her to bathe and change clothes, but at the same time, she is incontinent and spends hours in the bathroom cleaning herself. She causes the toilet to overflow a least once a week by using so much toilet paper." The daughter works full-time and has reluctantly decided to admit her mother to the memory care unit because Mrs. D's care is exceeding the family's abilities.

1. Drag and Drop

Scenario: Mrs. D needs an admission assessment. The experienced memory care team includes a registered nurse (RN), LPN/LVN, physical therapist, and assistive personnel (AP). There are many tasks that are part of this comprehensive assessment.

Which member of the memory care team would be **best** to assign or delegate to each task that contributes to the comprehensive assessment? **Instructions: Indicate which staff member listed in the left-hand column is appropriate for each task that is shown in the right-hand column. In the space provided, write in the letter of the best staff member for each task. Note that all responses will be used and may be used more than once.**

Members of the Memory Care Team

a. RN
b. LPN/LVN
c. AP
d. Physical therapist

Tasks

1. _____ Obtain weight and height measurements
2. _____ Ensure that the Long-Term Care Minimum Data Set (MDS) is correct and complete
3. _____ Assess memory and level of cognitive function
4. _____ Talk to Mrs. D and daughter about issues related to taking medications (e.g., fluid preferences)
5. _____ Collect and report data for the MDS
6. _____ Assess strength, balance, and movement
7. _____ Obtain vital signs and pulse oximeter readings
8. _____ Assess ability to use handrails in hallways and bathroom
9. _____ Perform medication reconciliation
10. _____ Assess daughter's risk for caregiver stress

2. Enhanced Hot Spot

History: Mrs. D is an 86-year-old woman with a history of mild confusion and forgetfulness. She started wandering several months ago, once at 2:00 a.m. Her hygiene has markedly deteriorated; frequency and time spent in the bathroom is excessive. **Assessment findings:** She is currently alert and cooperative. She is independently ambulatory with an unsteady gait and poor balance. She repeatedly asks for her daughter and attempts to go to the bathroom or exit the building, but she is easily redirected. She follows simple instructions but needs repetitive reminders for basic tasks, such as calling for help.

Which information from the from the history and assessment findings signals potential safety issues for Mrs. D?

Instructions:
Underline or highlight all of the information that relates to safety for Mrs. D.

3. Enhanced Multiple Response

Scenario: When a resident is admitted to a memory care unit, the nurse relies heavily on the APs to perform many of the routine tasks that help the residents to feel welcome and safe. These tasks include dealing with belongings, making the resident and family feel welcome, and familiarizing the resident and family with surroundings, routines, and other people in the environment.

Which tasks related to Mrs. D's admission could be safely delegated to AP? **Select all that apply.**

Instructions: Place an X in the space provided or highlight each task that can be delegated to the AP. Select all that apply.

1. _____Assist the daughter with labeling Mrs. D's personal belongings.
2. _____Assist Mrs. D with ambulating to the bathroom.
3. _____Orient the daughter to the services, activities, and programs.
4. _____Place the call light within reach.
5. _____Complete a clothing and personal belongings list.
6. _____Remind Mrs. D to use handrails in the hallways and bathroom.
7. _____Show Mrs. D how to use the hand soap dispenser near the bathroom sink.
8. _____Introduce Mrs. D to her roommate.
9. _____Place a personal sign on her door and show Mrs. D how to locate her room.

4. Enhanced Multiple Response

Scenario: Mrs. D is alert and conversant, but she is disoriented to time and place and she gets easily confused by the unfamiliar environment, activities, and staff at the memory care unit. She is pleasant, cooperative, and occasionally confabulates. She follows simple instructions, but her short-term memory is impaired.

Which communication techniques would the nurse use? **Select all that apply.**

Instructions: Place an X in the space provided or highlight each communication technique that the nurse would use with Mrs. D. Select all that apply.

1. _____Stand directly in front of Mrs. D.
2. _____Ask one question at a time and wait for a response.
3. _____Speak slowly and clearly.
4. _____Set firm boundaries and explain expectations.
5. _____Call Mrs. D by name and identify self.
6. _____Repeat complex questions in different ways until Mrs. D responds.
7. _____Give step-by-step instructions.
8. _____Use short, simple sentences.
9. _____During group activities, try to elicit opinions from everyone.
10. _____Touch Mrs. D before beginning to speak.

5. Which instruction related to environmental modifications for Mrs. D would the nurse give to the AP?
   1. Turn the lights off when Mrs. D is asleep.
   2. Put all personal items in an accessible drawer.
   3. Place a picture sign by the entrance and exit.
   4. Put family pictures in a visible area of the room.

6. Which tasks related to hygienic care can be delegated to AP? **Select all that apply.**
   1. Help Mrs. D to the bathroom first thing in the morning.
   2. Coach Mrs. D to wash her hands and face before breakfast.
   3. Lay out Mrs. D's clothes for the day in the order of donning.
   4. Assist Mrs. D with showering or bathing according to the care plan.
   5. Clip Mrs. D's toenails and smooth rough edges with a file.
   6. Determine if Mrs. D needs help to put on her clothes.

7. At 9:30 a.m., the AP tells the nurse that she tried to assist Mrs. D with taking a shower according to the schedule, but she said, "No dear, I shower at night before I go to bed." What would the nurse do **first**?
   1. Gently convince Mrs. D to cooperate with the AP.
   2. Ask Mrs. D about her nighttime shower routine.
   3. Tell the supervising RN that the schedule needs to be changed.
   4. Tell the AP to wait an hour and then help Mrs. D to shower.

8. Mrs. D is watching a television program about traveling in Hawaii and says, "I went to Hawaii last week. It was beautiful!" What is the **best** intervention?
   1. Report the comment to the supervising RN because it suggests delirium.
   2. Gently remind Mrs. D that she was admitted to the memory unit last week.
   3. Encourage Mrs. D to talk about traveling that she enjoyed in the past.
   4. Redirect the conversation to reality-based activities that are happening in the unit.

9. Mrs. D tells the nurse that she needs help to find and put on her coat and to locate her car keys. What would the nurse do **first**?
   1. Ask Mrs. D where she wants to go and what she plans to do.
   2. Report Mrs. D's comments and behavior to the supervising RN.
   3. Distract Mrs. D while the AP hides her coat and secures the keys.
   4. Invite Mrs. D to an activity and tell her that the coat and keys can wait.

10. Based on the principle of "least restrictive," which intervention would the nurse try **first** to address Mrs. D's tendency to wander?
    1. Give Mrs. D a mild antianxiety medication as needed (PRN).
    2. Ask the family to schedule times to sit at the bedside with Mrs. D.
    3. Allow Mrs. D to move freely about in a secure and monitored space.
    4. Ask the health care provider (HCP) to prescribe bed and chair alarms.

Mrs. D has been at the memory care unit for about 2 months. She continues to be confused about time and place, but she recognizes several day shift APs. Her queries about her daughter occur less frequently but are occasionally triggered by anxiety. She has an interest in activities that involve music and singing and she desires to attend church services on the unit. She frequently walks up and down the hallways and in the enclosed garden courtyard. She has triggered the exit alarm several times. Repeated reminders to avoid opening the door are ineffective; however, she is easily redirected.

11. On Saturday morning, the AP tells the nurse that during morning hygiene, Mrs. D was scratching at her perineal area and there was a strong urine odor on soiled linens and her underwear. Which instructions would the nurse give to the AP?
    1. Put mitts on Mrs. D's hands to prevent excoriation of the skin.
    2. Assess the skin in the perineal area and ask about pain during urination.
    3. Assist Mrs. D with taking a sitz bath and apply a thin layer of barrier cream.
    4. Assist with toileting every 2 hours and report urine qualities and discomfort.

12. Mrs. D usually wakes early and is eager for assistance with toileting and hygiene; however, on Sunday morning, the AP tells the nurse that Mrs. D is lethargic and irritable. What would the nurse do **first**?
    1. Instruct the AP to assist other residents and let Mrs. D sleep for a while.
    2. Tell the AP to remind Mrs. D that church will start in an hour.
    3. Assess Mrs. D's level of consciousness and response to normal stimuli.
    4. Check the medical record to see if Mrs. D had any issues during the night.

 Answer Key for this chapter begins on p. 183

13. Which signs or symptoms would suggest that Mrs. D is experiencing delirium rather than the baseline behavior that characterizes her dementia? **Select all that apply.**
   1. Sudden change in typical morning behavior.
   2. Confusion about where she is.
   3. Difficulty in reporting events that happened yesterday.
   4. Garbled and incoherent speech.
   5. Aggressive behavior during physical assessment.
   6. Attempts to independently walk to the bathroom.

14. The nurse reports the behavioral assessment findings to the supervising RN and expresses a concern that infection may be causing delirium. Based on suspicion of infection for Mrs. D, which physical assessment data is the RN **most** likely to expect the nurse to report? **Select all that apply.**
   1. Vital signs and pulse oximeter reading.
   2. Respiratory assessment and breath sounds.
   3. Daily weight and height measurement.
   4. Change in urinary patterns or urine quality.
   5. Bowel sounds and bowel habits.
   6. Evidence of pressure injuries.

15. The HCP is notified about Mrs. D's assessment findings and orders a urinalysis, urine culture, and oral trimethoprim-sulfamethoxazole for a probable medical diagnosis of urinary tract infection (UTI). In addition to the HCP prescriptions, which nursing measures will the nurse initiate? **Select all that apply.**
   1. Instruct AP that Mrs. D is likely to need frequent assistance to go to the bathroom.
   2. Instruct AP to help Mrs. D to don clean cotton underwear.
   3. Assess Mrs. D's willingness to try a sitz bath for symptom relief.
   4. Remind AP and Mrs. D to wipe the perineal area back to front.
   5. Encourage 12 large glasses of fluid throughout the day.
   6. Administer trimethoprim-sulfamethoxazole with orange juice.

16. Mrs. D has completed the full course of prescribed trimethoprim-sulfamethoxazole. Which objective data is the **best** indicator that the UTI has resolved?
   1. Vital signs: BP 130/82 mm Hg, P 92, R 20/min, T 98.06 °F (36.7°C).
   2. Urine is clear, pale, straw colored, with no strong odors.
   3. Follow-up urine culture shows: <10,000 bacteria per milliliter of urine.
   4. Mrs. D is alert, confused, and ambulating in hallways and garden courtyard.

Answers

1. **Ans: 1c, 2a, 3a, 4b, 5b, 6d, 7c, 8d, 9a, 10a** The RN is responsible for the initial assessment. Initial and ongoing assessment of cognitive functions would be particularly important for Mrs. D. The RN would perform medication reconciliation to identify and resolve problems with polypharmacy or drug–drug interactions. The RN must also assess for complex issues related to caregiver stress and family dynamics. The RN is generally responsible for the MDS. (Some states allow LPN/LVNs to certify for MDS. Be familiar with state and facility policies.) The LPN/LVN would collect and report initial and ongoing data for the MDS. (The MDS is a standardized screening and assessment tool. Long-term care facilities certified to participate in Medicare or Medicaid must complete this assessment on all residents.) The LPN/LVN is likely to be performing medication administration and knowing Mrs. D's routines and preferences will facilitate compliance. The physical therapist is responsible for assessing functions and planning therapies related to mobility and movement. The AP can weigh Mrs. D and take her vital signs. **Focus:** Assignment, Delegation; **QSEN:** TC; **Concept:** Care Coordination; **Cognitive Level:** Analyzing; **Cognitive Skill:** Generate Solutions; **IPEC:** R/R

2. **Ans:**

   History: Mrs. D is an **86-year-old** woman with a history of mild confusion and forgetfulness. She started **wandering** several months ago, **once at 2:00 a.m.** Her **hygiene has markedly deteriorated; frequency and time spent in the bathroom is excessive.**

   Assessment findings: She is currently alert and cooperative. She is **independently ambulatory with an unsteady gait and poor balance.** She **repeatedly asks for her daughter** and **attempts to go to the bathroom or exit the building,** but she is easily redirected. She follows simple instructions **but needs repetitive reminders for basic tasks, such as calling for help.**

   Mrs. D has several risk factors for falls: advanced age, getting out of bed at night, frequent and prolonged time in the bathroom (many fall incidents occur in the bathroom), independently ambulatory with unsteady gait and poor balance, restless behavior, seeking daughter, and an inability to remember instructions, such as the use of the call bell. Deterioration in hygiene increases the risk for infection. Wandering and attempts to exit the building suggest impaired judgment and these behaviors must be monitored to prevent elopement. **Focus:** Prioritization; **QSEN:** S;

   Concept: Safety; **Cognitive Level:** Analyzing; **Cognitive Skill:** Analyze Cues

3. **Ans: 1, 2, 4, 5, 6, 7, 8, 9** The AP can perform all of the tasks except orienting the daughter to the services and programs. A nurse should explain services, activities, and programs to the daughter, because these are frequently linked to the resident's care plan and the daughter may have questions about the therapeutic benefits and expected outcomes. **Focus:** Delegation; **QSEN:** TC; **Concept:** Clinical Judgment; **Cognitive Level:** Analyzing; **Cognitive Skill:** Generate Solutions; **IPEC:** R/R

4. **Ans: 1, 2, 3, 5, 7, 8** Standing directly in front, asking one question at a time, speaking slowly and clearly, calling Mrs. D by name, giving step-by-step instructions, and using short, simple sentences are good communication techniques to use with people who have dementia. Setting firm boundaries and explaining expectations are not useful when patients have dementia; however, these interventions are used for some mental health disorders, such as borderline personality disorder. Complex questions would be avoided; simple questions are a better choice. Soliciting opinions from all group members is a principle of small group communication, but for people with dementia, this could increase confusion or agitation. Touching a person before speaking violates a fundamental principle of communication. Permission to touch should always be obtained before touching. **Focus:** Prioritization; **QSEN:** PCC; **Concept:** Communication, Cognition; **Cognitive Level:** Analyzing; **Cognitive Skill:** Generate Solutions

5. **Ans: 4** The AP would be instructed to put family pictures in a visible area; familiar family references help with memory and orientation. Lights can be dimmed at night, but rooms should not be completely darkened. Personal items should be in view rather than in a drawer. Picture signs are placed by areas such as the bathroom and dining room. Exits would be marked for safety, but memory units would not call special attention to the building exits. **Focus:** Delegation, Supervision; **QSEN:** TC; **Concept:** Cognition; **Cognitive Level:** Applying

6. **Ans: 1, 2, 3, 4** The AP can be assigned to perform many of the tasks related to routine hygienic care. Nails are usually not clipped or cut by the APs. Facility policies will vary: filing nails is usually allowed, but foot/nail care may be done according to prescription by the RN or podiatrist. The nurse would assess Mrs. D's functional abilities; AP would then be instructed to assist with dressing as needed. **Focus:** Delegation; **QSEN:** TC; **Concept:** Care Coordination; **Cognitive Level:** Applying; **IPEC:** R/R

PART 3 Complex Health Scenarios

7. **Ans: 2**   First, the nurse would try to assess Mrs. D's statement. Even though Mrs. D has cognitive deterioration, lifelong habits may be retained, and the nurse would respectfully seek Mrs. D's preferences. People with dementia may also try to forego or resist hygienic care or they may confabulate (make up answers). Based on the assessment of Mrs. D's statement, the nurse may decide to use the other options. **Focus:** Prioritization; **QSEN:** PCC; **Concept:** Clinical Judgment, Communication; **Cognitive Level:** Analyzing

8. **Ans: 3**   Reminiscing about past happy times is the best intervention. People with cognitive disorders often comment on what is most obvious; however, the television program could have triggered a past memory of personal travel or other pleasurable events. Delirium and dementia can cause confusion, so Mrs. D's comment does not necessarily indicate delirium. Reminders about reality are not particularly useful and contradiction can increase anxiety; focusing on positive feelings is more therapeutic in most instances. Redirecting to reality-based activities is an intervention that is useful for patients who ruminate or perseverate over certain topics. **Focus:** Prioritization; **QSEN:** PCC; **Concept:** Communication, Cognition; **Cognitive Level:** Analyzing

9. **Ans: 1**   The priority is to assess the meaning of the behavior for Mrs. D. Often, the assumption is that persons with dementia are trying to follow old habits, such as going to work. However, there are multiple reasons that she may feel the need to leave. For example, she may be looking for family members, a familiar place, or a certain object. Trying to leave could be related to anxiety or stimulus overload. The nurse would report behavior and assessment findings to the RN so that interventions target Mrs. D's behavior. For example, if work is the underlying reason to leave, a "job" in the unit could fulfill that need. Putting coat and keys out of sight is an intervention that can be used if these items trigger wandering behaviors. Distraction is used when residents are readily redirected to other activities or topics. **Focus:** Prioritization; **QSEN:** S; **Concept:** Safety, Cognition; **Cognitive Level:** Analyzing; **Test Taking Tip:** The first step of the nursing process is assessment (data collection). The exception would be a life-threatening emergency, in which case the nurse may have to intervene immediately before gathering additional data.

10. **Ans: 3**   The least restrictive option is to allow Mrs. D to move about freely in a monitored space. This could be the hallways, a garden space, or an enclosed courtyard. Antianxiety medication could be considered a form of chemical restraint. Before administering an anxiolytic medication, the nurse must identify anxiety as a precipitating event, then other interventions, such as reassurance or distraction, would be tried first. Having a bedside sitter is an alternative, but it is expensive to hire someone and it is stressful for the family to maintain the sitting schedule. An exit door alarm would be a better choice than a bed and chair alarm to alert the staff about Mrs. D trying to leave the building. **Focus:** Prioritization; **QSEN:** EBP; **Concept:** Safety; **Cognitive Level:** Analyzing

11. **Ans: 4**   Toileting every 2 hours and tracking the quality of urine and discomfort address the nurse's concerns about possible urinary or vaginal infection or that Mrs. D's incontinence requires closer monitoring. Hand mitt restraints would not be a good choice; the reason for scratching must be identified and alleviated. The nurse would assess the perineum and ask about pain; this cannot be delegated to the AP. Sitz bath and barrier cream might provide relief, but these measures are not initiated until the problem is identified. **Focus:** Prioritization; **QSEN :** EBP; **Concept:** Elimination; **Cognitive Level:** Analyzing

12. **Ans: 3**   The nurse must assess and interpret Mrs. D's level of consciousness and response to normal stimuli. There are many possible explanations for Mrs. D to appear very sleepy and irritable. She may have had trouble sleeping during the night or the previous day's activities may have worn her out. However, there could be serious problems such as lack of oxygen, decreased tissue perfusion, medication side effects, infection, or problems with the glucose level. **Focus:** Prioritization; **QSEN:** EBP; **Concept:** Cognition; **Cognitive Level:** Analyzing

13. **Ans: 1, 4, 5**   Sudden changes in behavior (i.e., change in the morning routine, garbled speech, and aggressive behavior) are characteristic of delirium. Confusion about the place, short-term memory impairment, and attempts to independently walk are part of her baseline behavior associated with dementia. **Focus:** Prioritization; **QSEN:** S; **Concept:** Cognition; **Cognitive Level:** Analyzing. **Test Taking Tip:** The signs and symptoms of delirium, dementia, and depression can be similar. Review comparison charts of these disorders in your textbooks. When caring for older people with dementia or depression, knowledge of their baseline behavior can help you quickly identify delirium, which should be reported and treated as soon as possible.

14. **Ans: 1, 2, 4**   Whenever there is a change in status, vital signs and pulse oximeter reading should be obtained, compared to baseline measurements, and reported. Respiratory, urinary tract, and soft tissue infections are common among older people who live in nursing facilities. Respiratory assessment with breath sounds and a urinary assessment would be conducted. Mrs. D frequently walks and moves around independently; thus the nurse would not expect pressure injuries to be a likely source of infection. Weight loss can accompany illness, but this information does not help to identify

the source of infection. Abdominal infection could alter bowel sounds and bowel habits, for example, in peritonitis or gastroenteritis. (Abdominal pain or change in bowel patterns would prompt the nurse to conduct additional assessment on the gastrointestinal system as a possible source of infection.) **Focus:** Prioritization; **QSEN:** EBP; **Concept:** Infection; **Cognitive Level:** Analyzing; **Cognitive Skills:** Recognize Cues. **Test Taking Tip:** It is important to be aware of the most common problems that occur with selected patient groups. This will help you focus your study, because it is likely that NCLEX will test these topics.

15. **Ans: 1, 2, 3, 5** During a UTI, Mrs. D is likely to experience urinary frequency and urgency and will need frequent assistance to go to the bathroom. Clean cotton underwear, wiping front to back (not back to front), and increased fluid intake are measures to counter the UTI. Extra fluid is also needed to prevent crystallization that can occur with trimethoprim-sulfamethoxazole. Sitz bath is a comfort measure that would help to reduce dysuria. Orange juice is not a good choice because acid foods or fluids can irritate the bladder and worsen the subjective discomfort. **Focus:** Prioritization; **QSEN:** EBP; **Concept:** Infection; **Cognitive Level:** Analyzing; **Cognitive Skill:** Generate Solutions

16. **Ans: 3** All of the data suggests that Mrs. D's condition has improved; however, a normal urine culture (<10,000 bacteria/mL of urine) is the best evidence that the infection has resolved. Improvement in signs and symptoms can occur before the full course of antibiotics is completed. **Focus:** Prioritization; **QSEN:** EBP; **Concept:** Infection; **Cognitive Level:** Analyzing

QSEN Key: PCC, Patient-Centered Care; **TC,** Teamwork & Collaboration; **EBP,** Evidence-Based Practice; **QI,** Quality Improvement; **S,** Safety; **I,** Informatics.

IPEC Key: Domain 1 Values/Ethics (**V/E**); Domain 2 Roles/Responsibilities (**R/R**); Domain 3 Interprofessional Communication (**IC**); Domain 4 Teams/Teamwork (**T/T**).

PART 3

Complex Health Scenarios

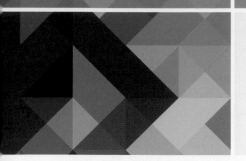

CASE STUDY 9

Patients With Incontinence

Questions

The nurse is working at a long-term care and rehabilitation center with a supervising registered nurse (RN) and several assistive personnel (APs). Among the patients assigned to the nurse and three APs are four patients with bladder and bowel incontinence.

1. Which factors contribute to the development of urinary incontinence for older adults? **Select all that apply.**
   1. Central nervous system (CNS) depressants.
   2. Dementia.
   3. Diuretic drugs.
   4. Anxiety.
   5. Arthritis.
   6. Parkinson disease.

2. Which questions will the nurse ask performing a focused assessment on a patient with urinary incontinence? **Select all that apply.**
   1. "What kind of problems are you having with your bladder?"
   2. "Has anyone else in your family had problems with incontinence?"
   3. "Do you have trouble holding your urine?"
   4. "When did you start having problems with leakage of urine?"
   5. "How often and when does the leakage occur?"
   6. "Do you have difficulty getting to the bathroom in time to void?"

 6. Nextgen. Enhanced Multiple Response.

Ms. C is a 68-year-old who had a right knee replacement and is admitted for 2 weeks of rehabilitation. She is alert and oriented. During admisassessment, she tells the nurse that she occasionally loses some urine when she coughs, sneezes, or laughs too hard. She reports that she wears pads when walking because she sometimes loses small amounts of urine when exercising.

3. Based on Ms. C's description, the nurse recognizes which type of urinary incontinence?
   1. Urge incontinence.
   2. Stress incontinence.
   3. Overflow incontinence.
   4. Functional incontinence.

4. Which factors increase the risk for the development of Ms. C's type of incontinence? **Select all that apply.**
   1. Being postmenopausal.
   2. Having an overactive bladder.
   3. Presence of urethral obstruction.
   4. History of three vaginal deliveries.
   5. Family history of Alzheimer's dementia.
   6. Consuming caffeinated beverages.

5. Which action or intervention will the nurse safely delegate to the AP when providing care for Ms. C?
   1. Teaching how to use vaginal weights.
   2. Assessing the ability to complete hygiene care.
   3. Assisting with ambulation to the bathroom.
   4. Creating a plan for rehabilitation.

Question	Instructions: Place an X into the space provided next to or highlight each item that applies to patient teaching about Kegel exercises.
The nurse is providing teaching for a patient with stress incontinence. Which important points will the nurse include when teaching about the performance of Kegel exercises?	_____ To locate the correct muscle, practice stopping the flow of urine while urinating on the toilet.
	_____ Practice once a day while urinating before beginning the exercise program.
	_____ While lying down, slowly count 1-2-3 while tightening your pelvic muscles.
	_____ Release the pelvic muscles rapidly to the count of 1-2-3, tightening and releasing slowly 15 times.
	_____ Repeat slowly tightening and releasing 15 times.
	_____ The exercise may be completed slowly 15 times while lying, sitting, or standing.
	_____ Start doing the exercises once a day and as you improve, increase to twice a day.
	_____ Improvement of ability to control loss of urine can occur in 6 to 8 weeks but may take up to 3 months.

Mr. M is an 84-year-old with type 2 diabetes and hypertension. He is overweight and describes his incontinence as occurring after a sudden strong need to urinate, followed by involuntary loss of urine. He states, "I just can't get to the toilet in time."

7. Which type of urinary incontinence does the nurse recognize for Mr. M?
   1. Urge incontinence.
   2. Stress incontinence.
   3. Overflow incontinence.
   4. Mixed incontinence.

8. Which medication will the nurse expect the health care provider to prescribe for Mr. M?
   1. Bethanechol.
   2. Tamsulosin.
   3. Oxybutynin.
   4. Furosemide.

9. Which type of behavioral intervention program would be **best** for the nurse to plan for Mr. M?
   1. Bladder training.
   2. Habit training.
   3. Prompted voiding.
   4. Medical therapy.

10. Which nutritional strategies will the nurse teach Mr. M to help avoid incontinence? **Select all that apply.**
    1. Avoiding foods that irritate the bladder (e.g., caffeine, alcohol, carbonated drinks).
    2. Consuming fluid-rich foods like fresh fruit and vegetables.
    3. Spacing fluids at regular intervals throughout the day.
    4. Teaching about potassium-rich foods such as bananas and broccoli.
    5. Limiting fluids after the dinner meal.
    6. Presenting strategies for weight loss.

Mrs. J who has Alzheimer's disease is incontinent of urine. Urination takes place in her bed, in the corner of her room, and in the bathtub.

11. Which type of urinary incontinence does the nurse recognize for Mrs. J?
    1. Stress incontinence.
    2. Urge incontinence.
    3. Overflow incontinence.
    4. Functional incontinence.

12. Mrs. J's incontinence is considered chronic and irreversible. What is the most appropriate outcome when planning her care?
    1. Patient rarely or never has urine leakage between voidings.
    2. Patient responds to signal to urinate in a timely manner.
    3. Patient uses urine containment to ensure dryness.
    4. Patient maintains a predictable pattern of voiding.

13. Which actions or interventions will the nurse delegate to an experienced AP for a patient when starting a habit training program? **Select all that apply.**
    1. Assessing the patient's 24-hour voiding pattern.
    2. Assisting the patient to the bathroom or providing a bedpan/urinal.
    3. Reminding the patient to void every 2 hours.
    4. Teaching staff to avoid using disposable briefs on the patient.
    5. Providing prompt patient and bed cleaning if incontinence occurs.
    6. Helping the patient to ambulate at least 10 minutes before bedtime.

14. What would be the nurse's **most** important concern when an alert older adult with incontinence who has recently had a stroke, refuses to call for help gets out of bed?
    1. Initiating fall precautions.
    2. Managing the incontinence.
    3. Accurately measuring intake and output.
    4. Assessing voiding pattern.

15. Which statement by a patient to the nurse indicates that treatment for urge incontinence has been successful?
    1. "I have been using bladder compression and it works."
    2. "I lose a little urine when I sneeze, but I wear a thin pad."
    3. "I had a little trouble at first, but now I go to the toilet every 3 hours."
    4. "I'm doing the exercises, but I think that surgery is my best choice."

Answer Key for this chapter begins on p. 188

Answers

1. **Ans: 1, 2, 3, 5, 6** Depression is a contributing factor, not anxiety. All of the other options are correct. CNS depressants such as opioid analgesics decrease the level of consciousness and urge to void. Dementia causes cognitive impairment with decreased awareness of the need to urinate and where to urinate. Diuretics cause frequent and large amounts of urination. Arthritis decreases mobility. Parkinson disease causes muscle rigidity with decreased ability to initiate movement. **Focus:** Prioritization; **QSEN:** PCC; **Concept:** Elimination; **Cognitive Level:** Analyzing; **Test Taking Tip:** During NCLEX, carefully consider the question in the context of the information provided. In this case, the emphasis is on incontinence in older adults. Anxiety can contribute to urinary problems for children

2. **Ans: 1, 3, 4, 5, 6** A family history of incontinence does not contribute to a focused patient history or to determining the type of incontinence; however, a history of a mother or sister's incontinence can increase the risk of incontinence for women. The nurse would need to ask a question specific to the patient's mother or sister with incontinence. The other options are appropriate to a focused assessment. The nurse would also ask about activities or situations associated with urine leakage (e.g., coughing, exercising, laughing, sneezing), soiling of clothes or bed linens, obstructions that prevent getting to the bathroom on time (e.g., stairs, extra furniture, distance), and the need for assistive devices (e.g., handrails). **Focus:** Prioritization; **QSEN:** PCC, S; **Concept:** Elimination; **Cognitive Level:** Analyzing

3. **Ans: 2** Stress incontinence occurs when the urethral sphincter fails and there is an increase in intraabdominal pressure. Evidence-based practice indicates that stress incontinence occurs with coughing, sneezing, laughing, or aerobic exercise. **Focus:** Prioritization; **QSEN:** PCC, EBP; **Concept:** Elimination; **Cognitive Level:** Analyzing; **Cognitive Skill:** Recognizing Cues

4. **Ans: 1, 4** Stress incontinence is common after childbirth when pelvic muscles are stretched and weakened. This form of incontinence often occurs in postmenopausal women because of low estrogen levels when vaginal, urethral, and pelvic floor muscles become thin and weak. Overactive bladder and urethral obstruction are associated with overflow incontinence. Consuming caffeinated beverages is a risk factor for urge incontinence. Forms of dementia with loss of cognitive function occur with functional incontinence. **Focus:** Prioritization; **QSEN:** PCC; **Concept:** Elimination; **Cognitive Level:** Applying; **Test Taking Tip:** Knowing the different forms of incontinence, their signs/symptoms, and their risk factors is important because treatment varies based on which type of incontinence is diagnosed

5. **Ans: 3** To safely delegate patient care, the nurse must be familiar with the scope of practice for an AP, which includes assisting with activities of daily living (ADLs), checking and recording vital signs and intake and output, and assisting with ambulation. Experienced APs may also be delegated more advanced actions or interventions if they have been taught and mastered the skills (e.g., checking oxygen saturation, checking fingerstick blood glucose). Teaching, assessing, and care planning require the skills and knowledge of professional nurses. **Focus:** Delegation, Supervision; **QSEN:** PCC, S; **Concept:** Care Coordination, Leadership; **Cognitive Level:** Applying

6. **Ans:**

Question	**Instructions**: Place an X next to or highlight each item that applies to patient teaching about Kegel exercises.
The nurse is providing teaching for a patient with stress incontinence. Which important points will the nurse include when teaching about the performance of Kegel exercises?	__X__ To locate the correct muscles, practice stopping the flow of urine while urinating on the toilet. _____ Practice once a day while urinating before beginning the exercise program. __X__ While lying down, slowly count 1-2-3 while tightening your pelvic muscles. _____ Release the pelvic muscles rapidly to the count of 1-2-3, tightening and releasing slowly 15 times. __X__ Repeat slowly tightening and releasing 15 times. __X__ The exercise may be completed slowly 15 times while lying, sitting, or standing. __X__ Start doing the exercises once a day and as you improve, increase to twice a day. __X__ Improvement of ability to control loss of urine can occur in 6 to 8 weeks but may take up to 3 months.

Practicing stopping the flow of urine on the toilet should be done several times a day to locate the correct muscles (not just once). When performing the Kegel exercises, both tightening and releasing the muscles should be done slowly to the 1-2-3 count. **Focus:** Prioritization; **QSEN:** PCC; **Concept:** Elimination, Patient Teaching: **Cognitive Level:** Applying; **Cognitive Skill:** Generating Solutions

7. **Ans: 1** Urge incontinence is characterized by an abrupt and strong urge to urinate followed by large loss of urine with each occurrence. A patient with urge incontinence is unable to suppress the signal of the need to urinate until in an appropriate place (e.g., bathroom or public restroom). Urge incontinence is also known as overactive bladder. **Focus:** Prioritization; **QSEN:** PCC; **Concept:** Elimination; **Cognitive Level:** Applying; **Cognitive Skill:** Recognizing Cues

8. **Ans: 3** Oxybutynin is a urinary antispasmodic drug that relieves spasms of the urinary bladder and is used to treat overactive bladder and incontinence. Bethanechol is a bladder stimulant used to treat urinary retention. Tamsulosin is used to treat benign prostatic hypertrophy. Furosemide is a loop diuretic that would make incontinence worse. **Focus:** Prioritization; **QSEN:** PCC; **Concept:** Elimination; **Cognitive Level:** Analyzing; **Test Taking Tip:** The nurse must be familiar with medications that may be prescribed for the treatment of incontinence. Knowledge of pharmacology is essential for passing the NCLEX examination

9. **Ans: 1** Bladder training is an educational program that helps a patient learn to control their bladder. For this program to work, the patient must be alert, aware, and able to resist the urge to urinate. Habit training or scheduled voiding is used for reducing incontinence in a patient with cognitive impairment. Caregivers remind the patient to void at specific times (e.g., every 2 hours). Prompted voiding is used with habit training to increase awareness of the need to urinate, which prompts the patient to ask for toileting assistance. Medical therapy is not a behavioral program. **Focus:** Prioritization; **QSEN:** PCC; **Concept:** Elimination; **Cognitive Level:** Analyzing

10. **Ans: 1, 3, 5, 6** Consuming fluid-rich foods may make Mr. M's incontinence worse, and teaching about potassium-rich foods will not decrease episodes of incontinence. Avoiding bladder-irritating foods, spacing fluids, and limiting fluids when nearing bedtime will decrease episodes of incontinence. Weight loss may help avoid incontinence by decreasing pressure on the bladder. **Focus:** Prioritization; **QSEN:** PCC; **Concept:** Patient Education; **Cognitive Level:** Applying

11. **Ans: 4** Functional incontinence is caused by cognitive inability to recognize the urge to urinate. Often the patient is also unaware that urination needs to occur in a socially accepted place (e.g., bathroom toilet, bedpan, bedside commode). Forms of dementia such as Alzheimer's disease often cause functional incontinence. **Focus:** Prioritization; **QSEN:** PCC; **Concept:** Elimination; **Cognitive Level:** Analyzing; **Cognitive Skill:** Recognizing Cues

12. **Ans: 3** An expected outcome for planning care for Mrs. J's incontinence is that she uses urine containment or collection measures to ensure dryness. An outcome of rarely to never having urine leakage would be for stress incontinence. An outcome for urge incontinence would be that the patient responds to signal (urge) to urinate in a timely manner. Maintaining a predictable pattern of voiding is appropriate for reflex urinary incontinence. **Focus:** Prioritization; **QSEN:** PCC, EBP; **Concept:** Elimination; **Cognitive Level:** Analyzing

13. **Ans: 2, 3, 5, 6** The nurse would not delegate assessing or teaching to an AP because these actions are not within their scope of practice and require the additional training and skills of professional nurses. Assisting with ambulation, providing a bedpan or urinal, reminding the patient about what has been taught, and providing cleaning of the patient and bed are within an AP's scope of practice. Helping the patient ambulate at least 10 minutes 1 to 2 hours before bedtime can help to mobilize fluid and decrease episodes of incontinence during the night. **Focus:** Delegation, Supervision; **QSEN:** PCC, S, TC; **Concept:** Elimination, Care Coordination; **Cognitive Level:** Analyzing; **IPEC:** IC

14. **Ans: 1** A common cause of falls in health care facilities is related to patient efforts to get out of bed unassisted to use the toilet. The nurse collaborates with all staff members, including APs, to consistently implement a toileting schedule and prevent incontinence. **Focus:** Prioritization; **QSEN:** PCC, S; **Concept:** Safety, Elimination; **Cognitive Level:** Analyzing.

15. **Ans: 3** For urge urinary incontinence, the best outcome is that the patient responds to the urge in a timely manner, gets to the toilet between urges, and passes urine. **Focus:** Prioritization; **QSEN:** PCC; **Concept:** Communication, Elimination; **Cognitive Level:** Analyzing

QSEN Key: PCC, Patient-Centered Care; **TC,** Teamwork & Collaboration; **EBP,** Evidence-Based Practice; **QI,** Quality Improvement; **S,** Safety; **I,** Informatics.

IPEC Key: Domain 1 Values/Ethics (**V/E**); Domain 2 Roles/Responsibilities (**R/R**); Domain 3 Interprofessional Communication (**IC**); Domain 4 Teams/Teamwork (**T/T**)

PART 3

Complex Health Scenarios

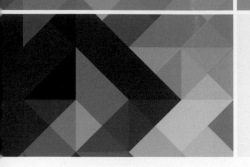

Patient With Altered Level of Consciousness

Questions

Mrs. J is a 73-year-old woman who is normally independent. Her daughter lives in another state and felt that assisted living was a safer option and would provide social opportunities for her mother. Mrs. J has high blood pressure that is well controlled with the combination losartan/hydrochlorothiazide (angiotensin II receptor blocker and diuretic). She takes warfarin to prevent the reoccurrence of deep vein thrombosis that occurred 3 months ago.

Staff checked on Mrs. J to see if she was ready to go on a field trip but discovered her sitting on the bathroom floor in a dazed condition. She thinks she might have fallen but is not exactly sure of the details as to when or how the accident occurred.

She is mildly confused and reports a slight headache, but she insists she is okay. There is no bleeding and no obvious wounds or external injuries.

1. Enhanced Multiple Response

Scenario: The on-call nurse assesses Mrs. J. Which risk factors and signs and symptoms indicate that Mrs. J needs medical evaluation for a possible concussion or traumatic brain injury (TBI)? **Select all that apply.**

Instructions: Place an X in the space provided or highlight risk factors and signs and symptoms of possible concussion or TBI. Select all that apply.

1. _____Age 73
2. _____Female gender
3. _____Dazed condition and mild confusion
4. _____Unsure about details of accident
5. _____No bleeding or obvious injuries
6. _____Anticoagulant medication (warfarin)
7. _____History of deep vein thrombosis
8. _____Hypertension

Mrs. J agrees to medical evaluation. During the ambulance ride, she becomes increasingly drowsy.

2. What is the **priority** concern with change of mental status when the cause is uncertain?
   1. Oxygenation.
   2. Cognition.
   3. Intracranial regulation.
   4. Perfusion.

3. On arrival at the hospital, which action does the nurse use **first** to assess the level of consciousness (LOC)?
   1. Use a loud tone of voice and give Mrs. J a simple command.
   2. Gently shake Mrs. J using an action similar to waking a child.
   3. Use a normal tone and pitch of voice and call Mrs. J by name.
   4. Firmly pinch and twist Mrs. J's trapezius muscle for 10 seconds.

4. The RN assesses Mrs. J and obtains a baseline Glasgow Coma Scale (GCS) score of 15, and then directs the LPN/LVN to recheck the GCS score every 15 minutes. For a score of 15, which behavior would the nurses expect to observe?
   1. Mild confusion, but able to localize painful stimuli.
   2. Oriented and able to follow simple commands.
   3. Extension posturing and incomprehensible speech.
   4. Opens eyes to painful stimuli and has flexion posturing.

5. The health care provider (HCP) orders magnetic resonance imaging (MRI). Which preprocedure task can be delegated to assistive personnel (AP)?
   1. Tell Mrs. J that she must remain motionless during the procedure.
   2. Apply the pulse oximeter to a finger on Mrs. J's nondominant hand.
   3. Ask Mrs. J if she has a pacemaker or implanted defibrillator.
   4. Help Mrs. J to remove jewelry or hairpins and safely store them.

Results of the MRI and laboratory tests are pending. Mrs. J's daughter has been notified, but it will be at least 24 hours before she can get to the hospital to be with Mrs. J. The daughter would like to be updated by phone or text. The HCP informs the nurse that Mrs. J will be admitted for 23-hour observation and should be treated for probable concussion with a possibility that a more serious TBI has occurred.

6. The AP places Mrs. J as depicted in the figure below. Which instruction would the nurse give to the AP?

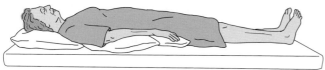

(Figure from Kostelnick C. [2015]. *Mosby's Textbook for Long-Term Care Nursing Assistants.* [7th ed]. Elsevier.)

   1. Tell the AP to raise the head of the bed slightly and keep neck in neutral alignment.
   2. Instruct the AP to remove the pillow from underneath Mrs. J's head and keep her flat.
   3. Tell the AP to put Mrs. J in a left-side-lying position with a pillow under the head.
   4. Ask the AP to position Mrs. J in a high Fowler's position and raise the knee gatch.

7. Which portion of vital signs and neuro checks for Mrs. J can be delegated to the AP?
   1. Ask Mrs. J to state full name and answer several questions.
   2. Check and report the size and reaction of the pupils.
   3. Ask Mrs. J to move extremities and demonstrate grip strength.
   4. Check and report and record a full set of vital signs.

8. During the 23-hour observation, the nurse is alert for which signs and symptoms as the **earliest** indicator of increased intracranial pressure (ICP)?
   1. Nausea and repetitive vomiting.
   2. Lethargy and increasing confusion.
   3. Pupils are equal but react slowly.
   4. Pulse is slow at 54 beats/min.

9. Mrs. J is intermittently drowsy but rouses readily to verbal stimuli. Which instruction would the nurse give to the AP about helping Mrs. J with toileting?
   1. "Keep Mrs. J in bed and help her with the bedpan."
   2. "She has fall risk; help her up; do not leave her alone."
   3. "She is normally independent; tell her to call if she needs help."
   4. "Help her to don incontinence pants and change as needed."

10. The AP reports that Mrs. J had pink-tinged urine and a faint pink stain on the toilet paper. Which action would the nurse take **first**?
    1. Ask the AP to watch for and report other problems with elimination.

   2. Ask Mrs. J about subjective symptoms related to a urinary tract infection.
   3. Assess Mrs. J for other signs/symptoms of bleeding or bruising.
   4. Check Mrs. J's chart for results of coagulation studies.

11. Baseline vital signs for Mrs. J are BP 125/72 mm Hg; P 78/min; RR 20/min; and T 98.3°F (36.8°C). The latest GCS score is 15. Which recent set of vital signs is the **most** concerning because of the risk for ICP?
    1. BP 130/80 mm Hg; P 98/min; R 20/min; T 99.3°F (37.4°C).
    2. BP 130/40 mm Hg; P 64/min; R 16/min; T 100.4°F (38°C).
    3. BP 118/60 mm Hg; P 70/min; R 20/min; T 97.6°F (36.4°C).
    4. BP 120/80 mm Hg; P 84/min; R 24/min; T 99.6°F (37.5°C).

12. The registered nurse (RN) is preparing to call the HCP and will use SBAR (situation, background, assessment, recommendation) to communicate the change of vital signs. Which task would the LPN/LVN be assigned to perform so that the **most** important data is included in the SBAR report?
    1. Call radiology to obtain a hard copy of the MRI results.
    2. Repeat the GCS and report the score to the RN.
    3. Perform a focused neuro assessment and report findings to RN.
    4. Examine the color, quality, and quantity of urine and record findings.

Based on the SBAR report, the HCP determines that while the vital signs are abnormal, Mrs. J's mental status and GCS are unchanged compared to the admission assessment. The HCP tells the nursing staff that it is possible that Mrs. J could have a urinary tract infection that contributed to the fall. So the HCP orders a straight catheter urine specimen for urinalysis and culture and sensitivity. Mrs. J's routine losartan/hydrochlorothiazide should be continued, but the warfarin is held. As-needed (PRN) acetaminophen is prescribed for a fever of 102° F (38.9° C) or as needed for discomfort. Vital signs and neuro checks every hour are continued. Mrs. J rests comfortably throughout the night and the remainder of 23-hour observation is uneventful.

Mrs. J's daughter arrives in the morning and is relieved to find Mrs. J eating breakfast and happily chatting with the AP.

13. The nurse is preparing to give the daughter and Mrs. J discharge instructions, when the daughter bursts out into tears. What is the **most** therapeutic response?
    1. "Let me give you privacy so that you and your mom can talk about what happened."
    2. "Your mom is going to be fine. She had a good night and all of the tests are negative."
    3. "You must be exhausted; sit down and we can review these instructions later."
    4. "This has been a very stressful experience; would you like to talk about it?"

Answer Key for this chapter begins on p. 193

PART 3   Complex Health Scenarios

14. Enhanced Multiple Response

Scenario: Mrs. J is being discharged. The HCP has advised that Mrs. J should not be left alone, until she has resumed her normal behavior and that older people have a greater risk for developing slow bleeding, which can manifest after several months. So her daughter plans to stay with Mrs. J for at least 2 months. The HCP informs them that nausea, mild headaches, dizziness, or poor concentration could continue for several weeks.

The nurse is reviewing the head injury instructions with Mrs. J and her daughter. Which signs or symptoms should be reported to the HCP if they occur within the first 48 hours? **Select all that apply.**

Instructions: Place an X in the space provided or highlight each sign or symptom that should be reported to the HCP.

1. _____Increasing confusion, restlessness, or agitation
2. _____Mild nausea after eating
3. _____Projectile vomiting
4. _____Unusual dizziness, loss of balance, or falls
5. _____Change in vision, such as blurred or double
6. _____Behaviors that are odd for Mrs. J
7. _____Headache, unrelieved with acetaminophen
8. _____Weakness in an arm or leg

15. Enhanced Multiple Response

Scenario: The daughter is happy that Mrs. J is being discharged. She is anxious for Mrs. J to go home, because family and friends are waiting at the house to welcome her. The daughter asks, "Would it be alright if I borrowed a wheelchair so that I can get mom to the lobby? We are packed and ready to leave."

The nurse informs the daughter that the staff is currently working to complete the discharge protocols and that within 30 to 40 minutes, they will be able to leave.

Which nursing actions should be performed because of the legal ramifications associated with discharging a patient who was treated for a head injury? **Select all that apply.**

Instructions: Place an X in the space provided or highlight the discharge actions that would be performed for a patient who had a head injury.

1. _____Transport Mrs. J in a wheelchair and assist her with getting into the daughter's car.
2. _____Call Mrs. J and her daughter to make sure that they arrived home safely.
3. _____Have daughter sign the discharge instruction form and ask if she has questions.
4. _____Give Mrs. J and her daughter a paper copy of follow-up instructions.
5. _____Take vital signs and perform a neuro assessment; then document findings.
6. _____Offer Mrs. J a nutritional snack and encourage clear fluids.
7. _____Have Mrs. J and the daughter complete a patient satisfaction survey.
8. _____Call Mrs. J's primary HCP and inform him or her that Mrs. J is being discharged.

Complex Health Scenarios

PART 3

Answers

1. **Ans: 1, 3, 4, 6, 8**   In older adults, the atrophied brain has more room to move within the skull, so the damage to blood vessels and brain tissue is potentially more severe during a head injury and harm could occur as the brain rebounds back and forth within the cranial vault. Changes in cognition and an inability to recall the accident may accompany a concussion, which is the mildest form of TBI. Anticoagulants increase the risk for intracranial bleeding. Although Mrs. J's hypertension is well controlled, an increase in systolic blood pressure could occur as a physiologic response to injury. Males have a greater risk for TBI. The presence or absence of visible injury cannot be used to confirm brain damage. Deep vein thrombosis is a potential concern *after* severe TBI because of immobility and coagulation issues **Focus:** Prioritization; **QSEN:** EBP; **Concept:** Intracranial Regulation; **Cognitive Level:** Analyzing

2. **Ans: 1**   Change of mental status can be caused by many things, but airway and oxygenation are the priorities. **Focus:** Prioritization; **QSEN:** S; **Concept:** Gas Exchange; **Cognitive Level:** Applying. **Test Taking Tip:** In emergency situations, use the ABCs (airway, breathing, circulation) to determine priorities.

3. **Ans: 3**   The first action is to try and arouse using normal stimuli. Progressive stimuli is used if there is no response: a loud voice and a simple command; gently shaking; and painful stimuli is the last option, with trapezius pressure being the least noxious of the physical methods. **Focus:** Prioritization; **QSEN:** EBP; **Concept:** Intracranial Regulation; **Cognitive Level:** Applying

4. **Ans: 2**   A GCS score of 15 means that the patient is fully alert. Spontaneous eye opening, obeying commands, and oriented conversation are expected. Confusion, localization of pain, posturing, incomprehensible speech, and opening eyes to painful stimuli indicate decreasing levels of consciousness. **Focus:** Prioritization; **QSEN:** N/A; **Concept:** Intracranial Regulation; **Cognitive Level:** Analyzing. **Test Taking Tip:** Develop a working knowledge of commonly used assessment tools and scales. The GCS is a standard tool that is used by other health care professionals and it applies to a variety of patient conditions where serial assessments of responsiveness and LOC must be performed.

5. **Ans: 4**   The AP can assist Mrs. J with removing jewelry and hairclips and safely storing them. The nurse should explain the need to remain very still; the patient may have additional questions or express concerns about tolerating the procedure. An experienced AP is frequently allowed to do routine pulse oximeter readings; however during an MRI a pulse oximeter can cause burns, if the device is not correctly applied. The nurse is responsibe for doing even simple tasks if there is an increased risk of injury for the patient. Metal implants and pacemakers may be a contraindication for MRI, so this task cannot be delegated. **Focus:** Delegation; **QSEN:** S, TC; **Concept:** Care Coordination; **Cognitive Level:** Analyzing; **IPEC:** R/R

6. **Ans: 1**   Raising the head of the bed and keeping the neck in a neutral (not slightly flexed) position facilitates venous drainage. The supine or side-lying position could cause increased ICP. High Fowler's position could cause hypoperfusion of the brain and hip flexion should be minimized. **Focus:** Delegation, Supervision; **QSEN:** TC, S; **Concept:** Intracranial Regulation; **Cognitive Level:** Analyzing; **IPEC:** IC

7. **Ans: 4**   The AP can take, report, and record the vital signs. The nurse should instruct the AP to report vital signs even if they are within normal limits, because the nurse needs to monitor trends and vital signs, which are part of the total assessment of neurological status. The other assessment actions cannot be delegated to the AP. **Focus:** Delegation; **QSEN:** TC; **Concept:** Intracranial Regulation; **Cognitive Level:** Applying; **IPEC:** R/R

8. **Ans: 2**   Change of mental status is the earliest sign of increasing ICP. Other signs can also be present. Slowing of the pulse is a late sign. **Focus:** Prioritization; **QSEN:** S; **Concept:** Intracranial Regulation; **Cognitive Level:** Analyzing

9. **Ans: 2**   The AP should be advised that Mrs. J has risk for falls and she should not be left alone. She needs help getting up to minimize straining, which can increase ICP. Keeping her in bed is not necessary and negotiating a bedpan causes awkward movements, which can increase ICP. She is normally independent in performing activities of daily living; however, the accident may have affected her strength and balance. She may not recognize the need to call for help, because she usually is capable of self-care. Incontinence pants are inappropriate for Mrs. J; she is able to get up with help and incontinence pants create an unnecessary risk for skin breakdown. **Focus:** Delegation, Supervision; **QSEN:** S; **Concept:** Safety; **Cognitive Level:** Applying; **IPEC:** IC

10. **Ans: 3**   The priority would be to assess for signs/symptoms of bleeding or bruising. Recall that Mrs. J takes an anticoagulant and this increases her risk for intracranial bleeding. Bleeding at other sites or recent bruising could suggest that she is having problems with coagulation. The nurse would also use the other options. The AP would be commended for reporting

PART 3 Complex Health Scenarios

the problem and instructed to watch for and report other problems. Assessing for urinary tract infection and checking for laboratory results would be done prior to notifying the supervising RN and the HCP. **Focus:** Prioritization; **QSEN:** S, TC; **Concept:** Perfusion, Clotting; **Cognitive Level:** Analyzing

11. **Ans: 2** A widening pulse pressure (subtract the diastolic from the systolic) is a sign of rising ICP, which occurs as the arterial pressure tries to overcome the increase in intercranial pressure. A slowing pulse is a later sign. Slowing or irregular breathing indicates a problem with neurological control. An increased temperature could be a sign of infection or damage to temperature control mechanisms. **Focus:** Prioritization; **QSEN:** S; **Concept:** Intracranial Regulation; **Cognitive Level:** Analyzing

12. **Ans: 3** All of this information would be included in the SBAR report; however, recall that the earliest sign of ICP is a change in LOC, so the neuro assessment is the most important. Emergency MRI results would be directly reported by the radiologist to the HCP who ordered the test. GCS score denotes trends; a nursing report on Mrs. J's current status would be more useful to the HCP. Mention of urine changes should be accompanied by a report of assessment findings associated with possible urinary tract infection and coagulation results. **Focus:** Prioritization; **QSEN:** TC; **Concept:** Intracranial Regulation, Communication; **Cognitive Level:** Analyzing; **IPEC:** IC

13. **Ans: 4** The nurse cannot be sure why the daughter has burst into tears but acknowledging the stress and giving her the opportunity to talk is the most therapeutic response. Giving privacy and allowing time for rest are possible options after the nurse allows the daughter to express feelings and concerns. "Going to be fine" is false reassurance; there are possible complications that could occur and negative test results do not guarantee a positive outcome. In addition, it is the HCP's responsibility to discuss test results with the patient and family. **Focus:** Prioritization; **QSEN:** PCC; **Concept:** Stress and Coping, Communication; **Cognitive Level:** Analyzing

14. **Ans: 1, 3, 4, 5, 6, 7, 8** The nurse recognizes the familiar indicators of a neurologic assessment and change of mental status: increasing confusion, restlessness or agitation, unusual dizziness, loss of balance, falls, change of vision, odd behaviors, severe or persistent headaches, and unilateral weakness. Projectile vomiting is sudden and forceful and occurs without nausea as a warning sign; it can be associated with increased ICP. Mild nausea is an expected symptom; however, progression to repetitive vomiting should be reported. **Focus:** Prioritization; **QSEN:** S; **Concept:** Intracranial Regulation; **Cognitive Level:** Applying; **Cognitive Skill:** Recognize Cues

15. **Ans: 1, 3, 4, 5** If discharge procedures are correctly followed, the patient is protected and there is a decreased chance that malpractice or negligence suits are brought against the staff or facility. Mrs. J has a risk for falls and transporting her via wheelchair to the car and helping her to get into the car reduces the risk. A responsible caregiver must be available to transport and take responsibility for follow-up care and observation. Getting a signature is legal proof that information was given. Paper copies help the caregiver and patient to recall complex and lengthy instructions. Taking vital signs and performing and documenting a final neuro assessment are important. If there is a lawsuit, this documentation shows that the nurse ensured that the patient was released in good condition. Follow-up courtesy calls are not legally required but may be done within a day or two to check on the patient's condition. (Courtesy calls vary by facility policy.) Offering foods and fluids to patients before discharge is not typical but may be done as a courtesy or in special circumstances, such as long-distance travel. Patient surveys are usually sent several days after discharge and they are not part of the nurse's legal obligation. The nursing staff is generally not required to inform the patient's primary HCP about a patient's discharge; however, the medical staff that were involved with Mrs. J's care may send a report or give recommendations to the primary HCP. **Focus:** Prioritization; **QSEN:** S; **Concept:** Intracranial Regulation, Health Care Law; **Cognitive Level:** Analyzing, **Cognitive Skill:** Generate Solutions

QSEN Key: PCC, Patient-Centered Care; **TC,** Teamwork & Collaboration; **EBP,** Evidence-Based Practice; **QI,** Quality Improvement; **S,** Safety; **I,** Informatics.

IPEC Key: Domain 1 Values/Ethics (**V/E**); Domain 2 Roles/Responsibilities (**R/R**); Domain 3 Interprofessional Communication (**IC**); Domain 4 Teams/Teamwork (**T/T**).

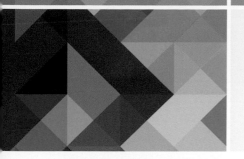

Questions

Jane W is a 24-year-old female who was seen in the clinic with a history of anxiety, depression, and hypomania. She has had many diagnoses in the past including bipolar disorder. Her history includes episodes of severe anxiety and depression alternating with elevated family conflict, substance abuse, and hypersexuality in her teen years. Jane has a high school education and although she has had jobs in the past, she is not presently employed. She lives with an aunt who is supporting her and has Jane's permission to be involved in her care. Jane has a husband, but they are currently estranged. Jane had been on mood stabilizers but lately has refused to take them because she says she is always tired and doesn't feel like herself. She is taking St. John's wort instead. Jane's mother was diagnosed with bipolar disorder and committed suicide when Jane was a teenager. Jane's aunt has brought her to the clinic for admission to the behavioral health unit at a private mental health hospital for treatment. Her aunt is concerned about her irrational behavior and is worried she too will commit suicide someday. Jane is anxious but agrees to be admitted voluntarily.

 1. **Nextgen.** Drag and Drop ——————————————————————————————

Case Study

Jane has arrived at the behavioral unit with her belongings.

1. ____Vital signs, height, and weight
2. ____Physical and psychological assessment
3. ____Search patient belongings for prohibited items
4. ____Explain patient rights and responsibilities
5. ____Orient Jane to the room and the unit
6. ____Introduce Jane to the day room patients
7. ____Obtain an admission history
8. ____Contribute to a nursing care plan
9. ____Obtain consent for voluntary admission

Question

Select the member of the team that would be **best** to assign or delegate to each task. (Letters may be used more than once).

A. Registered nurse (RN)
B. LPN/LVN
C. Assistive personnel (AP)
D. Health care provider (HCP)

2. The nurse assisting the therapist with an interview session finds both Jane and her aunt in the interview room. Which nursing intervention ensures the hospital will be in compliance with the Health Insurance Portability and Accountability Act (HIPAA)?
   1. Tell Jane's aunt the interview is only for Jane and accompany her to the visitor area.
   2. Have Jane sign an informed consent release form.
   3. Tell Jane the interview will need to be rescheduled.
   4. Allow Jane's aunt to stay in the interview session.

3. Nextgen. Matrix. _____

The HCP is conducting a physical exam for Jane. For each potential HCP order, place an X in the box to indicate whether essential, nonessential, or contraindicated.

Potential Order	Essential	Nonessential	Contraindicated
Toxicology screen			
Thyroid function studies			
Liver function studies			
Blood urea nitrogen (BUN), creatinine			
Urinalysis			
PAP/Pelvic			
Complete blood count (CBC), electrolytes			
Venereal disease research laboratory (VDRL)			
St. John's wort 300 mg three times a day			
Lithium 300 mg twice a day			

4. Which lab tests, if abnormal, would prevent the nurse from starting the lithium until the HCP is notified?
   1. Electrolyte levels.
   2. Kidney function studies.
   3. CBC.
   4. Liver function studies.

5. The nurse has assigned a new AP to care for Jane. The AP is upset and tells the nurse that Jane yelled at her and refused to leave her room to eat breakfast in the day room. Which nursing intervention is **most** therapeutic for patient care?
   1. Reassign Jane to a senior AP.
   2. Ask the AP if she might have said something that made Jane angry.
   3. Explain to the AP that irritability is a common response for hypomanic patients.
   4. Ask Jane why she is upset and actively listen to her reply.

6. Jane states, "I'm feeling really edgy. I need to stay in my room alone. I don't want to eat breakfast in the day room with all those patients. Please just let me stay in my room, I'm scared." Which statement by the nurse indicates a therapeutic intervention?
   1. "I will give you a medication to calm you so you will feel better about going out of your room."
   2. "Let's walk to the day room and I will sit with you while you eat breakfast."
   3. "I need you to come to the day room now to eat breakfast."
   4. "I will bring you breakfast this morning and we can talk about what you are feeling."

7. Jane is refusing to take lithium. She said she has been on lithium before and stopped taking it because it made her gain weight and she felt "dull." The HCP has discontinued the lithium and prescribed lurasidone hydrochloride 20 mg to her medical regimen. Which side effect of lurasidone is **most** important for the nurse to closely monitor?
   1. Sedation.
   2. Headache.
   3. Uncontrollable movements in the face, torso, and limbs.
   4. Nausea.

8. The therapist has given Jane a mood disorder questionnaire. Jane says it's difficult to see the print and asks the therapist for a pair of reading glasses. The HCP asked the nurse to arrange for an outpatient ophthalmology appointment using the hospital van. Who should the nurse assign to accompany Jane to the appointment?
   1. A female AP.
   2. A male AP.
   3. An LPN/LVN.
   4. Jane's husband.

9. The night nurs reports, "Patient averaged 4 hours of sleep and was walking the hallway at night. Patient states she is often tired during the day and nods off." Which nursing interventions will the nurse delegate to the AP?
   1. Interview Jane about her usual sleep habits.
   2. Remind Jane not to take naps during the day.
   3. Standardize wake and sleep times.
   4. Teach Jane to change thought patterns that prevent her from sleeping.

Answer Key for this chapter begins on p. 198

10. Jane is still unable to sleep despite limiting daytime naps and standardizing wake and sleep times. She continues to attend the cognitive behavioral therapy sessions offered by the RN. The HCP has ordered quetiapine 50 mg at Hour of Sleep (HS) for sleep. Which nursing interventions are **most** important when giving quetiapine? **Select all that apply.**
    1. Checking daily weights.
    2. Monitoring for increased thirst, urination, and hunger.
    3. Checking daily temperatures.
    4. Monitoring for muscle stiffness.
    5. Monitoring fasting venous blood glucose level.
    6. Performing a 12-lead EKG.

11. A patient in the dayroom states to the nurse, "When Jane and I are playing ping pong she tries to hit me with the ball instead of hitting it just over the net." Which activity would be more appropriate for Jane to engage in?
    1. Volleyball.
    2. Karaoke.
    3. Board games.
    4. Painting.

12. Jane is in her room throwing her clothes and pillows all around. She is shouting, "I'm sick of this place, the food is awful, there is nothing to do except talk, talk, talk. I want to go home." Which statement made by the nurse is **most** therapeutic to decrease Jane's aggravation and irritability?
    1. "Let's go to the dayroom and play a game of cards."
    2. "Let's get out of this room and take a walk together on the grounds."
    3. "The food isn't that bad and talking helps people understand themselves."
    4. "Until you can conduct yourself without outbursts, you won't be going anywhere."

13. The nurse notes that Jane's anxiety is decreasing and there have been no reports of angry outbursts. Jane tells the therapist and the nurse that she wants to learn how to use a computer because she wants to get a job and live independently. Which member of the staff is the **best** choice to show Jane how to use a computer?
    1. RN.
    2. Therapist.
    3. AP.
    4 LPN/LVN.

14. During her computer lesson, Jane can't stay on task and can't seem to remember what she had just learned. She becomes irritated and states, "They should fire you! I'll never learn anything from you; you are a lousy teacher." Which nursing interventions would be appropriate for the nurse to take? **Select all that apply.**
    1. Report Jane's change in behavior to the HCP.
    2. Tell Jane her behavior is unacceptable.
    3. Leave Jane alone in her room to think about her behavior.
    4. Ask the AP to observe Jane's behavior every 15 minutes for an hour.
    5. Administer an as-needed (PRN) sedative to Jane.
    6. Sit with Jane and ask her if she knows why she became so frustrated.

15. *The HCP increased Janes' dosage of lurasidone to 40 mg every day.* Which action should the nurse take to assure absorption of lurasidone?
    1. Give lurasidone an hour before the quetiapine.
    2. Give Jane a 350-calorie snack to eat with lurasidone at night.
    3. Give Jane lurasidone with a glass of grapefruit juice.
    4. Have Jane take lurasidone on an empty stomach in the morning.

16. During the family meeting, Jane's aunt asks for advice on foods that might help manage Jane's bipolar condition. Which foods will the nurse recommend? **Select all that apply.**
    1. Brown rice.
    2. Oatmeal.
    3. Salmon.
    4. Turkey.
    5. Red meats.
    6. Fruit juices.

17. *Jane is being discharged home with her aunt.* Which instructions will the nurse restate to Jane and her aunt? **Select all that apply.**
    1. Take medicine on time and as prescribed.
    2. Make sure to attend all your counseling sessions.
    3. Perform 30 minutes of activity a day such as walking, bike riding, or swimming.
    4. Be aware of early signs of mood disorder.
    5. Do not drink alcohol or do mind-altering drugs.
    6. Look for new opportunities to be involved in, like a new project or a group of friends.

    Answer Key for this chapter begins on p. 198

Answers

PART 3

Complex Health Scenarios

1. **Ans: 1 C, 2 D, 3 B, 4 A, 5 C, 6 B, 7 A, 8 B, 9 A**   The AP on a behavioral unit can take vital signs, measure and record height and weight, assist with ADLs and life skills, and assist the nurses and therapists. The AP can also orient the patient to the room and areas of the unit. The HCP completes a physical and psychological assessment and writes prescriptions and activity orders. The RN is responsible for management, supervision, and the majority of administrative duties such as explaining patient rights and responsibilities, obtaining a history from the patient for the admission assessment, and obtaining consent forms. The LPN/LVN on the unit is responsible for general patient care such as administering medications, providing emotional support, and supervising patient activities. The LPN/LVN does not start a nursing care plan but does contribute and suggest patient care elements for entry. **Focus:** Assignment, Delegation; **QSEN:** TC; **Concept:** Care Coordination; **Cognitive Level:** Applying; **IPEC:** R/R

2. **Ans: 4**   According to HIPAA, if a patient invites a family member or friend to be present in a treatment session, the HCP may assume that the person does not object to the disclosure of information, so obtaining a signed informed consent release before sharing information with a family member is not necessary. However, the nurse must follow any state laws or hospital policy related to mental health privacy that may be more encompassing than HIPAA. It is important for mental health nurses to become familiar with the laws in their state as well as hospital policy. **Focus:** Prioritization; **QSEN:** PCC; **Concept:** Health Care Law; **Cognitive Level:** Analyzing

3. **Ans:**

Potential Order	Essential	Nonessential	Contraindicated
Toxicology screen	X		
Thyroid function studies	X		
Liver function studies	X		
BUN, Creatinine	X		
Urinalysis		X	
PAP/Pelvic		X	
CBC, electrolytes	X		
VDRL	X		
St. John's wort 300 mg three times a day			X
Lithium 300 mg twice a day	X		

It's important to rule out physical illness before a mental illness diagnosis is made. A toxicology screen is needed to rule out drug-induced mental issues. Baseline labs are needed because many medications alter liver and kidney metabolism, and some medications cannot be given if liver and kidney function is not within normal limits. Thyroid disease can manifest as either hypomania or depression. A urinalysis is nonessential, as is a PAP/Pelvic. A CBC and electrolytes are done as baseline and also to check for sodium levels, which can manifest as mental illness. A VDRL is done to rule out syphilis, which in the late stages can cause personality changes, psychosis, and dementia. St. John's wort is contraindicated with many antidepressants. Lithium is often used for bipolar disorders. **Focus:** Prioritization; **QSEN:** EBP, S; **Concept:** Mood and Affect; **Cognitive Level:** Analyzing

4. **Ans: 2**   Lithium is a salt and is not metabolized by the liver. It is not protein bound and about 70% of the drug is reabsorbed by the proximal tubule in the kidneys. Lithium has a narrow therapeutic index, so blood levels are checked regularly at the beginning of therapy until the level is stabilized. After that, it is checked every 3 months. The therapeutic level of lithium is between 0.8 and 1.0 mmol/L. **Focus:** Prioritization; **QSEN:** S; **Concept:** Fluids and Electrolytes; **Cognitive Level:** Applying

5. **Ans: 4**   Reassigning Jane, asking if the AP said something wrong, or explaining that irritation is a common response is not a solution to Jane's problem of being irritated. The nurse needs to find out the source of Jane's irritation through active listening. **Focus:** Assignment, Prioritization; **QSEN:** PCC; **Concept:** Communication, Mood and Affect; **Cognitive Level:** Analyzing

6. **Ans: 4** This is the perfect time for the nurse to recognize Jane's anxiety and develop a trusting relationship with her. Giving an antianxiety medication might calm her but does little to establish trust. Being clear with Jane about expected behavior is a good response for manipulative behavior but not for someone with anxiety. Walking to the day room with or without Jane could worsen her anxiety because being with other patients is what is triggering the anxiety. The best intervention is to lessen Jane's anxiety by bringing breakfast to her room and encouraging her to talk about her feelings. **Focus:** Prioritization; **QSEN:** PCC; **Concept:** Communication, Anxiety; **Cognitive Level:** Analyzing

7. **Ans: 3** Although lurasidone can cause all of these side effect, those listed in option 3 indicate tardive dyskinesia. The patient should be closely monitored because this condition can remain permanent even after drug discontinuance or treatment. **Focus:** Prioritization; **QSEN:** S; **Concept:** Safety; **Cognitive Level:** Applying

8. **Ans: 1** It is neither necessary nor efficient for a nurse to accompany Jane as she is in stable condition and does not present a flight risk. Jane's husband is not a good candidate as they are estranged. A male candidate is not a good candidate because Jane's history of hypersexuality could put the male AP at risk for unwanted advances. A female AP who is familiar with Jane is the safest and best choice to accompany Jane to the appointment. **Focus:** Delegation, Assignment; **QSEN:** S; **Concept:** Safety; **Cognitive Level:** Analyzing

9. **Ans: 2** The AP can observe Jane during the day and remind her not to take naps. The nurse should interview Jane about her usual sleep habits and whether anything has changed since being on the unit. There may be something on the unit keeping her awake that can be adjusted so she will sleep better. The nurse should standardize the wake and sleep times for Jane based on the interview and the RN should educate Jane in cognitive-behavioral therapy techniques that can change her thought patterns for better sleep. **Focus:** Delegation; **QSEN:** PCC; **Concept:** Sleep; **Cognitive Level:** Applying

10. **Ans: 1, 3, 4, 5** Quetiapine (Seroquel) is an antipsychotic drug that is used at lower doses for insomnia in bipolar patients if nonpharmacological adjuncts do not work. It is associated with weight gain, hyperglycemia, dyslipidemia, and neuroleptic malignant syndrome (high temperature, irregular pulse, tachypnea, muscle rigidity, and altered mental status). Quetiapine can increase the risk for diabetes mellitus because of weight gain and increased glucose levels but does not cause the disease. A 12-lead EKG is not necessary before or after treatment unless cardiac issues occur. **Focus:** Prioritization; **QSEN:** S; **Concept:** Sleep; **Cognitive Level:** Analyzing

11. **Ans: 4** Jane is exhibiting aggressive social behavior, so her activities should be limited to endeavors she can pursue on her own until her behavior normalizes. **Focus:** Prioritization; **QSEN:** PCC; **Concept:** Mood and Affect; **Cognitive Level:** Applying

12. **Ans: 2** Taking Jane out of her present surroundings and walking with her will encourage her to talk about her feelings while providing an outlet for her tension. Going to the dayroom to play cards may escalate her outburst as other patients will be present and she is in too much of an aggravated state to be attentive to the rules of a card game. Arguing with Jane can accelerate her present behavior. The nurse needs to set limits on inappropriate behavior but telling Jane she won't be going anywhere until she can conduct herself appropriately is an angry response by the nurse and does not explain why her behavior is inappropriate. **Focus:** Prioritization; **QSEN:** PCC; **Concept:** Mood and Affect; **Cognitive Level:** Analyzing

13. **Ans: 3** Mental health APs assist in therapeutic activities and are able to teach daily life skills. Although RNs educate patients, using a computer is a daily life skill. Specialized health or medical knowledge is not required, so time and expertise of the licensed mental health staff can be best used in other tasks. **Focus:** Delegation; **QSEN:** PCC, T/C; **Concept:** Education; **Cognitive Level:** Applying

14. **Ans: 1, 4, 5, 6** Jane's behavior change should be reported to the HCP because Jane's treatment plan and medication may need to be adjusted. Jane is unable to control the angry impulses that go along with her bipolar diagnosis, so telling her it is unacceptable would cause shame. Jane should not be left alone in her room without observation because changes in behavior can indicate impending violence to herself or others. The AP should observe Jane's behavior every 15 minutes and report back to the nurse. Administering a sedative is within reason if the nurse feels it is most appropriate for the tenseness of the situation. Sitting with Jane and discussing her frustration in an empathetic manner is therapeutic. **Focus:** Prioritization; **QSEN:** PCC; **Concept:** Mood and Affect; **Cognitive Level:** Analyzing

15. **Ans: 2** Only 30% to 50% of lurasidone is absorbed if not taken with at least 350 calories of food. Lurasidone can be taken with quetiapine. Giving lurasidone with grapefruit juice increases its potency and can cause adverse effects from overdosage. Giving lurasidone on an empty stomach would decrease its efficacy. **Focus:** Prioritization; **QSEN:** S; **Concept:** Safety; **Cognitive Level:** Applying

16. **Ans: 1, 2, 3, 4** Whole grains and carbohydrates such as brown rice and oatmeal are thought to boost the production of serotonin, easing anxiety. Omega-3 fatty acids found in salmon are necessary for nerves to communicate with each other. Turkey is high in the amino acid tryptophan, which helps with sleep and

PART 3 Complex Health Scenarios

mood stabilization. Red meats are high in saturated fats, which increase the chances for heart disease and diabetes, and fruit juices are high in sugar, which can cause mood swings. Caffeine and alcohol should also be avoided by persons with bipolar disorder. **Focus:** Prioritization; **QSEN:** EBP; **Concept:** Mood and Affect, Nutrition; **Cognitive Level:** Analyzing

17. **Ans: 1, 2, 3, 4, 5** A hypomanic or manic mood change could occur if Jane searches out opportunities like a new project or new relationships. Jane will be attending counseling sessions every week and should talk to the therapist regarding the timing of any new endeavors she may be interested in.

Focus: Prioritization; **QSEN:** EBP; **Concept:** Mood and Affect; **Cognitive Level:** Analyzing

QSEN Key: PCC, Patient-Centered Care; **TC,** Teamwork & Collaboration; **EBP,** Evidence-Based Practice; **QI,** Quality Improvement; **S,** Safety; **I,** Informatics.

IPEC Key: Domain 1 Values/Ethics (**V/E**); Domain 2 Roles/Responsibilities (**R/R**); Domain 3 Interprofessional Communication (**IC**); Domain 4 Teams/Teamwork (**T/T**).

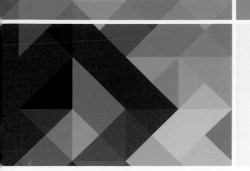

Questions

Anne is an 88-year-old female with mild cognitive impairment, end-stage heart failure, hypertension, and a history of strokes. Her adult son moved in with her recently when her husband, who had been taking care of her, died. He now has health care power of attorney. The last stroke left her paralyzed on the right side with mild memory loss and language problems. She is wheelchair bound and transfers to the chair, bed, toilet, and shower with one assist. She is continent of both urine and stool. She spends the day in her reclining chair, reading, watching TV, or looking out the window at the bird feeder. Her neighbor visits regularly for afternoon coffee and chats.

- Medications: Sacubitril/valsartan 49/51 mg QD, furosemide 40 mg QD, acetylsalicylic acid (ASA) 325 mg QD, famotidine 10 mg HS (bedtime), and hydrocodone/acetaminophen 5/325 mg QD and Q6 hours as needed for back pain. Oxygen per nasal cannula to maintain oxygen saturation of 94%.
- 5'4", 150 pounds.
- Allergy to penicillin.
- Catholic.
- Dual-chamber pacemaker.

1. Which sections of the hospice assessment are **most** important for the nurse to review before visiting the patient for the first time? **Select all that apply.**
   1. Level of pain.
   2. Emotional state.
   3. Spiritual needs.
   4. Caregiver support.
   5. Financial information.
   6. Medicare reimbursement.

2. Anne qualified for home health services as well as hospice services. She will have an assistive personnel (AP) that will help with aspects of personal care, housekeeping, laundry, and food preparation for two meals. The nurse will make a home visit to Anne twice a week. Which observation made by the nurse would cause the nurse to correct the AP?
   1. The AP transfers Anne using the right side of her body.
   2. The AP places the wheelchair extremely close to the patient.
   3. The AP locks the wheelchair.
   4. The AP bends her knees during the transfer.

3. Anne's son tells the nurse, "I feel so overwhelmed with all this; maybe it would be easier if she were in the hospital." Which response by the nurse would help Anne's son explore his feelings?
   1. "You are handling everything so well; I am impressed by the love and commitment you have for your mom."
   2. "There is quite a lot happening; how can I help relieve some of the burden?"
   3. "Tell me more about which parts of your mother's care overwhelms you the most."
   4. "The AP will be here during your work hours, which will lessen your burden."

4. Anne is complaining of shortness of breath. Vital signs are T 98.7°F (37°C), pulse 62 regular, R 28, BP 150/90, O₂ Sat 94% on room air, lung sounds crackles in both bases, 3+ pedal edema in both lower extremities. Which interventions will the nurse delegate to the AP?
   1. Measure Anne's legs for compression stockings.
   2. When Anne's son arrives home from work, remind him not to use salt when cooking dinner.
   3. Help Anne flex and extend both feet 10 to 20 times as tolerated three times a day.
   4. Assess the skin on Anne's legs for injury or signs of infection.

5. The AP tells the nurse it has become more difficult to transfer Anne to the toilet and shower. What is the **first** action of the nurse?
   1. Ask Anne about her level of pain.
   2. Make sure that the AP is using the gait belt when transferring Anne.
   3. Observe Anne closely as she is being transferred.
   4. Notify the RN case manager that Anne may need to be transferred to a nursing home.

6. Anne states, "I'm afraid I might go to hell when I die." Which response by the nurse is **most** appropriate?
   1. "I'm sure you never did anything in your life that would make you go to hell."
   2. "Why are you feeling so negative?"
   3. "Tell me more about your fears."
   4. "Did something happen that would make you feel that way?"

7. Anne is coughing up thick yellow sputum and her oxygen saturation levels have dropped to 86% on room air. Vital signs are T 101.4°F (38.5°C), pulse 62 regular, R 26, BP 120/70. Which medical intervention, if prescribed, should the nurse put into action?
   1. Send Anne to the hospital emergency department (ED) for treatment.
   2. Administer 2 mg morphine sublingual for pain as needed.
   3. Have Anne's priest come to anoint her with last rites.
   4. Apply oxygen by nasal cannula, administer levofloxacin 500 mg every day for 7 days.

8. Anne felt so much better after she finished her antibiotics that she began to give away her keepsakes. She asked the AP to pack several boxes of items for her grandchildren and great-grandchildren. Which end-of-life phase will the nurse prepare Anne and her family for?
   1. Transition phase.
   2. Preactive phase.
   3. Active phase.
   4. Late phase.

9. The AP reports to the nurse that Anne has what appears to be an abrasion on her right buttock that is not draining but that Anne says is painful. The nurse cannot see Anne until the next morning. Which instructions will the nurse give the AP? **Select all that apply.**
   1. Gently clean the wound with normal saline solution.
   2. Place a transparent dressing over the sore.
   3. Place a donut-shaped pillow in Anne's reclining chair.
   4. Keep the back of Anne's reclining chair in a 90-degree position.
   5. Assist Anne in taking a hydrocodone for pain.
   6. Offer Anne a protein drink in the afternoon after lunch.

10. Anne tells the nurse that the cardiologist called and said her pacemaker is due for a battery replacement. Anne asks the nurse if the pacemaker is keeping her alive. How should the nurse respond?
    1. "You should ask the cardiologist that question."
    2. "The pacemaker is not keeping you alive."
    3. "Without the pacemaker, your heart failure will quickly worsen."
    4. "Can you tell me why you are asking?"

11. Anne is too weak to brush her hair and teeth, and she often falls asleep while eating her breakfast. Which interventions for activity intolerance should the nurse delegate to the AP? **Select all that apply.**
    1. Allow Anne to rest after each activity of daily living (ADL).
    2. Talk with her during mealtime.
    3. Monitor and report increased sadness, sleeplessness, and negativism.
    4. Determine her spiritual needs.
    5. Encourage her to talk about her life.
    6. Monitor breath sounds and apply oxygen as ordered.

12. Which sign(s) in a family member indicates anticipatory grieving?
    1. Increasing use of alcohol/substances.
    2. Persistent anger.
    3. Distraction with daily life affairs.
    4. Sadness or tearfulness.

13. Which nursing actions and interventions are essential for a positive family outcome related to anticipatory grieving? **Select all that apply.**
    1. Facilitate a trusting relationship.
    2. Encourage relaxation techniques.
    3. Monitor for signs of hopelessness.
    4. Avoid giving false hope.
    5. Understand cultural expectations.
    6. Determine patient and family expectations of pain relief.

14. Anne is awake most of the night and is not eating well. The AP says she refuses to drink fluids during the day. Her pain is increasing and she feels cold all of the time. Her breathing is congested and her skin is pale. Anne tells the nurse she sees the death angel in the backyard and then cries as she states, "That angel is making me so nervous, tell her to leave."
A hospice comfort kit is available to the family with the following medications:
- *Morphine sulfate oral solution 20 mg per 5 mL. Give 2.5 to 10 mg every 3 hours as needed for pain.*
- *Lorazepam oral solution 2mg/mL. Give 0.5 to 1 mg sublingual every 4 hours as needed for anxiety.*
- *Atropine ophthalmic 1% drops 1 to 2 drops sublingual every 6 hours as needed for congestion.*
Which is the **priority** action for the nurse?
    1. Administering atropine for congestion.
    2. Assessing Anne's pain level.
    3. Administering 0.5 mg of lorazepam for anxiety.
    4. Notifying pastoral care.

Answer Key for this chapter begins on p. 204

15. Anne died with her family by the bedside. The nurse was present as well. What is the **first** action of the nurse?
    1. Notify the on-call RN.
    2. Stay and comfort the family.
    3. Ask the family members if they wish to help the nurse wash and dress the body after death.
    4. Notify the funeral home.

16. Which behaviors by Anne's family depict a normal period of mourning? **Select all that apply.**
    1. Putting family photos and music together for the funeral.
    2. Making funeral arrangements.
    3. Receiving visitors after the funeral.
    4. Declining to attend the funeral.
    5. Using alcohol and or drugs.
    6. Immediately relocating.

Answer Key for this chapter begins on p. 204

Answers

1. **Ans: 1, 2, 3, 4**   The nurse taking care of a hospice patient at home would need to review all aspects of a patient's physical, spiritual, and emotional functioning the first time she meets the patient. A patient's level of suffering is related not only to the medical diagnosis but to his or her emotional and spiritual health as well. Home hospice is not designed to provide 24-hour care, so the nurse needs to know what caregiver support is available when considering aspects of care continuity. Financial information and Medicare reimbursement are important, but the nurse does not need to review these for the first visit. If the patient were to express concern over financial issues, the nurse can notify the RN manager or social worker on the interdisciplinary team. **Focus:** Prioritization; **QSEN:** PCC; **Concept:** Palliative Care; **Cognitive Level:** Applying

2. **Ans: 1**   Anne is paralyzed on the right side. The transfer should take place on the left side, which is the stronger side of Anne's body. The rest of the actions are appropriate when transferring. **Focus:** Prioritization; **QSEN:** EBP; **Concept:** Safety; **Cognitive Level:** Applying

3. **Ans: 3**   When the nurse asks what overwhelms him the most, she is helping him explore and voice his feelings. The nurse shows respect when stating Anne's son is handling things well. The nurse is being understanding by asking if she can do anything to assist him. By stating he has some help during work hours, the nurse dismisses his feelings. **Focus:** Prioritization; **QSEN:** EBP; **Concept:** Communication; **Cognitive Level:** Analyzing

4. **Ans: 3**   Flexing and extending both feet will help pump the excess fluid back to the heart and is within the AP's scope of practice. The nurse should measure for compression stockings to ensure the correct size. If the stockings are too small, they can prevent blood circulation in the legs. Even though the AP will see Anne's son when he takes over care, it is the nurse who should alert him to a change in condition and actions to take. The nurse should complete a focused assessment on the skin of both legs. **Focus:** Assignment; **QSEN:** PCC/T/C; **Concept:** Fluid and Electrolytes; **Cognitive Level:** Applying; **IPEC:** R/R

5. **Ans: 3**   The nurse should first observe Anne and see what type of difficulty she is having during the transfer. Data collection and assessment is the first action of the nursing process. After observing Anne, the nurse can better understand what the problem is and then intervene accordingly. The nurse should ask about Anne's level of pain after she observes the transfer. The AP should be reminded to always wear the gait belt when transferring patients. It is premature to notify the RN that Anne may need to be transferred to a nursing home for continued care. **Focus:** Prioritization; **QSEN:** PCC, S; **Concept:** Mobility; **Cognitive Level:** Analyzing

6. **Ans: 3**   Asking Anne to tell the nurse more about her fear acknowledges she is afraid and opens the dialog. The first statement ignores Anne's feelings and is a closed statement, not allowing for further dialog. The second statement assumes that Anne is feeling negative rather than afraid. The fourth statement could be answered with a yes or no answer, which also does not lead to dialog. **Focus:** Prioritization; **QSEN:** PCC; **Concept:** Communication; **Cognitive Level:** Analyzing

7. **Ans: 4**   Hospice gives supportive and comfort care to people within a 6-month final phase of a terminal illness. Comfort care not only includes opioids for pain and spiritual care but medical care to reduce symptoms and maximize comfort. By sending Anne to the ED, she may no longer qualify for Medicare hospice services and would lose all her hospice benefits. Administering morphine might ease the pain of breathing but does nothing for her lung infection. Applying oxygen and administering an antibiotic maximizes comfort and addresses the underlying problem. **Focus:** Prioritization; **QSEN:** PCC; **Concept:** Palliative Care; **Cognitive Level:** Analyzing

8. **Ans: 2**   In the preactive phase, patients withdraw from social activities and begin to prepare to put affairs in order because they have accepted that they are dying. The transition phase is the phase immediately preceding the active phase when physical symptoms begin to appear. The active phase is very close to the end of life as evidenced by specific signs of imminent death. The late phase is when death occurs. **Focus:** Prioritization; **QSEN:** PCC; **Concept:** Palliative Care; **Cognitive Level:** Applying

9. **Ans: 1, 2, 5, 6**   The AP is allowed to clean a wound with normal saline and place a transparent dressing over the wound until the nurse can come to assess the injury. It's imperative to keep the wound clean to prevent infection. Donut pillows should **not** be used because they increase the risk of getting or making a pressure injury worse by reducing blood flow and causing increased edema to the area. Anne should be in a reclined position with the head of the bed or reclining chair at 30 degrees or less to decrease pressure on the buttock area. Unlicensed persons who work in home health cannot administer medications but they are allowed to assist the patient with taking medications without nursing supervision. **Focus:** Delegation; **QSEN:** PCC; **Concept:** Palliative Care, Tissue Integrity; **Cognitive Level:** Analyzing

10. **Ans: 3** Veracity means being honest with the patient and is related to the principle of autonomy. The pacemaker is not keeping Anne alive but without it, her heart failure will quickly worsen. This is important information to know for end-of-life decisions. Options 1 and 4 disregard the question. Option 2 does not tell the entire truth. **Focus:** Prioritization; **QSEN:** PCC, EBP; **Concept:** Palliative Care, Patient Education, Ethics; **Cognitive Level:** Analyzing; **IPEC:** Values/Ethics

11. **Ans: *1, 2, 3, 5*** Allowing time between ADLs, keeping Anne interested at mealtime, and talking with Anne about her life are therapeutic activities that allow for a small increase in activity tolerance. The AP can monitor for increasing signs of depression and report to the nurse. The nurse should ask Anne about her spiritual needs and engage pastoral care as necessary. The AP is allowed to apply oxygen as ordered but monitoring breath sounds is not within the AP scope of practice. **Focus:** Delegation; **QSEN:** PCC, T/C; **Concept:** Palliative Care; **Cognitive Level:** Analyzing

12. **Ans: 4** Anticipatory grief is grief that occurs before loss or death. Complicated grief occurs after death occurs and keeps the person grieving from moving through the five stages of grief: denial, anger, bargaining, depression, and acceptance. Options 1, 2, and 3 are signs of complicated grief. **Focus:** Prioritization; **QSEN:** EBP; **Concept:** Palliative Care, Mood and Affect; **Cognitive Level:** Applying

13. **Ans: 1, 2, 3, 4, 5** are all interventions that lead to positive outcomes related to anticipatory grieving. Determining patient and family expectations of pain relief is related to nursing interventions necessary for the relief of acute and or chronic pain. **Focus:** Prioritization; **QSEN:** EBP; **Concept:** Palliative Care; **Cognitive Level:** Applying

14. **Ans: 2** The priority action is to assess Anne's pain level. If Anne remains anxious over the hallucination of the death angel after being relieved of her pain, then lorazepam could be administered as well. Hallucinations are often part of the dying process and can either be disturbing or comforting for the patient. Pastoral care should be notified to provide spiritual comfort. Atropine dries secretions from the congestion that stays in the back of the throat, causing noisy breathing, otherwise known as the death rattle. The noisy breathing comes and goes and can also be relieved by position changes. **Focus:** Prioritization; **QSEN:** EBP; **Concept:** Palliative Care; **Cognitive Level:** Analyzing

15. **Ans: 1** Death must be pronounced by either the medical doctor (MD) or the RN. The LPN/LVN can declare death, but the MD or RN must pronounce death. The nurse would need to notify the supervising nurse to come to the home and pronounce the patient dead. The nurse should remain with the family and render comfort. After death is pronounced, the nurse can notify the funeral home. Washing and dressing the body can be accomplished while waiting for the funeral home to come and remove the body. **Focus:** Prioritization; **QSEN:** EBP; **Concept:** Palliative Care; **Cognitive Level:** Applying

16. **Ans: 1, 2, 3** Four tasks of mourning according to psychologist J. William Worden are as follows: accept the loss; acknowledge the pain of the loss; adjust to a new environment; and reinvest in the reality of a new life. Even though there may be a sense of denial and shock when death occurs, the family was still able to accept the loss, as indicated by putting together photos and music, making the funeral arrangements, and receiving visitors after the funeral. Declining to attend the funeral, using alcohol and drugs, and immediately relocating are examples of an abnormal response to grief and mourning. **Focus:** Prioritize; **QSEN:** EBP; **Concept:** Palliative Care; **Cognitive Level:** Applying

QSEN Key: PCC, Patient-Centered Care; **TC,** Teamwork & Collaboration; **EBP,** Evidence-Based Practice; **QI,** Quality Improvement; **S,** Safety; **I,** Informatics.

IPEC Key: Domain 1 Values/Ethics (**V/E**); Domain 2 Roles/Responsibilities (**R/R**); Domain 3 Interprofessional Communication (**IC**); Domain 4 Teams/Teamwork (**T/T**).

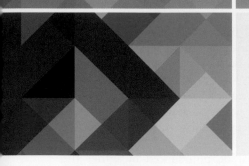

Questions

Mr. D is a cheerful and conversant 64-year-old male. He comes to the walk-in clinic for pain, urgency, and frequency of urination. He reports low back pain, body aches, and fever that started several days ago. He says, "I'd like to get a prescription for antibiotics. I had the same thing about 4 months ago and antibiotics cured me." After additional questioning, the nurse finds out that Mr. D has had at least two previous episodes of urinary tract infection (UTI) and experiences difficulty starting and a decreased strength of the stream. He states, "I'm healthy for my age and I usually go to one of those supermarket clinics." He does not have a primary health care provider (HCP). He recalls having a normal prostate-specific antigen (PSA) blood test at age 50 but has never been retested.

- Medications: Over-the-counter multiple vitamin
- 5'7", 250 pounds
- No known allergies
- Smoker for 40+ years
- Alcohol 2 to 3 drinks daily

1. Enhanced Hot Spot.

Scenario: While listening to Mr. D, the nurse becomes concerned, because he may have health problems that are beyond a simple uncomplicated UTI.

Which information from Mr. D's history suggests that he needs assistance with Health Promotion?

Instructions: Underline or highlight all of the information that indicates that Mr. D needs assistance with Health Promotion.

History: Mr. H is a cheerful and conversant 64-year-old male. He comes to the walk-in clinic for pain, urgency, and frequency of urination. He reports low back pain, body aches, and fever that started several days ago. He says, "I'd like to get a prescription for antibiotics. I had the same thing about 4 months ago and antibiotics cured me." With additional questioning, the nurse finds out that Mr. H has had at least two previous episodes of urinary tract infection (UTI). He states, "I'm healthy for my age and I usually go to one of those supermarket clinics." He does not have a primary HCP. He recalls having a normal PSA blood test at age 50 when but has never been retested.

- Medications: Over-the-counter multiple vitamin
- 5'7", 250 pounds
- No known allergies
- Smoker for 40+ years
- Alcohol 2 to 3 drinks daily

2. Drag and Drop.

Scenario: The HCP orders a midstream urine specimen to be sent for urinalysis and culture and sensitivity. The nurse instructs Mr. D on how to collect the specimen.

Instructions: In the left-hand column, write the number (1–9) that places the steps for midstream urine collection in the correct order.

Correct order of steps	Steps for a midstream urine collection
	a. Finish urinating; replace foreskin
	b. Repeat cleaning with a new swab
	c. Move the specimen cup into the stream and collect about 1 ounce
	d. With foreskin still retracted, begin urinating and pass a small amount
	e. Open cleaning swabs
	f. Perform hand hygiene
	g. Retract foreskin (if circumcised), start at tip of penis and clean outward with a circular motion; discard swab
	h. Open kit and place lid upside down; avoid touching inside of lid or specimen cup
	i. Secure lid on specimen cup; rinse and dry outside of cup; perform hand hygiene

3. The HCP orders a midstream urine specimen to be sent for urinalysis and culture and sensitivity. Which assessment finding is **most** likely to prompt the nurse to ask the HCP for an order to obtain the specimen with a catheter?
1. Mr. D lacks the manual dexterity required to clean and maintain retraction of foreskin.
2. Mr. D is unable to pass urine and says, "I went just before I came to the clinic."
3. Mr. D reports dribbling urine before the stream of urine begins to flow.
4. Mr. D tries repeatedly to pass urine and reports feelings of fullness and pain.

4. Which questions would the nurse ask to collect data about Mr. D's request for antibiotics for a probable UTI? **Select all that apply.**
1. Have you experienced any dribbling or leaking?
2. Have you noticed frank blood or pink-tinged urine?
3. How many times during the night do you have to get up to urinate?
4. Have you experienced any changes in concentration or memory?
5. Have you had or been exposed to a sexually transmitted infection (STI)?
6. Do you have any pain when starting the stream of urine?

Mr. D spends a significant amount of time talking to the HCP. As he is getting ready to leave the clinic, the nurse notices that he seems upset. He says, "The doctor won't give me a prescription.

He says I have to wait for culture results and he wants to do some other tests on my prostate. I really just want the antibiotics."

5. What is the **most** therapeutic response?
1. "Don't worry, I'll talk to the HCP and convince him to respect your wishes."
2. "Laboratory results will ensure that you get the best antibiotics to treat the UTI."
3. "So, how do you feel about the suggestion of getting some additional tests?"
4. "The HCP is looking out for you; repetitive episodes of UTI need follow-up."

Mr. D discloses that he has always been healthy and that the idea of diagnostic testing makes him feel old and vulnerable. "When the doctor said prostate problems or cancer, I just stopped listening. I must seem like a stupid coward." The nurse uses active listening and Mr. D tells her about his family, upcoming retirement, and future family plans. Finally, Mr. D says, "Well, I'll come back when you tell me to and get the test results and prescription. Would you be willing to give me more information about what I need to do to get tested?"

6. The nurse consults with the supervising registered nurse (RN) and they develop a teaching plan that the nurse will deliver when Mr. D returns for his test results and prescription. Below is the figure that the nurse will use to help Mr. D to visualize and understand where the obstruction is occurring. **Draw arrows and write in correct terms to indicate (1) the bladder, (2) enlarged prostate, and (3) compressed urethra.**

 Answer Key for this chapter begins on p. 210.

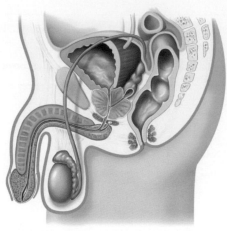

(Figure modified from Lewis S, Bucher L, Heitkemper MM, et al. [2017]. *Medical-Surgical Nursing*. [10th ed.] Elsevier.)

7. Which patient education brochure is the nurse **most** likely to prepare to help Mr. D to understand diagnostic testing related to bladder outlet obstruction?
   1. "Serum Creatinine Level: How Your Doctor Evaluates the Results."
   2. "How to Prepare for and What to Expect during Pressure Flow Studies."
   3. "Purpose and Procedure for a Digital Rectal Examination."
   4. "Ultrasound, a Noninvasive Test That Measures Urine in the Bladder."

8. Which task would be delegated to the assistive personnel (AP) that would contribute to patient education?
   1. Assist Mr. D with writing down questions that he would like to ask the HCP.
   2. Assist the RN, as instructed, in developing appropriate teaching strategies.
   3. Arrange chairs in a quiet room and obtain paper, pencils, and bottled water.
   4. Gather a variety of brochures about reproductive health that may interest Mr. D.

9. In addition to teaching about enlarged prostate and the diagnostic testing, the nurse sees that Mr. D is prescribed trimethoprim-sulfamethoxazole for a UTI. Which information is the **most** important to include in the teaching plan?
   1. Drink at least 12 large glasses of water every day to prevent crystallization in the urine.
   2. Take your temperature every day and take acetaminophen for fever and discomfort.
   3. If a red rash occurs, stop the antibiotic, and take an over-the-counter antihistamine.
   4. Measure and record all the fluid you drink and all of the urine that you pass each day.

Mr. D developed a good rapport with the nurse and appreciated the patient education information. Subsequently, he complied with all of the HCP recommendations. During the follow-up visit, the HCP informs Mr. D that the culture results show that the UTI has resolved after a full course of trimethoprim-sulfamethoxazole. Other diagnostic tests indicate that he has concurrent prostatitis and benign prostatic hyperplasia with no current evidence of complications. The HCP recommends a conservative approach as the first-line treatment.

10. Mr. D says to the nurse, "The doctor says I have concurrent prostatitis and benign prostatic hyperplasia (BPH) with no complications and we're going conservative. I have no idea what any of that means. Where do I start?" What is the **best** nursing action?
    1. Ask Mr. D what specifically he would like to work on first.
    2. Contact the HCP so that Mr. D can ask additional questions.
    3. Explain all of the unfamiliar terminology to Mr. D.
    4. Consult with the supervising RN to revise the teaching plan.

11. Mr. D says, "I was afraid that I might have prostate cancer and I requested a PSA test, but the doctor explained why PSA was not needed and I'm okay with his advice." Which explanation of the PSA is **most** accurate in Mr. D's case?
    1. Mr. D is past the age where PSA results would affect the treatment plan.
    2. The value of the PSA for cancer screening is currently being reexamined.
    3. The recommended conservative treatment decreases Mr. D's risk for cancer.
    4. Prostatitis, BPH, prostate cancer, and prostate biopsy cause elevations in PSA.

12. Which instruction related to the tamsulosin that was prescribed for Mr. D's prostatitis and BPH is the **most** important to give to the AP?
    1. Offer him extra fluids and remind him to drink fluids at home.
    2. Anticipate dizziness or orthostatic hypotension when he stands up.
    3. Expect that he will frequently desire to go to the bathroom to void.
    4. Place a box of tissues within reach because he is likely to have a runny nose.

13. Which self-care measures would the nurse recommend to Mr. D? **Select all that apply.**
    1. Urinate immediately when urge occurs.
    2. Urinate at regular timed intervals.
    3. Avoid food or drinks that contain caffeine.
    4. Restrict fluid if dribbling or leaking urine.
    5. Reduce retention of prostatic fluid by ejaculation.
    6. Avoid sexual intercourse.

14. The nurse is instructing Mr. D about signs and symptoms that should be reported to the HCP. Which sign/symptom is the **most** urgent?

1. Fever greater than 102°F (38.9°C).
2. Back pain that is unrelieved by acetaminophen.
3. Inability to pass urine for the past 6 hours.
4. Frank blood in urine with small clots.

Several months later, Mr. D has to go the emergency department in the middle of the night. He reports bladder fullness, progressively smaller amounts of urine, painful urination, and an inability to pass any urine for the past 5 hours. He is diaphoretic and appears distressed. He says, "I have been doing everything that the nurse at the clinic told me to do. If I could just pass a little urine, I think I'd feel better."

15. **Drag and Drop.**

Scenario: The emergency department HCP examines Mr. D and medical and nursing interventions are initiated to address Mr. D's discomfort and inability to urinate.

Which member of the emergency department staff would be **best** to assign or delegate each intervention?

Instructions: Staff members are listed in the far-left column. In the far-right column write in the best staff member for each intervention. Note that all responses will be used and each response may be used more than once.

Staff Member	Medical and Nursing Interventions	Best Staff Member for Each Intervention
RN	Report and record vital signs	
LPN/LVN	Accompany Mr. D to the bathroom and assess attempts to collect a midstream urine specimen	
AP	Perform admission physical assessment and obtain a medical and medication history	
	Administer prescribed medications	
	Attempt one time to insert an indwelling urinary catheter once inability to void is established	
	Assist Mr. D with changing into a patient gown	
	Obtain a coude catheter to have on standby for second attempt at catheterization	

Insertion of an indwelling catheter alleviated the immediate problem. The emergency department HCP tells Mr. D that he needs follow up care with a urologist to discuss possible surgical options to prevent potential complications. Mr. D is reluctant to consider surgery but agrees to make an appointment with a urologist.

16. **Enhanced Multiple Response.**

Scenario: Mr. D has already experienced some of the early symptoms of BPH and complied with the conservative treatment recommendations. The nurse recognizes that Mr. D needs help to identify and understand the potential complications.

Which potential complications are associated with BPH? **Select all that apply.**

Instructions: Place an X in the space provided or highlight each potential complication that is associated with BPH. Select all that apply.
_____ 1. Acute urinary retention
_____ 2. Urinary stasis
_____ 3. Renal failure
_____ 4. Pyelonephritis
_____ 5. Penile cancer
_____ 6. Bladder calculi (stones)
_____ 7. Recurrent UTIs
_____ 8. Erectile dysfunction
_____ 9. Hydroureter
_____ 10. Hydronephrosis

Answers

1. **Ans:** Mr. H is a cheerful and conversant **64-year-old male.** He comes to the walk-in clinic for pain, urgency, and frequency of urination. He reports low back pain, body aches, and fever that started several days ago. He says, "I'd like to get a prescription for antibiotics. I had the **same thing about 4 months ago** and antibiotics cured me." With additional questioning, the nurse finds out that Mr. H has had at least **two previous episodes of UTI.** He states, "I'm **healthy for my age** and **I usually go to one of those supermarket clinics.**" He **does not have a primary HCP.** He recalls having a normal PSA blood test at age 50 when but has **never been retested.**
   - Medications: Over-the-counter multiple vitamin
   - 5'7", **250 pounds**
   - No known allergies
   - **Smoker for 40+ years**
   - **Alcohol 2 to 3 drinks daily**

   Mr. D is at an age where he should have a primary HCP. He is having recurrent episodes of UTI but using a "supermarket clinic" limits continuity of care and follow-up. He believes that he is "healthy for my age," but he could have undetected health problems, such as high blood pressure, prediabetes, or (prostate) cancer. He is overweight, has smoked for a long time, and consumes more alcohol than the recommended limit (1 to 2 drinks/day for men, ideally with 2 to 3 days off/week) **Focus:** Prioritization; **QSEN:** EBP; **Concept:** Health Promotion; **Cognitive Level:** Analyzing; **Cognitive Skill:** Analyze Cues. **Test Taking Tip:** Health promotion begins with assessment of existing and potential health conditions, health behaviors, and health beliefs.

2. **Ans: 1 f, 2 h, 3 e, 4 g, 5 b, 6 d, 7 c, 8 a, 9 i** Collecting a midstream urine sample is a routine procedure for the nurse and many patients will know how to do this. Other patients may need to have the information repeated more than once or may require coaching or assistance during the process. **Focus:** Prioritization; **QSEN:** N/A; **Concept:** Patient Education; **Cognitive Level:** Applying; **Cognitive Skill:** Take Action. **Test Taking Tip:** First, visualize yourself doing the procedure; then look at the options. This should help you organize the process in the correct order. You can also use "mental rehearsal" during clinical rotations before you do a procedure on a patient.

3. **Ans: 4** Urinary retention with pain and an inability to pass urine suggests a blockage. Treatment would be to insert an indwelling catheter. The HCP may direct the nurse to attempt the insertion or the HCP may perform catheterization for patients with a confirmed blockage, because the catheter insertion may be difficult and painful. If a patient lacks manual dexterity to obtain a midstream urine sample, the staff would assist as needed. The urge to urinate is usually triggered by approximately 250 mL of urine. Waiting for urine to collect in the bladder is a better option than introducing a catheter. The nurse would reassure Mr. D that dribbling urine prior to starting the stream does not interfere with the midstream collection. **Focus:** Prioritization; **QSEN:** EBP; **Concept:** Infection, Elimination; **Cognitive Level:** Applying

4. **Ans: 1, 2, 3, 5, 6** The nurse is unlikely to ask about changes in mental status, such as decreased ability to concentrate or loss of memory. Urosepsis can cause delirium, but at this point, Mr. D shows no signs that the infection has progressed that far. The other questions contribute to the data collection for possible UTI. For young males, UTIs are more frequently associated with STIs, but the nurse would also pose the question to older males. **Focus:** Prioritization; **QSEN:** EBP; **Concept:** Infection, Elimination; **Cognitive Level:** Applying

5. **Ans: 3** First, the nurse encourages Mr. D to express what he is thinking and feeling. Based on Mr. D's response, the nurse could decide to advocate for Mr. D's desire for antibiotics, if he is making an informed choice. Giving information about the purpose of the laboratory tests and discussions about follow-up are appropriate when Mr. D shows readiness to hear the facts. **Focus:** Prioritization; **QSEN:** PCC; **Concept:** Communication; **Cognitive Level:** Applying. **Test Taking Tip:** Therapeutic communication is always patient centered. If the patient (or question) has an emotional or internal conflict, the nurse encourages expression of thoughts and feelings. After emotions are acknowledged, the patient is more receptive to information and in a better position to make decisions.

6

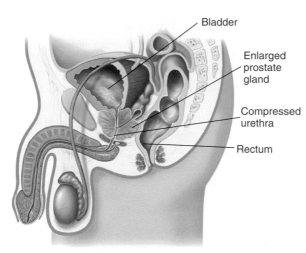

Bladder

Enlarged prostate gland

Compressed urethra

Rectum

(Figure from Lewis S, Bucher L, Heitkemper MM, et al. [2017]. *Medical-Surgical Nursing.* [10th ed.] Elsevier.)

Ans: Pictures are useful teaching tools that help the patient to understand terminology that the HCP will use and to visualize what is happening in the body. **Focus:** Prioritization; **QSEN:** PCC; **Concept:** Patient Education; **Cognitive Level:** Applying

7. **Ans: 2** The gold standard for suspected bladder obstruction is pressure flow studies or urodynamics to measure the increased bladder pressure relative to the urine outflow. Serum creatinine may be ordered if renal insufficiency is a concern. Digital rectal examination can be performed in the clinic as part of the physical examination and the HCP can detect enlargement of the prostate. An ultrasound is used to measure residual urine. **Focus:** Prioritization; **QSEN:** PCC; **Concept:** Elimination, Patient Education; **Cognitive Level:** Applying

8. **Ans: 3** A quiet, comfortable room with supplies contributes to the success of patient education. Creating a question list, developing teaching strategies, and identifying brochures that are relevant to Mr. D's needs should be done by the nurses. **Focus:** Delegation; **QSEN:** TC; **Concept:** Patient Education; **Cognitive Level:** Applying

9. **Ans: 1** Trimethoprim-sulfamethoxazole can cause crystal formation in the urine. Potentially, the crystals could enlarge and cause pain, discomfort, or blockage. The patient could monitor temperature and take acetaminophen, but fever is a normal response to an infection and should resolve within 48 hours of taking antibiotics. The patient would be instructed to notify the HCP if the fever is over 104°F (40°C), as well as notify the HCP for rash or other symptoms of an allergic reaction. Recommending over-the-counter medications is outside the nurse's scope of practice. Measuring and recording intake and output is usually not necessary for the outpatient treatment of

UTI. **Focus:** Prioritization; **QSEN:** PCC; **Concept:** Elimination; **Cognitive Level:** Applying

10. **Ans: 4**. It is the HCP's responsibility to explain the treatment; however, the supervising RN should be consulted because the teaching plan needs to be revised. The nursing staff can help the patient to understand terminology and coach the patient to ask the HCP focused questions. The multilayered nature of his condition, medication compliance, self-care measures, lifestyle modifications, and signs and symptoms of worsening would be included in the teaching plan. **Focus:** Prioritization; **QSEN:** PCC; **Concept:** Patient Education; **Cognitive Level:** Applying

11. **Ans: 4** Mr. D has diagnoses of prostatitis and BPH; both can cause an elevation of PSA, as does prostate cancer and prostate biopsy, so results would not be meaningful for cancer screening. For men over the age of 70, PSA may not be recommended, because prostate cancer develops slowly and the likelihood of life-threatening progression is low. The value of PSA for cancer screening is being reexamined. HCPs and patients are advised to discuss risk versus benefits before having the PSA test. Lifestyle modifications (e.g., smoking cessation, dietary changes and weight loss) and possibly treating prostatitis (research is ongoing) may decrease cancer risk. Other risk factors more strongly associated with risk for prostate cancer are nonmodifiable (e.g., age, ethnicity, genetics, family history). **Focus:** Prioritization; **QSEN:** PCC; **Concept:** Cellular Regulation; **Cognitive Level:** Applying. **Test Taking Tip:** Cancer screening guidelines are changed and updated as research findings become available. One resource for current information is the American Cancer Society (https://www.cancer.org/healthy/find-cancer-early/cancer-screening-guidelines/american-cancer-society-guidelines-for-the-early-detection-of-cancer.html).

12. **Ans: 2** Tamsulosin promotes relaxation of smooth muscles and decreased blood pressure, so the patient can experience dizziness and orthostatic hypotension and this increases the risk for falls. Fluid intake is not directly related to tamsulosin; however, increased fluid intake is recommended for patients who have frequent UTIs and UTI frequently accompanies prostatitis and BPH. Tamsulosin can affect voiding patterns because smooth muscle relaxation promotes urine flow. Runny or stuffy nose is a common side effect. For patient convenience, a box of tissue should be within easy reach. **Focus:** Prioritization, Supervision; **QSEN:** PCC; **Concept:** Safety, Perfusion; **Cognitive Level:** Applying

13. **Ans: 1, 2, 3, 5** Voiding at urge and regular voiding reduce urinary stasis, which contributes to UTI. Caffeine irritates the bladder and worsens UTI symptoms and urinary incontinence. Avoiding chocolate and tea helps to decrease prostatic secretions. Ejaculation reduces retention of prostatic fluid and

PART 3 Complex Health Scenarios

helps to clear the ducts. The patient should not be told to restrict fluids for dribbling or leakage; restricting fluids could worsen the problem because urine will be more concentrated. It is not necessary to avoid sexual intercourse; however, some men who have prostatitis may have pain with ejaculation and with BPH there may be reduced libido or erectile dysfunction. **Focus:** Prioritization; **QSEN:** PCC; **Concept:** Elimination, Self-Management, Patient Education; **Cognitive Level:** Applying; **Cognitive Skill:** Generate Solutions. **Test Taking Tip:** Notice that many of the self-care measures for BPH and prostatitis have similarities to measures for UTI and urinary retention.

14. **Ans: 3**   Inability to pass urine is a medical emergency. The symptoms are usually relieved by inserting an indwelling catheter. The HCP should also be notified about the other symptoms. High fever and unrelieved back pain are signs of worsening UTI with the possible complication of pyelonephritis. Pyelonephritis is inflammation of the kidneys that is caused by a bacterial infection; this condition requires urgent attention but is not an emergency. UTI can cause irritation of the bladder wall with bleeding. Bladder irrigation may be required to flush blood and clots if the problem is severe. **Focus:** Prioritization; **QSEN:** PCC; **Concept:** Elimination; **Cognitive Level:** Analyzing

15. **Ans:**

Staff Member	Intervention	Best Staff Member for Each Intervention
RN	Report and record vital signs	AP
LPN/LVN	Accompany Mr. D to the bathroom and assess attempts to collect a midstream urine specimen	LPN/LVN
AP	Perform admission physical assessment and obtain a medical and medication history	RN
	Administer prescribed medications	LPN/LVN
	Attempt one time to insert an indwelling urinary catheter once inability to void is established	RN
	Assist Mr. D with changing into a patient gown	AP
	Obtain a coude catheter to have on standby for second attempt at catheterization	AP

The AP can obtain vital signs, assist Mr. D with changing into a patient gown, and obtain a coude catheter from the storeroom. (The coude catheter is a specialized catheter with a curved tip that facilitates passage through narrow strictures or past obstructions. The HCP or urologist may perform the catheterization if a coude is required; however, facility policy may allow an RN or LPN/LVN to use the coude if it is ordered.) The RN should perform the initial assessment, which includes physical assessment and medical and medication history. The RN should also attempt the first catheter insertion. The procedure is not a routine catheterization because it is likely to be painful and difficult. If the first attempt is not successful, the RN would notify the HCP and obtain an order for coude insertion. The LPN/LVN should accompany Mr. D and observe attempts to urinate for a midstream specimen. An AP would normally perform this task; however, a nurse should be present to assess pain, anxiety, and Mr. D's method. Based on assessment, the nurse may be able to offer suggestions for relaxation, such as listening to running water or performing deep breathing exercises. The LPN/LVN can also administer medications as prescribed. **Focus:** Delegation, Assignment; **QSEN:** TC; **Concept:** Elimination; **Cognitive Level:** Analyzing; **Cognitive Skill:** Generate Solutions; **IPEC:** R/R

16. **Ans: 1, 2, 3, 4, 6, 7, 8, 9, 10**   Complications are preceded by some of the early symptoms that Mr. D experienced, such as pain, urgency, frequency of urination, difficulty starting the stream, and a decreased strength of the stream. Urinary retention and stasis contribute to UTIs and bladder calculi. Recurrent UTIs occur in BPH and prostatitis. Acute urinary obstruction causes pain and an inability to pass urine. This is an emergency situation that is usually relieved by the insertion of an indwelling catheter. Chronic obstruction eventually causes a backflow of urine, which creates favorable conditions for pyelonephritis and any infection creates the potential for sepsis. Backflow also causes hydroureter and hydronephrosis and decreases glomerular filtration. This can lead to renal failure. Penile cancer is not associated with BPH but is more associated with metastasis from adjacent areas (e.g., prostate cancer or testicular cancer). **Focus:** Prioritization; **QSEN:** PCC; **Concept:** Elimination; **Cognitive Level:** Analyzing; **Cognitive Skill:** Recognize Cues.

QSEN Key: PCC, Patient-Centered Care; **TC,** Teamwork & Collaboration; **EBP,** Evidence-Based Practice; **QI,** Quality Improvement; **S,** Safety; **I,** Informatics.
IPEC Key: Domain 1 Values/Ethics (**V/E**); Domain 2 Roles/Responsibilities (**R/R**); Domain 3 Interprofessional Communication (**IC**); Domain 4 Teams/Teamwork (**T/T**).

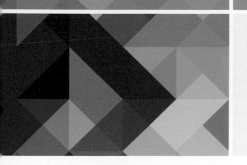

CASE STUDY 14
Patients With Sexually Transmitted Infections

Questions

The nurse is assisting the health care provider (HCP) at a community public health center that offers family planning, diagnosis, and treatment for sexually transmitted infections (STIs) and programs to help youth and adults develop healthy attitudes and behaviors that can reduce their risk for STIs.

1. Which statement made by a patient with a diagnosis of genital herpes will the nurse correct?
   1. "The valacyclovir will treat the herpes infection."
   2. "Herpes is transmittable only when I have lesions."
   3. "A condom must be worn when having sexual relations."
   4. "I will tell my partner that I have genital herpes."

2. A 16-year-old female asks to see the HCP for birth control pills. What is the **best** action of the nurse?
   1. Offer the patient an appointment to see the HCP.
   2. Tell the patient to bring a parent with her to the appointment.
   3. Tell the patient it is illegal to give birth control pills to a minor.
   4. Offer the patient free condoms and spermicidal jelly.

3. Which STIs cause few to no symptoms in women? **Select all the apply.**
   1. Human immunodeficiency virus (HIV).
   2. Human papillomavirus (HPV).
   3. Chlamydia.
   4. Gonorrhea.
   5. Trichomoniasis.
   6. Genital herpes (HSV-2).

4. Which questions should the nurse include when collecting data to assess risky behaviors that lead to STIs? **Select all that apply.**
   1. Do you have more than one sexual partner?
   2. Are your sex partners men or women or both?
   3. Do you have children and if so, did you have a normal delivery?
   4. What kinds of sexual contact do you engage in?
   5. Do you and your partners use protection?
   6. Have you ever had an STI?

5. Which tasks can be delegated to the assistive personnel (AP)? **Select all that apply.**
   1. Obtain a urine specimen.
   2. Prepare and set up equipment for a gynecology exam.
   3. Swab the mouth and throat of a patient.
   4. Chaperone a gynecological exam.
   5. Perform contact tracing.
   6. Provide a patient with condoms.

6. Which STIs must be reported to the local public health agency? **Select all that apply.**
   1. Chlamydia.
   2. HIV.
   3. Syphilis.
   4. Gonorrhea.
   5. HSV-2.
   6. HPV.

7. A male who had sex with a male (MSM) is complaining of flulike symptoms for 3 weeks and states that the rapid HIV test he purchased from the pharmacy is positive. What is the **first** action of the nurse?
   1. Have the patient see the counselor.
   2. Obtain a prescription for a repeat laboratory test.
   3. Give the patient pamphlets on safe sex practices.
   4. Have the patient seen for postexposure prophylaxis.

8. A female patient has been diagnosed with trichomoniasis and the HCP has prescribed metronidazole 500 mg twice a day for 7 days. Which instructions should the nurse review with the patient? **Select all that apply.**
   1. Metronidazole should be taken with food or a snack
   2. Do not have sex for 7 days after finishing the medication.
   3. Take the medication every 12 hours until the course is finished.
   4. Do not drink alcohol for 48 hours after finishing the medication.
   5. Make sure your sexual partners are also treated for trichomoniasis.
   6. If you get a metallic taste after taking, stop the drug and call the HCP.

9. Which tasks must be assigned to the registered nurse (RN) at the community public health center? **Select all that apply.**
   1. Design a school-based STI screening program.
   2. Gather self-collected swab specimens for gonorrhea and chlamydia at a screening.
   3. Provide posttest counseling on newly diagnosed persons with an STI.
   4. Dispense medication for persons testing positive for an STI.
   5. Collect urine specimens for chlamydia screening.
   6. Conduct a class on behaviors to reduce the risk of STIs.

10. A transgender male to female patient who was exposed to HIV 2 days ago is being seen in the clinic. Which drug does the nurse anticipate the HCP will prescribe?
    1. Emtricitabine and tenofovir alafenamide.
    2. Zidovudine.
    3. Nevirapine.
    4. Indinavir.

11. A 17-year-old female patient states she has symptoms of intense itching and burning with thick, white, odorless discharge of the vagina and vulva. Which prescription does the nurse anticipate the HCP will provide for the patient?
    1. A single dose of ceftriaxone 250 mg intramuscular (IM) and azithromycin 1 g orally.
    2. A single dose of benzathine penicillin G 2.4 million units IM.
    3. A single dose of metronidazole 2 g orally.
    4. A single dose of fluconazole 150 mg orally.

12. An 18-year-old female who is diagnosed with HPV tells the nurse she must have gotten it from a toilet seat because she has never had sexual intercourse. What is the **best** response by the nurse?
    1. "Research shows that HPV can be transmitted indirectly from other objects."
    2. "Intercourse is not the only way you can get HPV."

3. "HPV can be spread if your vagina touched someone else's genitals or mouth."
4. "HPV is the most commonly spread STI."

13. The nurse is reviewing instructions for a newly pregnant, HIV-positive patient. Which statements made by the patient will the nurse correct? **Select all that apply.**
    1. "I will continue to take all my medications exactly as prescribed."
    2. "I will get my blood drawn to check my viral load every month."
    3. "I won't need to use condoms now that I am pregnant."
    4. "I will be able to breastfeed my baby once he/she is born."
    5. "I may need to have a cesarean section if my viral load is high at delivery."
    6. "My baby will need to take antiretroviral drugs once he/she born."

14. Which factors influence awareness and beliefs regarding sexually transmitted diseases STIs in young adults? **Select all that apply.**
    1. Limited sex education in school.
    2. Confusion about how STIs are transmitted.
    3. Stigmatization of a gay and or transexual lifestyle.
    4. Knowledge deficits about different methods of STI prevention.
    5. Status as an emancipated minor.
    6. Adolescents being on parent's insurance.

15. The mother of an unemancipated adolescent asks for a copy of her daughter's medical record. Which statement will the nurse make?
    1. "The Health Insurance Portability and Accountability Act (HIPAA) assures her privacy."
    2. "I will ask the administrator to come and discuss the issue with you."
    3. "If you sign the medical records release, I will have it copied for you."
    4. "Due to privacy concerns, it is our policy not to copy medical records."

16. **Extended Multiple Response.** _____

The nurse and the RN director of the community health center are developing a program to decrease STIs in the adolescent population in their community.

Which behaviors/factors represent reasons why STIs may be high in the adolescent community? **Select all that apply.**
   ___ 1. Immature cervix
   ___ 2. Body piercing
   ___ 3. Substance use
   ___ 4. Multiple sex partners
   ___ 5. Use of dental dams
   ___ 6. Magical thinking
   ___ 7. Limited sex education
   ___ 8. Barriers to care
   ___ 9. Use of condoms

17. Cloze.

Instructions: Complete the sentences below by choosing the most probable option for the omitted information that corresponds with the same numbered list of options provided.

HPV infection is a common STI that is highly contagious. It is an infection that causes ___1_____. Some infections can cause cancer of the ___2_____ and___2___. HPV is spread by ___3____.

Options for 1	Options for 2	Options for 3
Smooth soft growths	Uterus	Indirect contact
Grainy rough growths	Penis	Direct contact
Draining pustules	Testicles	Fecal-oral contact
Benign tumors	Cervix	Parasites
Skin tags	Breast	Papanicolaou (Pap) test

18. Which STIs if left untreated in a woman who is giving birth can lead to blindness in the newborn? **Select all that apply.**
   1. Gonorrhea.
   2. Chlamydia.
   3. Syphilis.
   4. Hepatitis B.
   5. Genital herpes.
   6. Trichomoniasis.

19. A 45-year-old male who has an allergy to penicillin has a chancre on his penis. He states he had unprotected sex 3 weeks ago. Which medical interventions will the nurse expect the HCP to prescribe? **Select all that apply.**
   1. Venereal Disease Research Lab (VDRL) and Rapid Plasma Reagin (RPR) blood test.
   2. Microscopic view of chancre scrapings chancre.
   3. Fluorescent Treponemal Antibody Absorbed (FTA-ABS) blood test.
   4. Tetracycline 500 mg four times a day for 14 days.
   5. Single-dose benzathine penicillin G 2.4 million units IM.
   6. Metronidazole 2 g by mouth single dose.

20. Which interventions will the nurse implement out for a patient who is being diagnosed with syphilis? **Select all that apply.**
   1. Instructing the patient to withhold alcohol for 24 hours before the VDRL and RPR test.
   2. Asking the patient for the names of all sexual partners so that they can get treatment.
   3. Abstaining from sex for 7 days after the treatment is over.
   4. Returning to the clinic for repeat blood test as directed by the HCP.
   5. Giving the patient a Gardasil vaccination.
   6. Encouraging the use of condoms for future safe sex practice.

  Answer Key for this chapter begins on p. 216

Answers

1. **Ans: 2**   A person diagnosed with herpes simplex 1 (oral) or 2 (genital) who does not presently have lesions can still shed the virus and expose another person through contact with the area that is affected. Valacyclovir treats the infection and prevents it from spreading to other parts of the body but does not cure the virus. Wearing a condom is a safe sex practice for all persons who are not in a monogamous relationship. Although herpes is not a notifiable infection, it is best to be honest and inform a partner or potential partner of the infection's existence. **Focus:** Prioritization; **QSEN:** PCC, EBP; **Concept:** Infection; **Cognitive Level:** Applying

2. **Ans: 1**   Family planning services funded by Title X of the Public Health Service Act is a federal law that makes it legal for a practitioner to diagnose and treat sexually transmitted infection (STI) and provide prescription contraception to minors without requiring parental consent. The nurse should offer free condoms and spermicidal jelly until the birth control pills take effect, which can take 5 days or longer. **Focus:** Prioritization; **QSEN:** PCC, EBP; **Concept:** Health Care Law, Hormonal Regulation; **Cognitive Level:** Analyzing

3. **Ans: 2, 3, 4, 5, 6**   Some strains of HPV can cause genital warts but not all do. It is the most common STI and cannot always be prevented by condoms. Some strains of HPV can cause cervical cancer. Chlamydia is a silent infection mostly seen in women under the age of 25. Most women do not have symptoms but may experience burning or vaginal discharge several weeks after infection. Chlamydia can lead to pelvic inflammatory infection (PID). Gonorrhea does not cause symptoms in the majority of women and if left untreated can cause infections in other parts of the body such as the joints and brain and leads to PID and damage to the reproductive organs. Trichomoniasis is caused by a parasite and if left untreated can cause premature birth in pregnant women. It sometimes causes a fishy odor, burning and itching, and vaginal discharge. HSV-2 can be passed on with either oral or genital sex and does not always produce lesions. There is no cure. Herpes passed on to the neonate during delivery can spread and cause encephalitis and meningitis. **Focus:** Prioritization; **QSEN:** PCC, EBP; **Concept:** Infection, Health Promotion, Patient Education; **Cognitive Level:** Analyzing

4. **Ans: 1, 2, 4, 5, 6**   The nurse should ask about birth control measures being taken and also if the patient has a plan for becoming pregnant. Asking about children and type of delivery does not for assess

risky behavior. **Focus:** Prioritization; **QSEN:** EBP; **Concept:** Infection, Health Promotion; **Cognitive Level:** Analyzing. **Test Taking Tip:** The Centers for Disease Control and Prevention (CDC) created the five P's as a guide to asking questions that assess risky behavior. They are partners, practices, prevention of pregnancy, protection from STIs, and a past history of STIs.

5. **Ans: 1, 2, 4, 6**   An AP working in a STI clinic will be familiar with tasks such as obtaining a urine specimen, preparing and setting up equipment for an exam as well as chaperoning and assisting with gynecological exams and providing condoms. Swabbing the mouth, throat, or genital area must be done by either the nurse or the HCP. Contact tracing is done by public health registered nurses or unlicensed disease intervention specialists that require specialty training. **Focus:** Delegation; **QSEN:** TC; **Concept:** Care Coordination; **Cognitive Level:** Analyzing; **IPEC:** R/R

6. **Ans: 1, 3, 4**   Current reportable diseases according to the CDC are chlamydia, syphilis, and gonorrhea. Some states may mandate reporting of additional STIs, so nurses should be familiar with their own state and local reporting requirements. **Focus:** Prioritization; **QSEN:** EBP; **Concept:** Infection, Health Care Law; **Cognitive Level:** Applying

7. **Ans: 2**   If an HIV test is a rapid test or a self-test and it is positive, the person should get follow-up testing from a laboratory using a nucleic acid test (NAT), also known as an HIV viral load test, or an antibody/antigen test. Patients with HIV should see the counselor or the RN but not until the accuracy of the home test has been completed. The patient should be given information on safe sex practices but it is not the first action. The patient has had symptoms of HIV for 3 weeks, so postexposure prophylaxis (PEP) is not necessary because PEP needs to be started with in 72 hours of exposure to HIV. The patient should be seen as soon as possible to be started on antiretroviral drugs. **Focus:** Prioritization; **QSEN:** EBP, S; **Concept:** Infection; **Cognitive Level:** Analyzing

8. **Ans: 1, 2, 3, 4, 5**   Nausea and vomiting is common with metronidazole, so taking it with food or a snack is advised. Do not have sex with or without a condom for 7 days after the medication is finished to avoid reinfection. Antibiotic therapy twice a day works best if taken at equal intervals. Men left untreated can spread the infection, so all sexual partners need to be treated. It is common to get a metallic and taste with metronidazole. Hard candies, mints, and taking the medication

with chocolate can mask the taste. There is no need to stop the drug or call the HCP as this is a harmless side effect. **Focus:** Prioritization; **QSEN:** EBP, S; **Concept:** Infection; **Cognitive Level:** Analyzing

9. **Ans: 1, 3, 6** The RN provides education to patients and the public and can provide posttest counseling to a person newly diagnosed with an STI. Although the RN could gather self-collected vaginal/penile swabs or collect urine specimens, it is not economically practical as these tasks can be completed by the LPN/LVN. The RN or LPN/LVN can administer the medication but a pharmacist must dispense medications. Administration refers to providing a single dose of drug. Dispensing is defined as preparing, packaging, and labeling a prescription drug. **Focus:** Assignment; **QSEN:** TC; **Concept:** Care Coordination, Health Care Law; **Cognitive Level:** Analyzing

10. **Ans: 1** Emtricitabine and tenofovir alafenamide is used for HIV PEP and can be used by all patients exposed to HIV regardless of hormonal use. It should be started within 72 hours of exposure. Zidovudine is a nucleoside reverse transcriptase inhibitor (NRTI) that is used to prevent the passing of the HIV virus from pregnant women to the unborn child. Zidovudine is also used in newborns born to mothers with HIV to prevent infection in the newborn. It is usually given in combination with other HIV drugs. Nevirapine is a nonnucleoside reverse transcriptase inhibitor (NNRTI) that reduces HIV viral load and increases CD4 cell counts. It is taken in combination with other antiretroviral drugs and decreases estrogen levels in hormone therapy. Indinavir is a protease inhibitor (PI). PI's prevent viral replication and are used with other HIV drugs. **Focus:** Prioritization; **QSEN:** S; **Concept:** Infection; **Cognitive Level:** Analyzing

11. **Ans: 4** The patient has classic symptoms of a vaginal yeast infection. Although it is not considered an STI, if the infections are recurrent, it increases the risk of STIs in sexually active females. Yeast infections are caused by a change in vaginal pH from antibiotics, diabetes, douching, and contraceptives. **Focus:** Prioritization; **QSEN:** EBP; **Concept:** Infection; **Cognitive Level:** Applying

12. **Ans: 3** HPV is easily spread through skin-to-skin contact with someone else's vagina, penis, anus, or mouth. Research has not shown that HPV can be transmitted from a toilet seat but research has shown that HPV can be transmitted indirectly through certain fomites such as contaminated hospital equipment. HPV is the most commonly spread STI but that does not clarify the patient's statement. **Focus:** Prioritization; **QSEN:** EBP; **Concept:** Infection; **Cognitive Level:** Analyzing

13. **Ans: 3, 4** Condoms should still be used regardless of the partner's HIV status in order to prevent transmission of other STI's. Although HIV medications

reduce viral load, it is still possible to transmit the virus through breast milk. The majority of HIV drugs are safe to take during pregnancy. It is unusual for them to cause birth defects but not taking HIV drugs greatly increases the chance of the fetus getting HIV. If the mother's viral load is high when she is in labor, in order to decrease transmission to the infant, a cesarean section may be recommended. Zidovudine prophylaxis is recommended for infants for the first 6 weeks of life. **Focus:** Prioritization; **QSEN:** EBP; **Concept:** Infection; **Cognitive Level:** Analyzing

14. **Ans: 1, 2, 3, 4, 6** Status as an emancipated minor is not a factor. Emancipated or not, research has shown that young adults have the highest risk of contracting STIs. The risk is likely mediated by the social and cultural setting that impacts their awareness and beliefs and risk of contracting STIs. Lack of or limited sex education classes in school, misinformation that is spread among social media and peers, stigmatization of alternate lifestyles, and knowledge deficits of how to prevent STI are representative of such settings. Although adolescents can receive medical care for STIs privately, if an adolescent or young adult remains on their parent's insurance carrier, the information can be viewed by the primary insurance holder. This awareness may prevent treatment because the adolescent or young adult would not want their parents to know. **Focus:** Prioritization; **QSEN:** EBP; **Concept:** Infection, Health Disparity; **Cognitive Level:** Analyzing

15. **Ans: 2** Because the laws are complicated, the nurse should have the parent speak to the administrator of the clinic. If the adolescent was an emancipated minor, HIPAA applies and the parent cannot legally get a copy of the medical record. However, if the adolescent is unemancipated, it is more complicated. If the state or other law explicitly requires information to be disclosed to a parent, then the HCP must comply with the parental request for records. If there is no state or other law requiring information is to be disclosed to a parent, then HIPAA applies and records cannot be given to the parent without the adolescent's consent. If state law or other law permits but does not require information to be given to the parent, then the HCP can release or not release the records at their own discretion. **Focus:** Prioritization; **QSEN:** EBP; **Concept:** Health Care Law; **Cognitive Level:** Analyzing

16. **Ans: 1, 2, 3, 4, 6, 7, 8** Female adolescents have an immature cervix, which cultivates the growth of STIs. Body piercing if not done properly can lead to blood-borne pathogens. Genital body piercing can cause damage to condoms due to the inserted objects. Substance use affects judgment and leads to risky sexual behavior. Multiple sex partners increase exposure to many different STIs. Piaget proposed that magical thinking (continued through the concrete operation

period during childhood until the ages of 11 to 12) makes an adolescent think that an outcome can be influenced by doing something that is unrelated to the circumstances. Sex education in schools is sometimes not comprehensive enough and/or not allowed in some states because of parental disapproval. Barriers to care are embarrassment to seek services, cost, and clinic hours conflict with school. The use of dental dams and female condoms in a female and the use of condoms in a male help prevent STDs in adolescents. **Focus:** Prioritization; **QSEN:** EBP; **Concept:** Infection; **Cognitive Level:** Analyzing; **Cognitive Skill:** Prioritize Hypothesizes

17. **Ans:**   HPV infection is a common STI that is highly contagious. It is an infection that causes **grainy rough growths**. Some infections can cause cancer of the **cervix** and **penis**. HPV is spread by **direct contact**. **Focus:** Prioritization; **QSEN:** EBP; **Concept:** Infection; **Cognitive Level:** Analyzing; **Cognitive Skill:** Recognize Cues

18. **Ans: 1, 2**   A newborn who is exposed to either gonorrhea or chlamydia in the vaginal canal can contract neonatal conjunctivitis that can cause blindness. Prophylaxis with erythromycin eye ointment is currently recommended for all newborns within 24 hours of birth. **Focus:** Prioritization; **QSEN:** EBP; **Concept:** Infection; **Cognitive Level:** Applying

19. **Ans: 1, 2, 3, 4**   The VDRL and RPR may be negative in the primary stage of syphilis, which is likely when the patient states he had unprotected sex 3 weeks ago (the incubation period for syphilis). So the HCP will also scrape the chancre and send the scrapings to the lab for dark-field microscopy, which will visualize *Treponema*, the bacteria that causes syphilis. An FTA-ABS blood test will check for antibodies to *Treponema pallidum* bacteria. The patient will need to take tetracycline because he is allergic to penicillin. **Focus:** Prioritization; **QSEN:** EBP; **Concept:** Infection; **Cognitive Level:** Analyzing

20. **Ans: 1, 2, 3, 4, 6**   Alcohol intake can cause false-positive results and should be withheld for 24 hours before the test. All sexual partners should be treated for syphilis. The patient can call and tell their partners or the nurse can call them to keep the patient anonymous. Abstinence from sex for 7 days is necessary to assure the disease is cured. Test titers of the non *Treponemal* are done intermittently for 6 months after treatment. Gardasil vaccinations for HPV are recommended for boys and girls ages 9 to 26. Safe sex practices should be encouraged to prevent future infections. **Focus:** Prioritization; **QSEN:** EBP; **Concept:** Infection; **Cognitive Level:** Analyzing

QSEN Key: PCC, Patient-Centered Care; **TC,** Teamwork & Collaboration; **EBP,** Evidence-Based Practice; **QI,** Quality Improvement; **S,** Safety; **I,** Informatics.
IPEC Key: Domain 1 Values/Ethics **(V/E)**; Domain 2 Roles/Responsibilities **(R/R)**; Domain 3 Interprofessional Communication **(IC)**; Domain 4 Teams/Teamwork **(T/T)**.

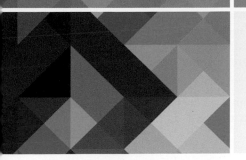

CASE STUDY 15

Patient With Parkinson Disease

Questions

Mr. V is a 69-year-old retiree who lives with his wife in a home they have owned in for 45 years. His medical history includes hypertension and gastroesophageal reflux disease (GERD). Over the past year, Mrs. V reports that she has noticed shaking in his hand and arm and that he moves a little slower when they go out to walk their dog in the mornings. Mr. V states that these changes are "just part of getting older." Mr. V is seen by his primary health care provider (HCP) for his annual checkup. The HCP instructs the nurse to check his weight and vital signs.

Vital signs: T 98.4°F (36.9°C), HR 88/min, RR 20/min, BP 102/76, SaO₂ 94% on room air.

Height: 67 inches (170.18 cm).

Weight: 178 pounds (80.7 kg). The nurse notes that Mr. V seemed to have some weakness on his right side when he steps on the scale.

His current medications include: amlodipine 10 mg every morning, famotidine 20 mg at bedtime, a multivitamin every morning, and acetaminophen 650 mg as needed.

1. The HCP suspects that Mr. V may have Parkinson disease (PD). What phase of the illness does the nurse suspect?
   1. Phase 1, Initial Stage.
   2. Phase 2, Mild Stage.
   3. Phase 3, Moderate Stage.
   4. Phase 4, Severe Disability.

2. Which additional change in vital signs will the nurse ask the assistive personnel (AP) to check and report results for?
   1. Increase in temperature.
   2. Decrease in heart rate.
   3. Increase in respiratory rate.
   4. Decrease in blood pressure with standing.

3. Which are the four cardinal signs of PD? **Select all that apply.**
   1. Tremor.
   2. Postural instability.
   3. Change in level of consciousness (LOC).
   4. Muscle rigidity.
   5. Bradykinesia.
   6. Vision loss.

4. **Nextgen. Enhanced Multiple Response. _____**
   Which questions will the nurse ask to collect information from a patient with symptoms of PD? **Instructions: Place an X next to or highlight the correct responses. Select all that apply.**
   1. _____ Have you ever had a head injury, meningitis, encephalitis, or cerebrovascular disorder?
   2. _____ Do you have a problem with restless energy or overactivity?
   3. _____ Have you been exposed to pesticides, metals, or carbon monoxide for extended periods?
   4. _____ Do you have any trouble with swallowing?
   5. _____ Do you experience constipation or urinary incontinence?
   6. _____ Have you been steadily gaining weight?
   7. _____ Have you noticed excessive salivation (drooling) and problems handling secretions?
   8. _____ Has your handwriting or dexterity decreased or deteriorated?
   9. _____ Do you have mood swings, hallucinations, or are you depressed?
   10. _____ Do you sweat excessively?

5. Which diagnostic test will the nurse expect the HCP to prescribe to confirm the diagnosis of PD for Mr. V?
   1. Magnetic resonance imaging (MRI) of the brain.
   2. Single-proton emission computed tomography (SPECT).
   3. Front and lateral x-rays of the brain.
   4. Deep brain stimulation (DBS).

6. What is the nurse's **best** response when Mr. V asks about the plan of care for his PD?
   1. "The primary cause for most cases of PD is unknown, but a secondary cause is exposure to pesticides."
   2. "The cure for PD is surgical treatment with DBS."
   3. "Nonsurgical care includes drugs that will slow the progression of the disease."
   4. "PD is slowly progressive and symptoms will worsen over time."

7. **Nextgen. Drag and Drop.** As the illness progresses, the HCP prescribes drug therapy for Mr. V. _____
   Instructions: Place the letter for the correct action in the second column next to the drug listed in the first column. Correct actions may be used more than once.

Column 1: Drug	Column 2: Correct Action
_____ Carbidopa-levodopa	A. Slows the breakdown of dopamine
_____ Selegiline	B. Used for motor symptom control
_____ Entacapone	C. Decreases tremor, rigidity, and bradykinesia
_____ Bromocriptine	D. Decreases rigidity and bradykinesia
_____ Amantadine	
_____ Rasagiline	

8. What precaution will the nurse be sure to teach Mr. and Mrs. V about when he is prescribed selegiline?
   1. Avoid all alcoholic beverages to prevent hypertension.
   2. The tremor may get worse before it improves.
   3. Avoid tyramine-containing foods and beverages.
   4. This drug may cause drowsiness and sedation.

9. As Mr. V's PD progresses, which additional symptoms will the nurse expect to observe? **Select all that apply.**
   1. Bilateral limb involvement.
   2. Increasingly elevated BP.
   3. Masklike face.
   4. Akinesia.
   5. Slow and shuffling gait.
   6. Postural instability.

After several months, Mr. V's Parkinson disease debilitating symptoms become too difficult for his wife to manage at home and he is admitted to a long-term care facility with stage 3 moderate PD.

10. Which instruction will the nurse provide to the AP responsible for Mr. V's morning care?
    1. "Provide equipment but encourage the patient to complete all of his bath and morning care."
    2. "Complete all of the patient's morning care so that he does not experience fatigue."
    3. "Allow the patient to do what he is able to complete, then help him with what he is unable to do."
    4. "Wait for Mrs. V to arrive and then let her assist with the patient's bath and mouth care."

11. The AP reports that Mr. V is losing weight and seems to have difficulty with swallowing. Which actions or interventions will the nurse take? **Select all that apply.**
    1. Request the supervising RN to submit consults with the registered dietician nutritionist (RDN) and speech-language pathologist (SLP).
    2. Always raise the head of the bed during feedings.
    3. Instruct the AP to make sure the patient consumes everything on his tray for all meals and snacks.
    4. Provide the patient with small, frequent meals and snacks.
    5. Have the AP weigh the patient every day at the same time, on the same scale, and wearing the same amount of clothes.
    6. Tell the AP to feed the patient faster to avoid fatigue while eating.

12. Mr. V appears withdrawn and irritable. He states, "It's hopeless. I don't know why I'm still alive. This is not life as I want to live it." What does the nurse suspect?
    1. Anxiety.
    2. Depression.
    3. Psychosis.
    4. Bipolar syndrome.

13. Which drug prescription does the nurse expect from the HCP at this time?
    1. Baclofen.
    2. Zolpidem.
    3. Venlafaxine.
    4. Atropine.

14. Mr. V has developed postural instability and a freezing gait (inability to move the feet forward despite the intention to walk). Which member of the health care team would be **best** to consult at this time?
    1. Physical therapist (PT).
    2. Occupational therapist (OT).
    3. RDN.
    4. SLP.

15. Mrs. V wants to help with feeding her husband. Which instructions will the nurse provide? **Select all that apply.**
    1. Keep the patient in an upright position.
    2. Give the patient small bites of food.
    3. Ensure that the patient eats all the food on his tray.
    4. Remind the patient to drop his chin while swallowing.
    5. Do not rush the patient while eating.
    6. Use a warming tray to keep the patient's food hot.

PART 3 Complex Health Scenarios

Answer Key for this chapter begins on p. 222

Answers

1. **Ans: 1** Phase 1 (initial stage) of PD is characterized by unilateral limb involvement, minimal weakness, and hand and arm trembling. PD is a progressive illness and as a patient goes through the phases, symptoms get worse. **Focus:** Prioritization; **QSEN:** PCC, S; **Concept:** Intracranial Regulation, Mobility, Clinical Judgment; **Cognitive Level:** Analyzing; **Cognitive Skill:** Recognizing Cues

2. **Ans: 4** With PD, there is reduced sympathetic nervous system influence on the heart and blood vessels, which results in orthostatic hypotension. **Focus:** Delegation, Supervision; **QSEN:** PCC, S, TC; **Concept:** Intracranial Regulation, Safety, Communication; **Cognitive Level:** Analyzing; **IPEC:** IC. **Test Taking Tip:** Remember that orthostatic hypotension is defined as a decrease in systolic blood pressure of 20 mm Hg or a decrease in diastolic blood pressure of 10 mm Hg within 3 minutes of standing when compared with blood pressure from the sitting or supine position.

3. **Ans: 1, 2, 4, 5** The four cardinal symptoms of PD are tremor, muscle rigidity, bradykinesia, and postural instability. While change in LOC occurs in some cases, it is not always present. Vision loss is also not common with PD. **Focus:** Prioritization; **QSEN:** PCC;

Concept: Intracranial Regulation; **Cognitive Level:** Analyzing; **Cognitive Skill:** Recognizing Cues

4. **Ans: 1, 3, 4, 5, 7, 8, 9, 10** A patient with PD would experience fatigue, not excess energy. They would also steadily lose weight, not gain weight. **Focus:** Prioritization; **QSEN:** PCC, EBP; **Concept:** Intracranial Regulation, Communication; **Cognitive Level:** Applying; **Cognitive Skill:** Recognizing Cues

5. **Ans: 2** SPECT is ordered because it can display the reduced uptake of dopamine, which occurs with PD. When dopamine levels are decreased, a person loses the ability to refine voluntary movement. **Focus:** Prioritization; **QSEN:** PCC, EBP; **Concept:** Intracranial Regulation; **Cognitive Level:** Applying; **IPEC:** IC

6. **Ans: 3** There is no cure for PD. Treatment includes prescribed drugs to slow the progression of the illness and control the symptoms. Physical therapy and emotional support are also important. Surgical treatment such a DBS does not cure the illness but can help treat many of the debilitating symptoms of PD. Options 1 and 4 are correct but do not answer the questions about the plan of care. **Focus:** Prioritization; **QSEN:** PCC; **Concept:** Patient Education; **Cognitive Level:** Applying

7. **Ans:**

Column 1: Drug	Column 2: Correct Action
__C__ Carbidopa-levodopa	A. Slows the breakdown of dopamine
__B/C__ Selegiline	B. Used for motor symptom control
__A__ Entacapone	C. Decreases tremor, rigidity, and bradykinesia
__C__ Bromocriptine	D. Decreases rigidity and bradykinesia
__D__ Amantadine	
__B__ Rasagiline	

Focus: Prioritization; **QSEN:** PCC; **Concept:** Intracranial Regulation; **Cognitive Level:** Applying; **Cognitive Skill:** Recognizing Cues

8. **Ans: 3** Selegiline is a monoamine oxidase inhibitor (MAOI). When a patient is prescribed this drug, they must be cautioned to avoid tyramine-containing foods (e.g., strong, aged cheeses; smoked processed meats; and pickled, fermented foods). Not all alcoholic beverages should be avoided; however, beer and red wine should be avoided to prevent severe headaches and hypertension. Selegiline does not cause tremors to worsen and mobility is improved. This drug causes difficulty

sleeping and insomnia, not drowsiness or sedation. **Focus:** Prioritization; **QSEN:** PCC, S; **Concept:** Safety, Patient Education; **Cognitive Level:** Analyzing

9. **Ans: 1, 3, 4, 5, 6** In stage 2 PD (mild) the patient is expected to develop bilateral limb involvement, a masklike face, and a slow shuffling gait. In stage 3 PD the patient will likely develop postural instability and increased gait disturbance. In stage 4 PD akinesia and rigidity develop. **Focus:** Prioritization; **QSEN:** PCC; **Concept:** Intracranial Regulation, Clinical Judgment; **Cognitive Level:** Analyzing; **Cognitive Skill:** Recognizing Cues

10. **Ans: 3** The best action would be to allow the patient to complete what he can for himself and then assist with what he is unable to do. With postural instability, it is not safe to expect the patient to complete all of his morning care (e.g., washing back or lower extremities). Expecting the patient to complete all of the care is unrealistic because of the fatigue associated with PD. Having the AP complete all of the care is not a good solution because a patient with PD should be encouraged to maintain flexibility and independence for self-care. Waiting for the patient's wife is not the best solution because the patient should be able to do mouth care and wash his face before breakfast and Mr. V was admitted because his wife was unable to manage his care at home. If Mrs. V makes a request and Mr. V is agreeable, the bath may be deferred until her arrival. **Focus:** Delegation, Supervision; **QSEN:** PCC, S, TC; **Concept:** Care Coordination; **Cognitive Level:** Applying; **IPEC:** IC

11. **Ans: 1, 2, 4, 5** Options 1, 2, 4, and 5 are appropriate for Mr. V's care at this time. Insisting that the patient consume all of the food on his tray and rushing with his feedings will increase his risk for aspiration when he is having trouble with swallowing. Instead, small meals and snacks, as well as slowly feeding, are appropriate. **Focus:** Delegation, Supervision; **QSEN:** PCC, S; **Concept:** Care Coordination, Safety; **Cognitive Level:** Analyzing; **Cognitive Skill:** Taking Action. **Test Taking Tip:** Remember that when a patient is having difficulty swallowing, the risk of aspiration is increased.

12. **Ans: 2** Depression is common among patients with PD as mobility and independence become severely limited and the disease progresses. Symptoms include feelings of guilt, worthlessness, and helplessness; pessimism and hopelessness; irritability; and withdrawing. **Focus:** Prioritization; **QSEN:** PCC, S; **Concept:** Mood and Affect; **Cognitive Level:** Analyzing; **Cognitive Skill:** Recognizing Cues

13. **Ans: 3** Venlafaxine is a serotonin-norepinephrine reuptake inhibitor (SNRI) antidepressant used to treat moderate to severe depression. Baclofen is used to relieve muscle spasms. Zolpidem is prescribed as a sleeping aid for insomnia. Atropine when given sublingually can help minimize drooling. **Focus:** Prioritization; **QSEN:** PCC; **Concept:** Care Coordination; **Cognitive Level:** Analyzing

14. **Ans: 1** A PT can provide nontraditional exercise programs such as yoga and tai chi, which can improve mobility and preserve flexibility. PT can also provide range-of-motion (ROM) exercises, muscle stretching, and out-of-bed activities with an individually designed program. An OT can provide assistive devices and provide training that will facilitate independence. The RDN can evaluate nutritional needs. An SLP can evaluate a patient's ability to swallow and assist with speech impairment. **Focus:** Prioritization; **QSEN:** PCC, S; **Concept:** Mobility, Clinical Judgment; **Cognitive Level:** Analyzing; **Cognitive Skill:** Generating Solutions; **IPEC:** R/R

15. **Ans: 1, 2, 4, 5, 6** All of these options are appropriate to teach Mrs. V when feeding her husband, except option 3. The patient should not be forced to continue eating until all of his food is consumed. Eating too much food can increase the risk for aspiration, especially if Mr. V experiences any difficulty with swallowing. It is best to give the carbidopa-levodopa 30 minutes before meals to control symptoms of gagging and aspiration. Offering frequent and smaller meals and snacks is a better option. **Focus:** Prioritization; **QSEN:** PCC, S; **Concept:** Nutrition, Safety, Patient (Family) Teaching; **Cognitive Level:** Applying; **Cognitive Skill:** Taking Action

QSEN Key: PCC, Patient-Centered Care; **TC,** Teamwork & Collaboration; **EBP,** Evidence-Based Practice; **QI,** Quality Improvement; **S,** Safety; **I,** Informatics.
IPEC Key: Domain 1 Values/Ethics (**V/E**); Domain 2 Roles/Responsibilities (**R/R**); Domain 3 Interprofessional Communication (**IC**); Domain 4 Teams/Teamwork (**T/T**).

PART 3 Complex Health Scenarios